# Recent Results in Cancer Research

Fortschritte der Krebsforschung

Progrès dans les recherches sur le cancer

## 39

*Edited by*





*Editor in chief*
*P. Rentchnick, Genève*

*Sponsored by the Swiss League against Cancer*

# Current Problems in the Epidemiology of Cancer and Lymphomas

*Edited by*

E. Grundmann and H. Tulinius

*With 80 Figures*

Springer-Verlag Berlin Heidelberg GmbH 1972

Professor Dr. E. Grundmann
Institute of Pathology, University of Münster, D-44 Münster, Germany

Dr. H. Tulinius
World Health Organization, International Agency for Research on Cancer, Lyon, France

Symposium of the „Gesellschaft zur Bekämpfung der Krebskrankheiten Nordrhein-Westfalen, e. V." Düsseldorf, 4th—6th November, 1971

ISBN 978-3-662-40553-6 ISBN 978-3-662-41032-5 (eBook)
DOI 10.1007/978-3-662-41032-5



Originally published by Springer-Verlag Berlin · Heidelberg · New York in 1972
Softcover reprint of the hardcover 1st edition 1972

Library of Congress Catalog Card Number 72-81166.

# Contents

# List of Participants


BAIKIE, A. G., University of Oxford, Radcliffe Infirmary, Oxford, Great Britain

CHAN, W. C., Department of Pathology, University of Hong Kong, Queen Mary Compound, Hong Kong

DAVIES, J. N. P., Department of Pathology, Albany Medical College of Union University, Albany, NY, USA

DHOM, G., Pathologisches Institut der Universität des Saarlandes, Homburg, Germany

DÖRKEN, H., I. Medizinische Universitätsklinik, Hamburg, Germany

FRANKS, L. M., Imperial Cancer Research Fund, Department of Cellular Pathology, Lincoln's Inn Fields, London, Great Britain

FRANSSILA, K., Third Department of Pathology, University of Helsinki, Helsinki Finland

GRUNDMANN, E., Pathologisches Institut der Universität Münster, Münster, Germany

HOHBACH, M., Pathologisches Institut der Universität des Saarlandes, Homburg, Germany

KRÜGER, G., National Institutes of Health, National Cancer Institute, Laboratory of Pathology, Bethesda, MD, USA

LIAVÅG, I., Diakonissehusets sykehus, Department of Surgery, Oslo, Norway

LINSELL, C. A., International Agency for Research on Cancer, Nairobi Regional Centre, Nairobi, Kenya

MACMAHON, B., Department of Epidemiology, Harvard University, School of Public Health, Boston, MA, USA

MUÑOZ, N., Unit of Biological Carcinogenesis, International Agency for Research on Cancer, Lyon, France

PIKE, M., University of Oxford, Radcliffe Infirmary, Oxford, Great Britain

RAMOT, B., Department of Haematology, Government Hospital Tel-Hashomer, Tel Hashomer, Israel

ROTKIN, I. D., Department of Preventive Medicine and Community Health, University of Illinois at the Medical Center, Chicago, IL, USA

SCHMAUZ, R., Deutsches Krebsforschungszentrum, Institut für Dokumentation, Information und Statistik, Heidelberg, Germany

SOBIN, L. H., Cancer Unit, WHO, Geneva, Switzerland

STASZEWSKI, J., Instytut Onkologii, Wybrzeże Armii Czerwonej, Gliwice, Poland

STEINITZ, R., Ministry of Health, Division of Chronic Diseases and Rehabilitation, Jerusalem, Israel

DE-THÉ, G. B., WHO, International Agency for Research on Cancer, Lyon, France

Tulinius, H., WHO, International Agency for Research on Cancer, Lyon, France

Tuyns, A. J., WHO, International Agency for Research on Cancer, Lyon, France

Wagner, J. C., Medical Research Council, Pneumoconiosis Research Unit, Llandough Hospital, Penarth, Glamorgan, Wales, Great Britain

Wang, D., Department of Endocrinology, Imperial Cancer Research Fund, Lincoln's Inn Field, London, Great Britain

Watanabe, S., Pathology Division, National Cancer Center, Research Institute, Tokyo, Japan

# Opening Remarks

Ladies and Gentlemen!

I welcome you in Düsseldorf on behalf of the Gesellschaft zur Bekämpfung der Krebskrankheiten Nordrhein-Westfalen e.V. As a representative of this society it is a great honour to me to see you in this city. Some of you had to make long and inconvenient journeys, not only from foreign countries, but also from remote continents. I thank you all for your coming and the trouble you had to take.

The "Gesellschaft zur Bekämpfung der Krebskrankheiten" is, as we call it in German, an "eingetragener Verein", that is a registered society. That means that it consists of a private organization. It has been established by the initiative of doctors in practises, in sciences and last not least in the Public Health Service. — Some months ago we celebrated the 20th birthday of our society.

Though the society is a private one, it is supported mainly by the State Government of our Federal State Nordrhein-Westfalen and in particular by the Health Department of the Ministry of Labour and Social Affairs under the charge of Dr. Studt. Our mutual work lies in the Public Health Service to which we contribute with different cancer problems. Naturally, we cannot do this work on our own. The public, which grants us the financial means has the right to be regularly informed by us on the results of the research. In Germany, however, as well as in the whole western world, some newspapers take advantage of the subject of cancer by printing articles with thrilling headlines. This bears, of course, the danger that the layman, i.e. the potential patient with cancer, receives scientifically wrong information, which results in many cases in a delusive hope for quite a lot of people who suffer from this disease. It should not be kept secret that even doctors often give misleading instructions. So, one of the main tasks of our society is the public enlightenment on the subject of cancer for the doctors on one side and the laymen on the other.

Those of you, ladies and gentlemen, who have come from foreign countries and continents may ask themselves why the Federal State Nordrhein-Westfalen has her own Society for Cancer Research. Well, perhaps I shall have the opportunity tonight to report some more facts and details on this subject. At this stage, let me only point out that, on the foundation of the Federal Republic of Germany in 1948/49, all fields belonging to culture, education and science were regarded as competence of the different states due to the federal formation. That's why all our universities are 'Länder'-universities and even the Public Health Service is still a part of the Ministries of the 'Länder'. Likewise, in the early fifties, private societies were founded in all German Federal States aiming at bringing together specialists in medical science and organisators in order to give way to modern cancer-campaign. Only one year had passed since the first centralized German Cancer Research Society was established.

According to the constitution of our society the support of cancer research, cancer delection, cancer prophylaxis and public enlightenment on cancer for doctors and laymen are the most important tasks of our society. You all, ladies and gentlemen, contribute to this work and you have been invited to this Symposium to speak about your experience and achievements in the various fields of cancer research with special regard to the "Epidemiology of Cancer" as the heading of our Symposium. Most people tend to combine the term "epidemiology" with the spreading of an infectious disease. We all know, however, that this definition isn't correct at this time with regard to cancer. If, however, in spite of this, the term "epidemiology" should prevail in the linguistic usage, there might be the hope that more details of the nature of cancer may be established by examinations of the geographical distribution of malignant tumors — we pathologists would call this: geographical pathology. — When, in 1954, as a young assistant pathologist I got familiar with the results of the 5th Congress of the International Society for Geographical Pathology in Washington, I was fascinated by the possibilities of learning much more about the causes of human cancer and lymphomas in this way, than by means of the experimental pathology closely connected with my own work. Due to the concentration of scientific work, especially within the scope of the WHO, new important facts have been worked out in the meantime, some of which will be discussed today and tomorrow.

We have intentionally kept the number of participants rather small, since we have experienced that on all international symposia the success of a congress does not depend on the number of participants. Accordingly a thorough selection of the subjects in question was necessary for us. In the meantime some questions have already been settled or been in discussion on other symposia as e.g. the importance of air-pollution for lung-cancer. Our intention, with regard to the selection of the participants and presentations, was to offer a vast variety of topics. Owing to the co-operation with my old friend from our years in Freiburg, Dr. H. Tulinius, many problems could be solved more easily, especially the selection of the participants, which is, as you all know, an ungrateful and difficult task. I thank you, Dr. Tulinius, very much indeed for your efforts and in particular for your readiness to act as Chairman in these two days.

I thank you, ladies and gentlemen, for your kind attention.

# The World Health Organization's Programme for the Histopathological Definition and Classification of Tumours [1]

L. H. Sobin

World Health Organization, Geneva, Switzerland

Since 1957, the World Health Organization has been involved in a programme aimed at developing a uniform, internationally acceptable morphological classification of tumours, which would facilitate communications between those engaged in studies on cancer.

In general, the following procedure has been carried out for drafting the classifications and testing their applicability.

For each tumor site, a tentative histopathological typing and classification is drawn up by a group of experts.

An International Reference Centre (IRC) and a number of collaborating laboratories are then designated by WHO to evaluate the proposed classification. These laboratories exchange histological preparations in the form of microscope slides and paraffin blocks, accompanied by clinical information. The histological typing is then made in accordance with the proposed classification. Subsequently, one or more technical meetings are called by WHO to facilitate an exchange of opinions. If necessary, the classification is then amended to take account of criticisms.

The IRC then prepares sets of microscope slides covering all the proposed histological types and sends these with the revised classification to other pathologists, usually not more than ten, for their comments and suggestions. When replies have been received from all these reviewers, the classification is again revised in accordance with their comments.

A publication is then prepared for the series "International Histological Classification of Tumours" consisting of the classification and nomenclature, brief explanatory notes, and colour photomicrographs. These are not intended to serve as textbooks but rather as guides to the typing of tumours. Also available are sets of 35 mm colour transparencies of the photomicrographs, designed for teaching purposes. English, French and Spanish editions are produced.

Sets of transparencies with the book are distributed free to the directors of pathology departments of all medical schools throughout the world. These may also be purchased from WHO or its distributors.

---

1 This article is based on a paper that was published in *Meth. Inform. Med.*, 1971, 10, 120—122 and appears by kind permission of the editor of that journal.

The IRC also prepares sets of histological slides from its collection for distribution to national societies of pathology to serve as reference material. This distribution is carried out by the International Council of Societies of Pathology.

Training facilities are usually available at the IRC or collaborating centres for pathologists to become more familiar with the classifications by studying the slide collections.

Table 1. WHO international reference centres for nomenclature and classification of tumours

| Subject | Location | Date of establishment | State of work |
|---|---|---|---|
| Lung | Oslo | 1958 | Classification published 1967[a] |
| Breast | London | 1958 | Classification published 1968[b] |
| Soft tissues | Washington | 1958 | Classification published 1969[c] |
| Haematopoietic/lymphoid | Villejuif | 1962 | Publication in preparation |
| Oral | Agra | 1963 | Classification published 1971[d] |
| Bone | Buenos Aires | 1963 | Publication in preparation |
| Ovary | Leningrad | 1963 | Publication in preparation |
| Thyroid | Zurich | 1964 | Work in progress |
| Salivary glands | London | 1964 | Publication in preparation |
| Skin | Perth | 1965 | Publication in preparation |
| Male urogenital | Washington | 1965 | Work in progress |
| Odontogenic | Copenhagen | 1966 | Classification published 1971[e] |
| Comparative oncology | Washington | 1966 | Work in progress |
| Uterus | Copenhagen | 1967 | Work in progress |
| Oral precancer | Copenhagen | 1967 | Work in progress |
| Gastro-oesophageal | Tokyo | 1968 | Work in progress |
| Intestinal | London | 1968 | Work in progress |
| Exfoliative cytology | Geneva | 1968 | Publication in preparation |
| Central nervous system | Cologne | 1970 | Work in progress |

[a] KREYBERG, L., LIEBOW, A. A., and UEHLINGER, F. A.: Histological typing of lung tumours, Geneva 1967. World Health Organization (International Histological Classification of Tumours, No. 1).

[b] SCARFF, R. W. and TORLONI, H.: Histological typing of breast tumours, Geneva 1968. World Health Organization (International Histological Classification of Tumours, No. 2).

[c] ENZINGER, F. M., LATTES, R., and TORLONI, H.: Histological typing of soft tissue tumours, Geneva 1969. World Health Organization (International Histological Classification of Tumours, No. 3).

[d] WAHI, P. N., COHEN, B., LUTHRA, U. K., and TORLONI, H.: Histological typing of oral and oropharyngeal tumours, Geneva 1971. World Health Organization (International Histological Classification of Tumours, No. 4).

[e] PINDBORG, J., KRAMER, I., and TORLONI, H.: Histological typing of odontogenic tumours, jaw cysts, and allied lesions, Geneva 1971. World Health Organization (International Histological Classification of Tumours, No. 5).

Since 1958, 19 IRCs have been established to deal with the morphological classification and nomenclature of tumours. Their subjects, locations, dates of establishment, and state of work are given in Table 1.

Five classifications have been published; six more IRCs have reached final agreement and are preparing their publications; and eight IRCs are still testing their tentative classifications.

The IRC for male urogenital tract tumours has completed the classification of urinary bladder tumours and is continuing work on other sites. The IRC responsible for the nomenclature in exfoliative cytology has completed its work on the female genital tract and is proceeding with the study of extragenital cytology.

In addition to IRCs responsible for the major sites of tumours in man, an IRC for Comparative Oncology was established to deal with tumours of domestic animals.

It is intended to establish IRCs for tumours of the liver, biliary tract and pancreas, eye, upper respiratory tract, and endocrine glands.

Up to the present, this programme has involved the collaboration of over 200 pathologists in 48 countries.

# Investigation on the Epidemiological Significance of Detailed Cancer Data — Preliminary Results [1]

RUTH STEINITZ and CORINA COSTIN

Ministry of Health, Division of Chronic Diseases, Jerusalem, Israel

## Purpose

Published reports of cancer registries' data so far confined themselves to the categories of the International Classification of Diseases. Epidemiological conclusions pointed to differences in morbidity. Most workers feel that more light might be shed on the nature of these differences, if the categories could be subdivided by anatomical specification and/or by morphological diagnosis including behaviour, and by survival experience.

Some attempts in this direction have been made, for example by BIGNALL [1] for Lung Tumours and by the End Results Group [2] for various selected sites. Many cancer registries have provisions for coding the histological diagnosis. The Israel Cancer Registry added to this a very detailed code for anatomical subsites and for including "behaviour" in the histology code.

Therefore, we proposed to the International Agency for Research on Cancer a study on the epidemiological significance of detailed cancer data. The established differences in morbidity by ICD categories among the various population groups in Israel serve as background [3].

Another, not less important question was whether cancer registry data as they are collected today are sufficiently and reliably detailed for such an intensive workup. It is evident that reliable and homogenous material, which may answer the rigorous requests of conscientious pathologists can only be had from certain selected hospitals. However, this material can never be used for epidemiological studies.

The population-based cancer registry has at its disposal a very heterogonous material. Both, habits and fashions in the use of medical terms, and various degrees of accuracy and thorouhgness of description, lead to a vast range of quality of data, from excellent and complete information to outright uncertain cases which can not be excluded unless proven to be erroneous.

Our study may shed some light on whether the results are worth the effort of detailed coding and work-up. If the answer should be negative—do the results, so far, support an attempt to improve the quality of the data?

---

1 Supported by Research Agreement IARC S2/2 M.E. Israel.

## Methods and Material

Cancer incidence in the 7 years' period 1960—1966 was published in the conventional way as the Israel Cancer Registry's contribution to "Cancer Incidence in 5 Continents", Vol. II [4]. The same material was submitted one year later, after updating, to detailed coding of selected sites diagnosed in the Jewish groups: born in Europe or America, born in Asia, born in Africa, and Israel born. Data were used as they were achieved by ordinary cancer registry procedures (e.g. case summaries from hospitals, pathology reports, death notifications etc.). No attempt was made —at this stage—to improve them by going back to the hospital files.

Following the way of presentation of "Cancer Incidence in 5 Continents", levels of morbidity for each site and population group are expressed as World Population Standardized Rates (W.S.R.) with the addition of both, the percentage of microscopic confirmation and the percentage of cases known from death certificates only. This is the background for our detailed investigation.

"Survival" in our case should be termed more correctly "reported mortality", as the Israel Cancer Registry is not able to get routine confirmation of the living status at a certain date, but has to confine itself to death notifications by any of the sources mentioned. Four periods of length of survival were chosen: 1) 3 months (early death), 2) from 4 to 12 months, 3) up to 3 years, and 4) more than 3 years.

This preliminary report refers to the investigation of Cancer of Stomach, of Lung, of Female Breast and of Ovary, by anatomical subsites, histological types, behaviour and "reported mortality".

## Results

### Stomach

There is a striking difference of incidence among the three main male population groups, and a lesser but still discernable difference among females. It is evident that these observed differences can not be due to various degrees of diagnostic achievement, as the percentage of microscopic confirmation and the percentage of data based on death notifications only show small variations (Table 1).

*Anatomical Subsites:* The desired anatomical subdivisions of the Stomach as Upper Part (excepting Cardiac Region if confirmed as Squamous Cell Ca., which belongs to Oesophagus) and Lower Part, with still more specification as Curvatura Minor, Curvatura Major and Pyloric Region, were available in a range of 63.9% for Europe and America born males to 44.5% for Israel born females (Table 2 and 3). Documentation for females, in all population groups, is less accurate.

Among the cases with subdivisions stated the dominant location is the Lower Part of the Stomach, in all population groups and in both sexes, but with females showing significantly less Upper Part involvement (Table 4). An attempt was made for further subdivision of the Lower Part. Something similar is suggested in the proposal for the Ninth Revision of the International Classification of Diseases, Injuries and Causes of Death [5]. As far as data are available, "Curvatura Minor" occupies the highest percentage in males for all population groups, with the exception of Asia born males in whom the Pyloric Region is dominant.

Table 1. Malignant Neoplasms of Stomach. Israel, 1960—1966[a], Jewish Population. All ages, by Origin and Sex. Number of Cases (N); World Population Standardized Rate per 100,000 (W.S.R.)[b]; Microscopic Confirmation (%) and Registered on Death Certificates only (%)

| Origin | N | W.S.R. | % Microscopic confirmation | % Death certificates only |
|---|---|---|---|---|
| *Males* | | | | |
| All Jews | 1745 | 27.0 | 70.0 | 7.1 |
| Europe and America | 1339 | 31.4 | 71.6 | 6.0 |
| Africa | 122 | 20.1 | 68.3 | 11.4 |
| Asia | 204 | 16.7 | 62.3 | 7.7 |
| Israel born | 35 | 11.4 | 63.6 | 15.2 |
| *Females* | | | | |
| All Jews | 1095 | 16.4 | 67.7 | 8.7 |
| Europe and America | 803 | 18.8 | 68.9 | 8.0 |
| Africa | 92 | 13.8 | 62.8 | 8.5 |
| Asia | 128 | 10.2 | 63.0 | 9.5 |
| Israel born | 27 | 8.2 | 74.1 | 11.1 |

[a] Cancer Incidence in 5 Continents, Vol. II, p. 184—197; 384—386.
[b] Idem p. 334, 346, 348.

Table 2. Malignant Neoplasms of Stomach. Israel, 1960—1966, Jewish Population. All ages by Origin and Sex. Number of Cases (N). Availability of subsite and histology: percentage

| Origin | N | % Subsite available | % Histology available |
|---|---|---|---|
| *Males* | | | |
| All Jews | 1799 | 61.0 | 66.9 |
| Europe and America | 1349 | 63.9 | 69.6 |
| Africa | 123 | 66.1 | 56.9 |
| Asia | 207 | 56.0 | 56.0 |
| Israel born | 33 | 60.6 | 51.5 |
| *Females* | | | |
| All Jews | 1114 | 51.6 | 59.5 |
| Europe and America | 808 | 54.3 | 59.4 |
| Africa | 99 | 42.4 | 52.5 |
| Asia | 127 | 45.7 | 44.9 |
| Israel born | 27 | 44.4 | 70.3 |

*Morphology:* More specified histological diagnosis than just "Carcinoma" in those microscopically confirmed is available in range of 69.6% for males born in Europe/America, to 51.5% in Israel-born, and for females, between 70.4% in the Israel-born and 44.9% in the Asian group (Table 5). "Adenocarcinoma" reaches the highest percentage of specified histology throughout.

*Behaviour:* Females of all population groups are outstanding for a higher degree of anaplasia for all morphological types (Table 6).

Interestingly, the more specified diagnosis for anatomical subsites and for morphology appears in the group with the highest incidence.

Table 3. Malignant Neoplasms of Stomach. Israel, 1960—1966, Jewish Population. Subsites, all ages, by origin and sex. Number of cases and percentage

| Origin and Sex | | All cases: Total | | Upper part | | Lower part | | Whole organ + multiple | | St. p. partial gastrectomy | | N.A. | |
|---|---|---|---|---|---|---|---|---|---|---|---|---|---|
| | | N | % | N | % | N | % | N | % | N | % | N | % |
| Total Jews | M | 1799 | 100.00 | 273 | 15.17 | 682 | 37.91 | 120 | 6.67 | 39 | 2.17 | 685 | 38.07 |
| | F | 1114 | 100.00 | 94 | 8.43 | 421 | 37.79 | 50 | 4.48 | 10 | 0.89 | 539 | 48.38 |
| Europe and America | M | 1349 | 100.00 | 219 | 16.23 | 517 | 38.32 | 94 | 6.98 | 32 | 2.37 | 487 | 36.10 |
| | F | 808 | 100.00 | 71 | 8.78 | 322 | 39.85 | 37 | 4.57 | 9 | 1.11 | 369 | 45.66 |
| Africa | M | 123 | 100.00 | 11 | 8.94 | 47 | 38.21 | 10 | 8.13 | 1 | 0.81 | 54 | 43.90 |
| | F | 94 | 100.00 | 6 | 6.38 | 29 | 30.85 | 6 | 6.38 | 1 | 1.06 | 52 | 55.31 |
| Asia | M | 207 | 100.00 | 26 | 12.56 | 75 | 36.23 | 11 | 5.31 | 4 | 1.93 | 91 | 43.96 |
| | F | 127 | 100.00 | 12 | 9.44 | 41 | 32.28 | 5 | 3.93 | — | — | 69 | 54.33 |
| Israel | M | 33 | 100.00 | 6 | 18.18 | 13 | 39.39 | 1 | 3.03 | — | — | 13 | 39.39 |
| | F | 27 | 100.00 | 1 | 3.70 | 10 | 37.03 | 1 | 3.70 | — | — | 15 | 55.55 |

N.A. = Not Available. — = Rate not calculated for less than 5 cases.

Table 4. Malignant Neoplasms of Stomach. Israel, 1960—1966, Jewish Population. Subsites, all ages, by origin and sex. Number of cases and percentage

| Origin and sex | | Cases with sub-sites stated | | | | | | | | | |
|---|---|---|---|---|---|---|---|---|---|---|---|
| | | Total | | Upper part | | Lower part | | Whole organ +multiple | | St. post partial gastrect. | |
| | | N | % | N | % | N | % | N | % | N | % |
| Total Jews | M | 1114 | 100.00 | 273 | 24.50 | 682 | 61.22 | 120 | 10.77 | 39 | 3.50 |
| | F | 575 | 100.00 | 94[a] | 16.34 | 421 | 73.21 | 50 | 8.69 | 10 | 1.73 |
| Europe and America | M | 862 | 100.00 | 219 | 25.40 | 517 | 59.97[b] | 94 | 10.90 | 32 | 3.71 |
| | F | 439 | 100.00 | 71 | 16.17 | 322 | 73.34 | 37 | 8.42 | 9 | 2.05 |
| Africa | M | 69 | 100.00 | 11 | 15.94 | 47 | 68.11[b] | 10 | 14.49 | 1 | 1.44 |
| | F | 42 | 100.00 | 6 | 14.28 | 29 | 69.04 | 6 | 14.28 | 1 | 2.38 |
| Asia | M | 116 | 100.00 | 26 | 22.41 | 75 | 64.65 | 11 | 9.48 | 4 | 3.44 |
| | F | 58 | 100.00 | 12 | 20.68 | 41 | 70.68 | 5 | 8.62 | — | — |
| Israel | M | 20 | 100.00 | 6 | 30.00 | 13 | 65.00 | 1 | 5.00 | — | — |
| | F | 12 | 100.00 | 1 | 8.33 | 10 | 83.33 | 1 | 8.33 | — | — |

[a] $\chi^2 = 14.88$ ($P = 0.01$); [b] $\chi^2 = 1.62$ ($P > 0.05$).

Table 5. Malignant Neoplasms of Stomach. Israel, 1960—1966, Jewish Population. All subsites with histological diagnosis by sex and origin. Number of cases and percentage

| Origin | Total | | Mucoid Ca. | | Papillar-Ca. | | Adeno-Ca. | | Linitis plastica | | Others[a] | | N.A. | |
|---|---|---|---|---|---|---|---|---|---|---|---|---|---|---|
| | N | % | N | % | N | % | N | % | N | % | N | % | N | % |
| *Males* | | | | | | | | | | | | | | |
| Total Jews | 1799 | 100.00 | 133 | 7.39 | 29 | 1.61 | 904 | 50.25 | 102 | 5.67 | 35 | 1.94 | 596 | 33.13 |
| Europe and America | 1349 | 100.00 | 97 | 7.19 | 22 | 1.63 | 746 | 55.30 | 63 | 4.68 | 11 | 0.81 | 410 | 30.40 |
| Africa | 123 | 100.00 | 10 | 8.13 | 1 | 0.81 | 45 | 36.58 | 8 | 6.50 | 6 | 4.87 | 53 | 43.08 |
| Asia | 207 | 100.00 | 14 | 6.76 | 5 | 2.41 | 82 | 39.61 | 11 | 5.31 | 4 | 1.93 | 91 | 43.96 |
| Israel born | 33 | 100.00 | 1 | 3.03 | — | — | 12 | 36.36 | 1 | 3.03 | 3 | 9.09 | 16 | 48.48 |
| *Females* | | | | | | | | | | | | | | |
| Total Jews | 1114 | 100.00 | 91 | 8.17 | 19 | 1.77 | 494 | 44.34 | 46 | 4.13 | 13 | 1.17 | 451 | 40.48 |
| Europe and America | 808 | 100.00 | 60 | 7.42 | 14 | 1.24 | 379 | 46.90 | 17 | 2.11 | 10 | 1.24 | 328 | 40.59 |
| Africa | 99 | 100.00 | 15 | 15.15 | — | — | 33 | 33.33 | 4 | 4.04 | — | — | 47 | 47.47 |
| Asia | 127 | 100.00 | 6 | 4.73 | 1 | 0.80 | 44 | 34.66 | 6 | 4.73 | — | — | 70 | 55.09 |
| Israel born | 27 | 100.00 | 4 | 14.81 | 1 | 3.70 | 14 | 51.85 | — | — | — | — | 8 | 29.62 |

[a] Including few cases of lymphoma. (—) No percentage calculated for less than 5 cases.

Table 6. Malignant Neoplasms of Stomach. Israel, 1960—1966, Jewish Population. All Subsites, all ages, histology and behaviour, by sex and origin. Number of cases and ratio well differentiated (W)/Anaplastic type (A) = (W/A)

| Origin and sex | | Total | | | Mucoid Ca. | | | Papillary Ca. | | | Adeno Ca. | | | Linitis plastic. | Others[a] | | | N.A. |
|---|---|---|---|---|---|---|---|---|---|---|---|---|---|---|---|---|---|---|
| | | Well differ. | Ana-plast. | Ratio W/A | Well differ. | Ana-plast. | Ratio W/A | Well differ. | Ana-plast. | Ratio W/A | Well differ. | Ana-plat. | Ratio W/A | | Well differ. | Ana-plast. | Ratio W/A | |
| Total Jews | M | 818 | 385 | 2.38 | 105 | 28 | 3.75 | 22 | 7 | 3.14 | 663 | 241 | 2.58 | 102 | 28 | 7 | 4.00 | 596 |
| | F | 433 | 230 | 1.88 | 70 | 21 | 3.33 | 15 | 4 | 3.75 | 335 | 159 | 2.11 | 46 | 13 | — | — | 451 |
| Europe and America | M | 649 | 290 | 2.24 | 79 | 18 | 4.34 | 18 | 4 | 4.50 | 543 | 203 | 2.67 | 63 | 9 | 2 | 4.50 | 410 |
| | F | 311 | 169 | 1.84 | 31 | 29 | 1.07 | 11 | 3 | 3.66 | 259 | 120 | 2.16 | 17 | 10 | — | — | 328 |
| Africa | M | 48 | 22 | 2.18 | 6 | 4 | 1.50 | — | 1 | — | 37 | 8 | 4.62 | 8 | 5 | 1 | 5.00 | 53 |
| | F | 29 | 23 | 1.26 | 11 | 4 | 2.75 | — | — | — | 18 | 15 | 1.20 | 4 | — | — | — | 47 |
| Asia | M | 85 | 31 | 2.74 | 12 | 2 | 6.00 | 5 | — | — | 64 | 18 | 3.55 | 11 | 4 | — | — | 91 |
| | F | 31 | 26 | 1.19 | 5 | 1 | 5.00 | 1 | — | — | 25 | 19 | 1.32 | 6 | — | — | — | 70 |
| Israel born | M | 13 | 4 | 3.25 | 1 | — | — | — | — | — | 10 | 2 | 5.00 | 1 | 2 | 1 | 2.00 | 16 |
| | F | 13 | 6 | 2.17 | 4 | — | — | 1 | — | — | 8 | 6 | 1.33 | — | — | — | — | 8 |

[a] Including 9 male and 2 female cases of lymphoma.

Table 7. Malignant Neoplasms: Selected Sites. Incidence 1960—1966, Jewish Population. Reported deaths by sex and origin. All ages

| *Males* | | | | | | *Females* | | | | | | | |
|---|---|---|---|---|---|---|---|---|---|---|---|---|---|
| Origin | | *Stomach* | | *Lung* | | *Stomach* | | *Lung* | | *Breast* | | *Ovary* | |
| | | All cases | Deaths | All cases | Deaths | All cases | Deaths | All cases | Deaths | All cases | Deaths | All cases | Deaths |
| Total Jews | | 1799[d] | 1480 | 2010[d] | 1649 | 1114[d] | 945 | 665[d] | 516 | 3867[d] | 1496 | 980[d] | 673 |
| Europe and America | N | 1349 | 1164 | 1349 | 1207 | 808 | 723 | 475 | 383 | 2817 | 1124 | 730 | 563 |
| | % | 100.00 | 86.29 | 100.00 | 89.47 | 100.00 | 89.48 | 100.00 | 80.63 | 100.00 | 39.90 | 100.00 | 77.12 |
| Africa | N | 123 | 105 | 176 | 146 | 94 | 86 | 35 | 27 | 232 | 124 | 40 | 31 |
| | % | 100.00 | 85.36 | 100.00 | 82.95 | 100.00 | 91.49 | 100.00 | 77.14 | 100.00 | 53.44 | 100.00 | 77.50 |
| Asia | N | 207 | 180 | 267 | 247 | 127 | 111 | 90 | 80 | 316 | 160 | 74 | 51 |
| | % | 100.00 | 86.96 | 100.00 | 92.51 | 100.00 | 87.40 | 100.00 | 88.89 | 100.00 | 50.63 | 100.00 | 68.92 |
| Israel born | N | 33 | 31 | 55 | 49 | 27 | 25 | 29 | 26 | 183 | 88 | 44 | 28 |
| | % | 100.00 | 93.94 | 100.00 | 89.09 | 100.00 | 92.59 | 100.00 | 89.65 | 100.00 | 48.09 | 100.00 | 63.64 |

*Chi-Square* Lung males: Europe/Africa — 2.41; Europe/Africa — 6.37[b]; Africa/Israel — 1.63; Africa/Asia —11.54[c]

Lung females: Europe/Asia —4.24[a]; Africa/Asia —2.75

Breast: Europe/Africa —17.40[c]; Europe/Asia —13.97[c]; Europe/Israel — 5.44[b]

Ovary: Europe/Asia — 2.00; Europe/Israel — 3.20

[a] Significant with P = 0.05; [b] Significant with P = 0.02; [c] Significant with P = 0.01; [d] Total Jews cases include Jews origin unknown.

Table 8. Malignant Neoplasms of Stomach. Incidence 1960—1966, Jewish population. "Reported Mortality" by origin and sex. All ages; length of survival in months

| Origin and sex | | Length of Survival | | | | | |
|---|---|---|---|---|---|---|---|
| | | Total | | | | | |
| | | N | % | —3 m. | 4—12 m. | 13—35 m. | 36+ m. |
| Total Jews | M | 1480 | 100.0 | 52.1 | 30.1 | 14.5 | 3.3 |
| | F | 945 | 100.0 | 50.4 | 33.5 | 13.0 | 3.1 |
| Europe and America | M | 1164 | 100.0 | 50.0 | 31.5 | 15.1 | 3.4 |
| | F | 723 | 100.0 | 49.9 | 32.6 | 13.8 | 3.6 |
| Africa | M | 105 | 100.0 | 61.0 | 22.9 | 15.2 | 1.0 |
| | F | 86 | 100.0 | 53.5 | 32.6 | 10.5 | 3.5 |
| Asia | M | 180 | 100.0 | 60.0 | 25.0 | 11.0 | 4.4 |
| | F | 111 | 100.0 | 50.5 | 40.5 | 9.0 | — |
| Israel born | M | 31 | 100.0 | 54.8 | 29.0 | 12.9 | 3.2 |
| | F | 25 | 100.0 | 52.0 | 32.0 | 16.0 | — |

Chi square: Europe/Africa-males (—3 m.) —4.14[a]; Europe/Asia-males (—3 m.) —5.75[b].
[a] Significant with P = 0.05; [b] Significant with P = 0.02.

*Reported Mortality:* The overall high mortality in the observed period surveyed —about 90% for both sexes (Table 7)—does not show any appreciable differences among the various population groups. "Early" mortality is especially prevalent in African and Asian males (statistically significant—Table 8). The expectation that anaplasia is correlated with a higher and earlier mortality is not consistently confirmed for Stomach cancer.

## Lung

This is a site where the overall morbidity in the various population groups in Israel shows less differences than for Stomach cancer. The previously noted low male/female ratio [3], especially for Israel born and born in Europe/America is again observed. The percentage of microscopic confirmation reaches approximately the same level in all population groups, but shows clearly the decline with age, described also by Bignall [1]. The reverse is seen for the cases available from death notifications only (Table 9).

*Anatomical Subsites:* The subsites investigated are right and left, upper, middle and lower lobe, and central versus peripheral location. Specified localization is stated in about three quarters of the cases (Table 10). Registry data are in agreement with findings of clinical and pathology series [1] that central, right side, and upper lobes are the most frequent sites of the malignancy (Table 11). However in our material in males, age 45—54, the tumour appears more often on the left side. That the right middle lobe is a more frequent location than the Lingula had to be expected in accordance with the mass of available lung tissue.

*Morphology:* Squamous cell carcinoma occurs more frequently in males and Adenocarcinoma in females, a well-known fact. However, the low male/female ratio for Squamous cell carcinoma 6.6 : 1 and for Adenocarcinoma 2.0 : 1 are out-

Table 9. Malignant Neoplasms of Lung. Israel, 1960—1966[a], Jewish Population. All ages, by Origin and Sex. Number of Cases (N); World Population Standardized Rate per 100,000 (W.S.R.)[b]; Microscopic Confirmation (%) and Registered on Death Certificates only (%)

| Origin | N | W.S.R. | % Microscopic confirmation | % Death certificates only |
|---|---|---|---|---|
| *Males* | | | | |
| All Jews | 1871 | 27.8 | 60.8 | 5.0 |
| Europe and America | 1321 | 30.4 | 62.7 | 4.0 |
| Africa | 168 | 17.9 | 56.3 | 8.0 |
| Asia | 262 | 21.4 | 56.2 | 7.1 |
| Israel born | 54 | 15.4 | 65.5 | — |
| *Females* | | | | |
| All Jews | 612 | 9.1 | 58.4 | 6.0 |
| Europe and America | 441 | 8.6 | 58.1 | 5.3 |
| Africa | 29 | 4.7 | 48.6 | 2.9 |
| Asia | 88 | 6.9 | 55.6 | 12.2 |
| Israel born | 28 | 7.3 | 82.8 | 8.5 |

[a] Cancer Incidence in 5 Continents, Vol. II, p. 184—197; 384—386.
[b] Idem, p. 334, 354, 356.

Table 10. Malignant Neoplasms of Lung. Israel, 1960—1966, Jewish Population. All ages by origin and sex. Number of cases (N). Availability of subsite and histology: percentage

| Origin | N | % Subsite available | % Histology available |
|---|---|---|---|
| *Males* | | | |
| All Jews | 2010 | 74.4 | 58.7 |
| Europe and America | 1349 | 76.3 | 61.7 |
| Africa | 176 | 72.7 | 58.0 |
| Asia | 267 | 77.2 | 54.7 |
| Israel born | 55 | 78.2 | 60.0 |
| *Females* | | | |
| All Jews | 665 | 73.2 | 53.1 |
| Europe and America | 475 | 74.5 | 53.3 |
| Africa | 35 | 82.9 | 34.3 |
| Asia | 90 | 83.3 | 56.7 |
| Israel born | 29 | 65.5 | 72.4 |

standing and may be correlated with the above mentioned low sex ratio for lung cancer in Israel (Table 12).

*Behaviour:* In general, there is more anaplasia in males than in females, except for the Asian-born and Israel-born; but the highest percentage of anaplasia is found in females with Squamous cell carcinoma (Table 13).

*Reported mortality:* An amazing finding in our survey is the significantly lower mortality experience of African-born males. The same seems to hold true for African-born females (Table 7). As to subsite—in males, centrally located tumours of the

Table 11. Malignant Neoplasms of Lung. Israel, 1960—1966, Jewish Population. Sub-sites by origin, sex. All ages. Number of cases and percentage

| Origin and sex | | | | Central | | | | | | | | | | | |
|---|---|---|---|---|---|---|---|---|---|---|---|---|---|---|---|
| | | Total | | Right | | Left | | S.N.S. | | Peripheral | | Others[a] | | N.A. | |
| | | N | % | N | % | N | % | N | % | N | % | N | % | N | % |
| Total Jews | M | 2010 | 100.00 | 762 | 37.91 | 656 | 32.63 | 5 | 0.24 | 21 | 1.04 | 51 | 2.53 | 515 | 25.62 |
| | F | 665 | 100.00 | 252 | 37.89 | 178 | 26.76 | — | — | 19 | 2.85 | 38 | 5.71 | 178 | 26.76 |
| Europe and America | M | 1349 | 100.00 | 523 | 38.76 | 446 | 33.06 | 2 | 0.14 | 17 | 1.26 | 41 | 3.03 | 320 | 23.72 |
| | F | 475 | 100.00 | 187 | 39.36 | 127 | 26.73 | — | — | 16 | 3.36 | 24 | 5.05 | 121 | 25.47 |
| Africa | M | 176 | 100.00 | 67 | 38.06 | 53 | 30.11 | — | — | 1 | 0.56 | 7 | 3.97 | 48 | 27.27 |
| | F | 35 | 100.00 | 13 | 37.14 | 8 | 22.85 | — | — | 1 | 2.85 | 7 | 20.00 | 6 | 17.13 |
| Asia | M | 267 | 100.00 | 109 | 40.83 | 91 | 34.08 | 2 | 0.74 | 2 | 0.74 | 2 | 0.74 | 61 | 22.84 |
| | F | 90 | 100.00 | 43 | 47.77 | 25 | 27.77 | — | — | 1 | 1.11 | 6 | 6.66 | 12 | 16.66 |
| Israel born | M | 55 | 100.00 | 26 | 47.27 | 16 | 29.09 | — | — | — | — | 1 | 1.81 | 10 | 21.81 |
| | F | 29 | 100.00 | 10 | 34.48 | 9 | 31.03 | — | — | — | — | — | — | 15 | 34.48 |

[a] Includes upper and middle lobe, lower and middle lobe, lung and mediastinum, multiple.

Table 12. Lung Cancer. Squamous Cell Carcinoma and Adeno Cell Carcinoma, by age. Sex ratio M/F = 1

| Source | All ages | | 45—54 | | 55—64 | | 65—74 | |
|---|---|---|---|---|---|---|---|---|
| | Squam. | Adeno | Squam. | Adeno | Squam. | Adeno | Squam. | Adeno |
| Clinical series DOLL and HILL[a] 1948—1952 | 26.4 | 3.3 | 31.0 | 4.3 | 32.7 | 2.6 | 8.8 | 2.6 |
| Cancer registry Israel, 1960—1966 | 6.6 | 2.0 | 4.3 | 1.27 | 12.3 | 3.4 | 7.4 | 1.7 |

[a] Source: From BIGNALL, J. R., "Carcinoma of the Lung". Edinburgh-London: Livingstone 1958, p. 185.

right side carry a higher mortality than the left ones. In those female groups, where the number of cases seems reasonable for evaluation, anaplasia is associated with early mortality.

## Female Breast

Differences in Breast cancer morbidity among the various Jewish groups—high rates for Jews born in Europe/America and low rates for Asian and African born—were so striking that they were observed by clinicians long before the establishment of the Cancer Registry. In Breast cancer too, as in the other sites, levels of microscopic confirmation, and known from death notifications only, are the same for all population groups (Table 14).

*Anatomical Subsites:* Specified information—which side, quadrant etc., is not available in about 60% (Table 15). This is in agreement with the Working Party for the Ninth Revision of the ICD [5]. For all ages and origins, the statement that the tumour is lateral, is more frequent. However, it can be assumed, that the percentage of the lateral location is still underestimated, as "Medial" and perhaps also "Central" are more likely to be expressively stated because of the therapeutic implications. Interestingly, in the age group 35—44, Israel-born and African-born have a higher percentage of medial location. The same applies in the age group 45—54, but for African-born only. In other words, our figures indicate that in the lower incidence population groups there may be a higher percentage of medially located tumours (Table 16).

As reported also by CLEMMESEN [6], left-sided tumours are in excess, for all ages and all population groups, except for Asian-born.

*Morphology:* There are great differences in preference for certain terms used by pathologists for malignancies of the breast, and also, whether only the dominant histology is mentioned or all morphological variations within one neoplasm are described. With this reservation in mind, the following results should be interpreted. No differences in histology are observed whether the tumour is right or left sided (Table 17). In central tumours Ductal carcinoma is prevalent, as expected. In others, Scirrhous, Lobular and Adenocarcinoma are the most frequent.

Table 13. Malignant Neoplasms of Lung. Israel, 1960—1966, Jewish Population. Subsites, histological diagnosis including behaviour by sex: all ages. Number of cases and ratio well differentiated (W)/anaplastic (A)

| Origin and sex | | Total | | | Central | | | | | | | | | | | | Peripheral | | | N.A. | | |
|---|---|---|---|---|---|---|---|---|---|---|---|---|---|---|---|---|---|---|---|---|---|---|
| | | | | | Right | | | Left | | | S.N.S. | | | Total | | | | | | | | |
| | | Well differ. | Ana-plastic | Ratio W/A | W | A | Ratio W/A | W | A | Ratio W/A | W | A | Ratio W/A | W | A | Ratio W/A | W | A | Ratio W/A | W | A | Ratio W/A |
| Total Jews | M | 717 | 463 | 1.55 | 298 | 201 | 1.48 | 278 | 169 | 1.64 | 2 | — | — | 578 | 370 | 1.56 | 14 | 6 | 2.33 | 125 | 87 | 1.44 |
| | F | 234 | 119 | 1.96 | 95 | 63 | 1.50 | 63 | 29 | 2.17 | — | — | — | 158 | 92 | 1.72 | 12 | 3 | 4.00 | 64 | 24 | 2.70 |
| Europe and | M | 495 | 338 | 1.46 | 210 | 150 | 1.40 | 192 | 120 | 1.60 | 1 | — | — | 403 | 270 | 1.49 | 10 | 6 | 1.67 | 82 | 62 | 1.32 |
| America | F | 166 | 87 | 1.91 | 73 | 45 | 1.62 | 33 | 20 | 1.65 | — | — | — | 106 | 65 | 1.63 | 9 | 3 | 3.00 | 51 | 19 | 2.68 |
| Africa | M | 66 | 36 | 1.83 | 29 | 13 | 2.23 | 20 | 16 | 1.25 | — | — | — | 49 | 29 | 1.69 | 1 | — | — | 16 | 7 | 2.28 |
| | F | 10 | 2 | 5.00 | 3 | 2 | 1.50 | 5 | — | — | — | — | — | 8 | 2 | 4.00 | 1 | — | — | 1 | — | — |
| Asia | M | 101 | 45 | 2.24 | 34 | 21 | 1.62 | 46 | 17 | 2.70 | 2 | — | — | 82 | 38 | 2.16 | 1 | — | — | 18 | 7 | 2.57 |
| | F | 35 | 16 | 2.19 | 12 | 9 | 1.33 | 10 | 6 | 1.67 | — | — | — | 22 | 15 | 1.47 | 1 | — | — | 12 | 1 | 12.00 |
| Israel born | M | 22 | 11 | 2.00 | 16 | 6 | 2.67 | 3 | 5 | 0.60 | — | — | — | 19 | 11 | 1.73 | — | — | — | 3 | — | — |
| | F | 13 | 8 | 1.62 | 5 | 3 | 1.67 | 3 | 1 | 3.00 | — | — | — | 8 | 4 | 2.00 | — | — | — | 5 | | 1.25 |

Table 14. Malignant Neoplasms of Female Breast. Israel, 1960—1966[a], Jewish Population. All ages, by Origin. Number of Cases (N); World Population Standardized Rate per 100,000 (W.S.R.)[b]. Microscopic confirmation (%) and Registered on death Certificates only (%)

| Origin | N | W.S.R. | % Microscopic | % Death |
|---|---|---|---|---|
| All Jews | 3763 | 52.1 | 89.7 | 1.1 |
| Europe and America | 2978 | 63.6 | 91.0 | 1.1 |
| Africa | 239 | 27.0 | 86.2 | 1.3 |
| Asia | 343 | 26.6 | 89.2 | 0.6 |
| Israel born | 203 | 47.9 | 88.5 | 1.6 |

[a] Cancer incidence in 5 Continents, Vol. II, p. 184—197; 384—386.
[b] Idem, p. 356.

Table 15. Malignant Neoplasms of Female Breast. Israel, 1960—1966, Jewish Population. All ages by Origin. Number of Cases (N). Availability of Subsite and Histology: percentage

| Origin | N | % Subsite available | % Histology available |
|---|---|---|---|
| All Jews | 3867 | 37.4 | 86.7 |
| Europe and America | 2817 | 39.0 | 87.6 |
| Africa | 232 | 37.5 | 83.6 |
| Asia | 316 | 37.3 | 85.1 |
| Israel born | 183 | 39.9 | 83.6 |

*Behaviour:* Jews born in Asia and Africa seem to have more anaplastic tumours. Again, as in Stomach cancer, the lower incidence groups have the higher anaplasia, in this case correlated with the medial location.

*Reported Mortality:* Breast cancer patients of African origin are dying significantly earlier than other groups (Table 18 and 19). However, we could not confirm from

Table 16. Malignant Neoplasms of Female Breast. Israel, 1960—1966, Jewish Popula-

| Origin | | Total | | | | Right | | | | | |
|---|---|---|---|---|---|---|---|---|---|---|---|
| | | Total | Right | Left | N.O.S. | Total | Medial | Later. | Centr. | Others | N.A. |
| Total Jews | N | 3575 | 1515 | 1610 | 450 | 1515 | 117 | 352 | 93 | 57 | 896 |
| | % | 100.00 | 42.38 | 45.03 | 12.59 | 100.00 | 7.72 | 23.23 | 6.14 | 3.76 | 59.14 |
| Europa a. America | N | 2619 | 1118 | 1212 | 289 | 1118 | 86 | 274 | 65 | 42 | 651 |
| | % | 100.00 | 42.69 | 46.28 | 11.03 | 100.00 | 7.69 | 24.50 | 5.81 | 3.75 | 58.22 |
| Africa | N | 214 | 86 | 104 | 24 | 86 | 11 | 20 | 4 | 3 | 48 |
| | % | 100.00 | 40.18 | 48.59 | 11.21 | 100.00 | 12.79 | 23.25 | 4.65 | 3.48 | 55.81 |
| Asia | N | 300 | 144 | 125 | 31 | 144 | 7 | 26 | 11 | 6 | 94 |
| | % | 100.00 | 48.00 | 41.66 | 10.33 | 100.00 | 4.86 | 18.05 | 7.63 | 4.16 | 65.27 |
| Israel born | N | 172 | 70 | 82 | 20 | 70 | 11 | 13 | 4 | 5 | 37 |
| | % | 100.00 | 40.69 | 47.67 | 11.62 | 100.00 | 15.71 | 18.57 | 5.71 | 7.14 | 52.85 |

[a] Excludes bilateral and subsites not stated.

our material that there is a correlation between histological type and length of survival, as found by INGLEBY and GERSHON-COHEN [7] (Scirrhous-fastest growing and Duct. Ca.-slowest).

### Ovary

The great difference in incidence between Jews born in Europe/America and the other population groups is obvious. This is true for all age groups, starting at age 34, and this again despite the equality in percentage of microscopic confirmation and of percentage of data based on death certificates only (Table 20).

*Laterality:* A statement on side is available in appr. 60%, for all population groups (Table 21). Right is mentioned more often, consistently in all groups except the Israel-born (Table 22). We have not been able to find whether difference in size of the organ, e.g. the amount of available tissue, could serve as anatomical explanation of this finding.

*Morphology:* Percentage distribution of the various histological types of malignancies is the same for right and left. An exception is malignant Granulosa cell Carcinoma, which in our series is more often found in the left ovary.

*Behaviour:* There is more anaplasia in the population group with a higher incidence, e.g. Europe/America born, a finding which is not consistent with that encountered in the other examined sites (Table 23).

Bilateral tumours seem to be associated with higher anaplasia—this was also found by KOTTMEIER [8].

*Reported Mortality:* Africa-born Jews with Ovarian cancer have a higher percentage of early deaths (Table 24), but this was not found to be correlated with anaplasia. Bilateral tumours carry a higher mortality, as expected.

## Discussion and Conclusions

One of the most annoying features of our investigation is the amount of "unavailables" in the desired categories. On the other hand we think that the "available"

tion. Laterality by subsites[a] and origin, all ages. Number of cases and percentage

| Left | | | | | | N.O.S. | | | | | |
|---|---|---|---|---|---|---|---|---|---|---|---|
| Total | Medical | Lateral | Cent. | Others | N.A. | Total | Med. | Later. | Centr. | Others | N.A. |
| 1610 | 142 | 372 | 73 | 66 | 957 | 450 | 8 | 10 | 19 | 7 | 406 |
| 100.00 | 8.81 | 23.10 | 4.53 | 4.09 | 59.44 | 100.00 | 1.77 | 2.22 | 4.22 | 1.55 | 90.22 |
| 1212 | 107 | 288 | 53 | 49 | 715 | 289 | 4 | 7 | 15 | 5 | 258 |
| 100.00 | 8.83 | 23.76 | 4.37 | 4.04 | 59.00 | 100.00 | 1.38 | 2.42 | 5.19 | 1.73 | 89.27 |
| 104 | 11 | 20 | 7 | 2 | 64 | 24 | 1 | — | — | — | 23 |
| 100.00 | 10.57 | 19.23 | 6.75 | 1.92 | 61.53 | 100.00 | 4.16 | — | — | — | 95.83 |
| 125 | 10 | 35 | 5 | 7 | 68 | 31 | 1 | 3 | 2 | — | 25 |
| 100.00 | 8.00 | 28.00 | 4.00 | 5.60 | 54.40 | 100.00 | 3.22 | 9.67 | 6.45 | — | 80.64 |
| 82 | 11 | 16 | 2 | 5 | 48 | 20 | — | — | — | — | 20 |
| 100.00 | 13.41 | 19.51 | 2.43 | 6.09 | 58.53 | 100.00 | — | — | — | — | 100.00 |

Table 17. Malignant Neoplasms of Female Breast. Israel, 1960—1966, Jewish Population. Laterality[a] by histology, all ages. Number of cases and percentage

| Laterality | | Total | Ductal Ca. | Mucinous a. papillary Ca. | Medullary Ca. a. Ca. solidum | Inflammatory Ca. | Scirrhous Lobular and Adeno Ca. | Carcinoma N.O.S. | Cysto-sarcoma | Others | N.A. |
|---|---|---|---|---|---|---|---|---|---|---|---|
| Total | N | 3575 | 823 | 92 | 216 | 11 | 1206 | 799 | 23 | 45 | 360 |
| | % | 100.00 | 23.02 | 2.57 | 6.04 | 0.31 | 33.73 | 22.34 | 0.64 | 1.26 | 10.06 |
| Right | N | 1515 | 350 | 45 | 92 | 5 | 560 | 312 | 12 | 15 | 124 |
| | % | 100.00 | 23.10 | 2.97 | 6.07 | 0.33 | 36.96 | 20.59 | 0.79 | 0.99 | 8.18 |
| Left | N | 1610 | 370 | 35 | 110 | 6 | 571 | 372 | 10 | 23 | 113 |
| | % | 100.00 | 22.99 | 2.18 | 6.83 | 0.37 | 35.46 | 23.10 | 0.62 | 1.42 | 7.01 |
| N.O.S. | N | 450 | 103 | 12 | 14 | — | 75 | 115 | 1 | 7 | 123 |
| | % | 100.00 | 22.89 | 2.66 | 3.11 | — | 16.66 | 25.55 | 0.22 | 1.55 | 27.33 |

[a] Excludes bilateral and subsites not stated.

Table 18. Malignant Neoplasms of Female Breast. Incidence 1960—1966, Jewish population. "Reported Mortality" by origin. All ages; length of survival in months

| Origin | Length of survival | | | | |
|---|---|---|---|---|---|
| | N | % | — 12 m. | 13—35 m. | 36 + m. |
| Total Jews | 1496 | 100.0 | 23.6 | 41.9 | 34.5 |
| Europe and America | 1124 | 100.0 | 32.3 | 41.0 | 36.4 |
| Africa | 124 | 100.0 | 22.6[a] | 46.0 | 21.8 |
| Asia | 160 | 100.0 | 23.8 | 45.0 | 31.3 |
| Israel born | 88 | 100.0 | 23.9 | 42.0 | 34.1 |

[a] Chi-Square: Europe/Africa (—12 m.) —4.87; Significant with P = 0.05.

Table 20. Malignant Neoplasms of Ovary. Israel, 1960—1966[a], Jewish Population. All ages, by Origin. Number of Cases (N); World Population Standardized Rate per 100,000 (W.S.R.)[b]; Microscopic Confirmation (%) and Registered on death certificates only (%)

| Origin | N | W.S.R. | % Microscopic confirmation | % Death certificates only |
|---|---|---|---|---|
| All Jews | 877 | 12.4 | 86.5 | 1.5 |
| Europe and America | 677 | 15.2 | 86.0 | 1.6 |
| Africa | 33 | 4.0 | 80.0 | 2.5 |
| Asia | 65 | 4.9 | 85.1 | 2.7 |
| Israel born | 40 | 7.7 | 88.6 | — |

[a] Cancer Incidence in 5 Continents, Vol. II, p. 184—197; 384—386.
[b] Idem, p. 360.

Table 21. Malignant Neoplasms of Ovary. Israel, 1960—1966, Jewish Population. All ages by origin. Number of cases (N). Availability of subsite and histology: percentage

| Origin | N | % Subsite available | % Histology available |
|---|---|---|---|
| All Jews | 980 | 96.3 | 87.8 |
| Europe and America | 730 | 96.0 | 87.8 |
| Africa | 40 | 95.0 | 70.0 |
| Asia | 74 | 97.3 | 82.4 |
| Israel born | 44 | 95.5 | 86.4 |

findings must not be discarded as useless. Compared with autopsy series, the population-based registry has the definite advantage of an unselected population and can document the disease at the time of first diagnosis. Therefore, the following conclusions are suggested:

1. A higher percentage of more specified diagnosis, as to subsite and to morphology, appears in the population group with the highest incidence (Stomach, Lung).

2. The preponderance of the Lower part of Stomach as site of tumour, as against the Upper part, is greater for females.

Table 19. Malignant Neoplasms of Females Breast. Incidence 1960—1966, Jewish Population. "Reported Mortality" by origin and histological behaviour. All ages; length of survival in months

| Behaviour | | Total | | | | | —12 months | | | | | 13—35 months | | | | | 36+ months | | | | |
|---|---|---|---|---|---|---|---|---|---|---|---|---|---|---|---|---|---|---|---|---|---|
| | | Total Jews | Europe and America | Africa | Asia | Israel born | Total Jews | Europe and America | Africa | Asia | Israel born | Total Jews | Europe and America | Africa | Asia | Israel born | Total Jews | Europe and America | Africa | Asia | Israel born |
| Well | N | 703 | 536 | 62 | 63 | 42 | | | | | | | | | | | | | | | |
| different. | % | 100.0 | 100.0 | 100.0 | 100.0 | 100.0 | 21.5 | 20.7 | 29.1 | 20.6 | 21.4 | 42.2 | 41.4 | 45.2 | 50.8 | 35.7 | 36.3 | 37.9 | 25.8 | 28.6 | 42.9 |
| Ana- | N | 547 | 414 | 38 | 66 | 29 | | | | | | | | | | | | | | | |
| plasia | % | 100.0 | 100.0 | 100.0 | 100.0 | 100.0 | 20.1 | 18.8 | 29.0 | 21.2 | 24.1 | 43.7 | 42.5 | 50.0 | 43.9 | 51.7 | 36.2 | 38.6 | 21.1 | 34.8 | 24.1 |
| Not | N | 246 | 174 | 24 | 31 | 17 | | | | | | | | | | | | | | | |
| available | % | 100.0 | 100.0 | 100.0 | 100.0 | 100.0 | 37.4 | 37.4 | 45.8 | 35.5 | 29.4 | 37.0 | 36.2 | 41.7 | 35.5 | 41.2 | 25.6 | 26.4 | 12.5 | 29.0 | 29.4 |

Table 22. Malignant Neoplasms of Ovary. Israel, 1960—1966, Jewish Population. Subsites by origin, all ages. Number of cases and percentage

| Origin | All Subsites | | | | | | | | | | | | | | Ovary: Subsites stated | | | | | | | |
|---|---|---|---|---|---|---|---|---|---|---|---|---|---|---|---|---|---|---|---|---|---|---|
| | Total | | Ovary | | | | | | | | Fallopian tubes | | Others and N.A. | | Total | | Right | | Left | | Bilateral | |
| | | | Right | | Left | | Bilat. | | S.N.S. | | | | | | | | | | | | | |
| | N | % | N | % | N | % | N | % | N | % | N | % | N | % | N | % | N | % | N | % | N | % |
| Total Jews | 980 | 100.00 | 190 | 19.38 | 145 | 14.79 | 180 | 18.36 | 409 | 41.73 | 20 | 2.04 | 36 | 3.67 | 515 | 100.00 | 190 | 36.89 | 145 | 28.15 | 180 | 34.95 |
| Europe/America | 730 | 100.00 | 133 | 18.21 | 105 | 14.38 | 146 | 20.00 | 304 | 41.64 | 13 | 1.78 | 29 | 3.96 | 384 | 100.00 | 133 | 34.63 | 105 | 27.34 | 146 | 38.02 |
| Africa | 40 | 100.00 | 10 | 25.00 | 8 | 20.00 | 4 | 10.00 | 16 | 40.00 | — | — | 2 | 5.00 | 22 | 100.00 | 10 | 45.45 | 8 | 36.36 | 4 | 18.18 |
| Asia | 74 | 100.00 | 22 | 29.72 | 8 | 10.81 | 9 | 12.16 | 32 | 43.24 | 1 | 1.35 | 2 | 2.70 | 39 | 100.00 | 22 | 56.41 | 8 | 20.51 | 9 | 23.07 |
| Israel born | 44 | 100.00 | 5 | 11.36 | 8 | 18.18 | 12 | 27.27 | 17 | 38.63 | — | — | 2 | 4.54 | 25 | 100.00 | 5 | 20.00 | 8 | 32.00 | 12 | 48.00 |

Table 23. Malignant Neoplasms of Ovary. Israel, 1960—1966, Jewish Population. Behaviour stated by subsites and origin, all ages. Number of cases and ratio well differentiated (W)/anaplastic type (A)

| Origin | Total | | | Ovary | | | | | | | | | | | | | | | Fallopian Tubes | | | Others and N.A. | | |
|---|---|---|---|---|---|---|---|---|---|---|---|---|---|---|---|---|---|---|---|---|---|---|---|---|
| | | | | Right | | | Left | | | Bilateral | | | S.N.S. | | | Total | | | | | | | | |
| | Well diff. | Ana-plasia | Ratio W/A | W | A | Ratio W/A | W | A | W/A | W | A | W/A | W | A | W/A | W | A | W/A | W | A | W/A | W | A | W/A |
| Total Jews | 736 | 124 | 5.93 | 134 | 23 | 5.83 | 113 | 19 | 5.94 | 123 | 31 | 3.96 | 328 | 46 | 7.13 | 698 | 119 | 5.86 | 16 | 2 | 8.00 | 22 | 3 | 7.33 |
| Europe/America | 566 | 110 | 5.14 | 101 | 23 | 4.39 | 82 | 18 | 4.55 | 111 | 27 | 4.11 | 242 | 40 | 6.05 | 536 | 108 | 4.96 | 13 | 1 | 13.00 | 17 | 1 | 17.00 |
| Africa | 25 | 3 | 8.33 | 5 | — | — | 7 | — | — | 1 | 2 | 0.50 | 12 | 1 | 12.00 | 25 | 3 | 8.33 | — | — | — | — | — | — |
| Asia | 55 | 6 | 9.16 | 15 | 1 | 15.00 | 6 | — | — | 7 | 1 | 7.00 | 24 | 4 | 6.00 | 52 | 6 | 8.66 | 1 | — | — | 2 | — | — |
| Israel | 33 | 5 | 6.60 | 3 | 1 | 3.00 | 6 | — | — | 9 | 1 | 9.00 | 14 | 2 | 7.00 | 32 | 4 | 8.00 | — | — | — | 1 | 1 | 1.00 |

Table 24. Malignant Neoplasms of Ovary. Incidence 1960—1966, Jewish population. "Reported mortality" by origin. All ages; length of survival in months

| Origin | Length of survival | | | | | |
|---|---|---|---|---|---|---|
| | Total | | | | | |
| | N | % | —3 m. | 4—12 m. | 13—35 m. | 36+ m. |
| Total Jews | 673 | 100.0 | 24.5 | 37.3 | 30.8 | 7.4 |
| Europe and America | 563 | 100.0 | 23.1 | 38.0 | 31.4 | 7.5 |
| Africa | 31 | 100.0 | 41.9[a] | 25.8 | 25.8 | 6.5 |
| Asia | 51 | 100.0 | 27.5 | 37.3 | 27.4 | 7.8 |
| Israel born | 28 | 100.0 | 28.6 | 35.7 | 28.6 | 7.1 |

[a] Chi Square — Europe/Africa (—3 m.) —4.43. Significant with P = 0.05.

3. Anaplasia is higher in females than in males for all morphological types of Stomach cancer, and for Squamous cell ca. in Lung cancer.

4. A positive correlation of anaplasia to early mortality is not found consistently for Stomach and for Ovarian and Breast Cancer, but seems probable for Lung cancer in females.

5. The low male/female ratio for Lung cancer in Israel is correlated with a low sex ratio for Squamous cell ca.

6. African-born Jews are outstanding for a lower mortality in Lung cancer, and, on the other hand, for a higher mortality in Breast cancer, the latter correlated with a medial location of the tumor.

Discontinuation of detailed coding seems not indicated. We would rather try to improve the quality of the data and to extend the investigation to other sites.

## Summary

On the background of differences in morbidity levels in the main Jewish population groups in Israel, the significance of anatomical subsites, of histology including behaviour, and of survival data were investigated. The sites chosen were Stomach, Lung, Female Breast and Ovary, for the 7 years' incidence 1960—1966, a total of 10, 435 cases. In spite of the amount of "unavailables" in the desired categories, the epidemiological significance of detailed data is suggested by the findings of this investigation. It is proposed to carry on with detailed coding of cancer registry information and to extend the method to other cancer sites.

## References

1. Bignall, J. R. (editor): Carcinoma of the Lung. Edinburgh and London: E. and S. Livingstone Ltd. 1958, p. 153—202.
2. Cutler, S. J., *et al.*: End Results in Cancer. Report No. 3. Bethesda: National Cancer Institute 1968, p. 1—3.
3. Steinitz, R.: 5-Year's Morbidity From Neoplasms in Israel's Population Groups, 1964. Published by the Ministry of Health, Jerusalem, Oct. 1967, p. 7—10.
4. Doll, R., Muir, C., Waterhouse, J. (editors): Cancer Incidence in Five Continents. Vol. II. Berlin-Heidelberg-New York: Springer 1970, p. 183—197.

5. International Agency for Research on Cancer: Draft Proposal for the Cancer Chapter of the Ninth Revision of the International Classification of Diseases, Injuries and Causes of Death. Typescript 1971.
6. CLEMMESEN, J.: Statistical Studies in Malignant Neoplasms. Vol. I. Copenhagen: Munksgaard 1965, p. 266—267.
7. INGLEBY, H., GERSHON-COHEN, J.: In: Comparative Anatomy, Pathology and Roentgenology of the Breast. University of Pennsylvania Press, 1960 — cited by J. S. MACDONALD; in: Clinical Evaluation in Breast Cancer, ed. by J. L. HAYWARD and R. D. BULBROOK. London-New York: Academic Press 1966, p. 11—12.
8. KOTTMEIER, H. J.: Clinical Staging in Ovarian Carcinoma. In Ovarian Cancer, edited by F. GENTIL and A. C. JUNQUEIRA. UICC Monograph Series, Vol. 11. Berlin-Heidelberg-New York: Springer 1968, p. 146—155.

# Multiplicity of Lung Tumour Classifications

L. H. Sobin

World Health Organization, Geneva, Switzerland

## Introduction

"Classification is fundamental to the quantitative study of any phenomenon. It is recognized as the basis of all scientific generalization and is therefore an essential element in statistical methodology. Uniform definitions and uniform systems of classification are prerequisites in the advancement of scientific knowledge."[1]

Histological classifications of tumours are used in four main types of studies:

1. to determine the nature of tumours
2. to elucidate their causes
3. to describe their biological behaviour
4. to assess the value of medical intervention

The first is directed at determining the histogenesis of a tumour and its relations to other tumours; the second seeks relationships between occurrence and geography, occupation, habits, etc.; the third examines clinical, pathogenetic and prognostic aspects; and the fourth measures effects of therapy on the third.

Meaningful comparisons depend largely on comparability of data, which in turn requires a reasonable degree of uniformity in definitions and systems of classification.

The purpose of this study is to examine the histological classifications currently in use in the English language literature, taking as an example lung cancer, in order to determine to what extent uniformity and diversity exist.

## Methods

A review was made of classifications of lung cancer used in English language articles in the recent medical literature. Most of the articles were obtained by searching the *Index Medicus* and several specialty journals dealing with cancer. Selection was generally at random but also depended largely on the availability of particular journals. This was not intended to be an exhaustive survey but rather to illustrate the varieties of classifications that are in use today.

In order to present a general picture, broad categories of classification were tabulated without major concern for finer points of distinction and definition. Epidermoid and squamous carcinomas were grouped together regardless of criteria

1 World Health Organization, 1967.

employed for inclusion. (These criteria were usually not noted in the papers reviewed.) The category "small cell carcinoma" includes oat-cell and related tumours whether specified or not. The category "adenocarcinoma" is used if no distinction is made between bronchiolo-alveolar and bronchogenic adenocarcinoma. "Large cell carcinoma" applies only when mentioned as such, regardless of definition. The heading "undifferentiated/anaplastic carcinoma" includes any tumours so named. Uncommonly used terms, such as clear cell, solid, polygonal, simplex, etc. are noted under the category "others".

## Results

Of the 57 papers reviewed, 34 were concerned with clinical investigations on the treatment and survival of patients with different forms of lung cancer. These are tabulated as "Therapy Studies" in Table 1. The 23 remaining reports dealt with the following subjects (number of papers per subject in brackets): clinical diagnosis (2), cytology (4), epidemiology (3), etiology (3), genetics (1), occupation (3) and pathology (7). They are tabulated as "Other studies".

A total of 13 distinct systems of classification were used in the 57 studies. The "therapy studies" used 12 different classifications and the "other studies" used 7.

The epidermoid/squamous carcinoma group was used in all of the studies, 40 specifying squamous, 16 epidermoid and 1 cancroid. Most of the papers did not distinguish degrees of differentiation among these tumours.

About half of the studies did not distinguish between bronchiolo-alveolar and bronchogenic adenocarcinomas. Three classifications, representing 28% of the papers, distinguished small cell from undifferentiated/anaplastic carcinomas. The others appeared to make no distinction. Those systems using the category large cell carcinoma always used the small cell category as well and never the undifferentiated group. One study separated undifferentiated and anaplastic tumours, but they are here tabulated together. Only a few papers actually defined the criteria used for inclusion of cases in particular histological classes.

The two most frequently used systems may be described as the "lumpers" (24%) and the "splitters" (21%), the former dividing the tumours into epidermoid, undifferentiated and adenocarcinomas and the latter grouping them into epidermoid, small cell, large cell, bronchiolo-alveolar and bronchogenic adenocarcinomas. The third largest group (14%) also divided the tumours into 5 categories somewhat similar to those of the second classification.

## Discussion

It is clear that there is no uniformity in the classifications used to analyse data from studies on lung cancer. The most obvious differences are in the extent to which distinctions are made between the types of undifferentiated tumours and between the two forms of adenocarcinoma.

The multiplicity of classifications used is even more striking when one considers that the classification of lung tumours is not one of the most controversial fields of nosology. A mere comparison with the classifications of central nervous system or ovarian tumours will make this point obvious. The main cell types of lung tumours are clearly recognized by most pathologists so that they nearly all know what is meant by the major headings in Table 1. But these main types are used in different combinations of "lumping" and "splitting" to produce a variety of systems for presenting otherwise comparable data.

Less obvious differences among the classifications concern the actual definitions of categories. Merely citing the use of epidermoid carcinoma as a type in a classification does not indicate at what level of differentiation one includes tumours in this category. A strict definition limits this type to tumours showing signs of keratinization or intercellular bridges. Mere stratification of cells is not sufficient for a tumour to enter the group and results in such tumours being assigned to an undifferentiated or small cell or large cell category. A less strict definition for this type would include some of these less differentiated tumours as epidermoid.

One cannot expect every paper on lung cancer to define all the criteria used in delineating each histological group. In the studies summarized in Table 1, very few did. The use of a standardized classification with widely known definitions allows the investigator to reasonably expect his readers to already know, or be able to find, the criteria.

Since the foundation of tumour classification is microscopy, the histopathologist is in the key position of determining what type of classification and nomenclature will be used. He not only determines this for his own department but often for his other colleagues concerned with oncology. The pathologist's terms of diagnosis become part of the patient's record and from there find their way into tumour registries, death certificates, etc. Thus do radiologists, surgeons and statisticians become dependent. If the pathologist of a particular hospital is a "lumper" it is most likely that papers describing clinical trials from that institution will present histopathological classifications in this fashion. If the particular pathologist does not appreciate the value of international comparability of data his clinical colleagues may have to appear likewise when they publish data on their patients.

The pathologist may base his reluctance to accept a standardized classification on the fear that it may indicate that this is a definitive work thus stifling curiosity and further attempts to elucidate nosological problems. This danger exists and must be considered, particularly in regard to periodic revisions of classifications in the light of new knowledge. Acceptance may also create fear of being forced to use a particular system rather than having the free choice to select one's own means of classification. This too is a valid objection but weak as an excuse for not utilizing a common format in the interests of international communication, just as we have accepted a common system of measurement.

The following quotation, written by a pathologist, illustrates these fears of unification of tumour classification:

"While cooperation ... would seem desirable, I cannot give my support to the imposition of a uniform classification of ... tumours on pathologists throughout the world. Such uniformity can only serve statistical purposes at the cost of stifling the individual study of tumours on which advances in their classification and understanding depend. Is statistical uniformity of such importance that individual interpretations must be suppressed?"

The use of 13 classifications to express data on lung tumours (Table 1) has not apparently promoted nosological perfection nor communication. In fact, none of

Table 1. Categories enumerated in classifications used for studies on carcinoma of the lung

| Reference no.[a] | Types of Carcinomas: Epidermoid Squamous | Small Cell | Bronchogenic Adenocarcinoma | Adenocarcinoma | Alveolar | Large Cell | Undifferentiated Anaplastic | Others | Number of Therapy Studies | Number of Other Studies | % Total Studies |
|---|---|---|---|---|---|---|---|---|---|---|---|
| 1 | + | | | + | | | + | | 10 | 5 | 24 |
| 2 | + | + | + | | + | + | | | 6 | 6 | 21 |
| 3 | + | + | + | | + | | + | | 4 | 4 | 14 |
| 4 | + | + | | + | | | + | | 4 | 3 | 12 |
| 5 | + | + | | + | | + | | | 2 | 3 | 9 |
| 6 | + | | + | | + | | + | | 2 | 1 | 5 |
| 7 | + | + | + | | + | | | | 1 | — | 2 |
| 8 | + | + | | + | | | | | 1 | — | 2 |
| 9 | + | | | + | | | + | Simplex | — | 1 | 2 |
| 10 | + | | | | | | | + | 1 | — | 2 |
| 11 | + | + | | + | | | | Polygon. | 1 | — | 2 |
| 12 | + | + | + | | + | | | Cylindrical, Solid | 1 | — | 2 |
| 13 | + | + | + | | + | | + | Clear Cell | 1 | — | 2 |
| | | | | | | | | | 34 | 23 | 100 |

[a] Numbers refer to the references below using the corresponding classifications.

1 Bignall and Moon, 1955; Gifford and Waddington, 1957; Sensening, Rossi and Ehrenhaft, 1963; Rasmussen, 1964; Belcher and Anderson, 1965; Shimizu, 1967; Ashley, 1968; Nasiel, 1968; Ashley, 1969; Ashley and Davies, 1969; Brett, 1969; Neyazaki, Ikeda, Seki, Egawa and Suzuki, 1969; Weiss, Cooper and Boucet, 1969; Abramson and Cavanaugh, 1970; Deaner and Trummer, 1970.

2 Galofre, Payne, Woolner, Clagett and Gage, 1964; Yesner, Gerstl and Auerbach, 1965; de la Garza, Carr, Bisel, 1968; Roswit, Patno, Rapp, Veinbergs, Feder, Stuhlbarg and Reid, 1968; Cahansky, Pauzner and Kalter, 1969; Hinds and Hitchcock, 1969; Razzuk, Race, Lynn, Martin, Urschel and Paulson, 1970; Uys, 1970; Weiss, Boucot and Cooper, 1970; Yesner, Feinstein and Gelfman, 1970; Saccomanno, Archer, Auerbach, Kuschnev, Saunders and Klein, 1971; Berraya, Polk, Raju and Bailey, 1971.

3 Andrews and Rosser, 1964; Thorarinsson, Hallgrimsson, Bjarnason and Petersen, 1967; Watson and Schottenfeld, 1968; Bennett, 1969; Collaborative Study (USA), 1969; Guttmann, 1969; Snider and Placik, 1969; Limas, Japaze and Garcia Bunuel, 1971.

4 Nohl, 1956; Hinson and Kuper, 1963; Goldman, 1965 (a); Goldman, 1965 (b); Gibbons and Baker, 1969; Croxatto and Barcat, 1970; Bates, 1970.

5 Simecek, 1966; Frable, 1968; Byrd, Carr, Miller, Payne and Woolner, 1969; Smith and Parnsingha, 1969; Goldberg, Glicksman, Khan and Nickson, 1970.

6 Bolooki and Minkowitz, 1967; Steensberg, 1968; Wanebo, Johnson, Sato and Thorslund, 1968.

7 Watson, 1965.

8 Caldwell and Bagshaw, 1968.

9 Warren and Gates, 1964.

10 Holsti, 1969.

11 Sellors, 1955.

12 Madey, 1968.

13 Abbey Smith, 1970

these 13 classifications is obviously any closer to the "truth" than some of the others. They are all variations on the same theme.

It is clear that we are not yet at the stage where enough knowledge is at hand to classify all tumours in a completely logical, systematic and definitive manner. Until that state is attained we should have the means by which we can efficiently communicate our data to one another. This can be done by accepting the use of a single classification and nomenclature for the sake of comparability. It is with this in mind that WHO has pursued its programme "International Histological Classification of Tumours"[2]. These classifications and nomenclatures[3] are developed by multinational groups of pathologists collaborating with international reference centres for particular tumour sites. Their primary task is not to solve all nosological problems nor impose classifications, but to elaborate means to facilitate communication in this field. They try to overcome national and linguistic preferences in order to achieve general acceptance, thus promoting statistical uniformity.

Recognizing the degree of diversity that currently exists, one cannot expect all pathologists and oncologists to be completely satisfied with any standardized classification, but in the face of the alternatives and in the interests of improved communications it is hoped that use of the WHO system will be widely accepted.

## References


Abbey Smith, R.: Long-term clinical follow-up after operation for lung carcinoma. Thorax **25**, 62—76 (1970).

Abramson, N., Cavanaugh, P. J.: Short-course radiation therapy in carcinoma of the lung. Radiology **96**, 627—630 (1970).

Andrews, G. S., Rosser, T.: Clinical value of exfoliative cytology in neoplasia of the lung. Thorax **19**, 279—286 (1964).

Ashley, D. J. B.: Lung cancer in miners. Thorax **23**, 87—91 (1968).

Ashley, D. J. B.: Blood groups and lung cancer. J. Med. Genet. **6**, 183—186 (1969).

Ashley, D. J. B., Davies, H. D.: Lung cancer in women. Thorax **24**, 446—450 (1969).

Bates, M.: Results of surgery for bronchial carcinoma in patients aged 70 and over. Thorax **25**, 77—78 (1970).

Berraya, R. B., Polk, J. W., Raju, P., Bailey, A. H.: Concurrent pulmonary tuberculosis and primary carcinoma. Thorax **26**, 384—387 (1971).

Belcher, J. R., Anderson, R.: Surgical treatment of carcinoma of the bronchus. Brit. med. J. **1**, 948—954 (1965).

Bennett, D. E.: Adenocarcinoma of the lung in men: A clinicopathological study of 100 cases. Cancer **23**, 431—439 (1969).

Bignall, J. R., Moon, A. J.: Survival after lung resection for bronchial carcinoma. Thorax **10** 183—190 (1955).

Bolooki, H., Minkowitz, S.: Evaluation of primary carcinoma of the lung and survival rate after curative resection in a large city hospital. Dis. Chest. **52**, 680—682 (1967).

Brett, G. Z.: Earlier diagnosis and survival in lung cancer. Brit. med. J. **4**, 260—262 (1969).

Byrd, R. B., Carr, D. T., Miller, W. E., Payne, W. S., Woolner, L. B.: Radiographic abnormalities in carcinoma of the lung as related to histological cell types. Thorax **24**, 573—575 (1969).


---

2 Sobin, L. H.: 1971.

3 Kreyberg, L., Liebow, A. A., Uehlinger, E. A., 1967.
Scarff, R. W., Torloni, H., 1968.
Enzinger, F. M., Lattes, R., Torloni, H., 1969.
Wahi, P. N., Cohen, B., Luthra, U. K., Torloni, H., 1971.
Pindborg, J. J., Kramer, I., Torloni, H., 1971.

Cahansky, G., Pauzner, Y., Kalter, Y.: Five-year post-surgical follow-up of 100 cases of malignant lung tumours. Harefuah **77**, 547—550 (1969).
Caldwell, W. L., Bagshaw, M. A.: Indications for and results of irradiation of carcinoma of the lung. Cancer **22**, 999—1004 (1968).
Collaborative Study (USA): Preoperative irradiation of cancer of the lung. Cancer **23**, 419—430 (1969).
Croxatto, O. C., Barcat, J. A.: Lymph node metastases in bronchogenic carcinoma. Study on its role in dissemination. Johns Hopk. Hosp. Rep. **126**, 121—129 (1970).
Deaner, R. M., Trummer, M. J.: Carcinoma of the lung in women. J. thorac. cardiovasc. Surg. **59**, 551—554 (1970).
Enzinger, F. M., Lattes, R., Torloni, H.: International Histological Classification of Tumours No. 3. Histological Typing of Soft Tissue Tumours. Geneva: WHO 1969.
Frable-William, J.: The relationship of pulmonary cytology to survival in lung cancer. Acta cytol. (Philad.) **12**, 52—56 (1968).
Galofre, M., Payne, W. S., Woolner, L. B., Clagett, O. T., Gage, R.: Pathological classification and surgical treatment of bronchogenic carcinoma. Surg. Gynec. Obstet. **119**, 51—61 (1964).
de la Garza, J. G., Carr, D. T., Bisel, H. F.: Hexamethylmelanine (NSC-13875) in the treatment of primary cancer of the lung with metastases. Cancer **22**, 571—575 (1968).
Gibbons, J. R. P., Baker, R.: Treatment of carcinoma of the bronchus by interstitial irradiation. Thorax **24**, 451—456 (1969).
Gifford, J. H., Waddington, J. K. B.: Review of 464 cases of carcinoma of the lung treated by resection. Brit. med. J. **1**, 723—730 (1957).
Goldberg, E. M., Glicksman, A. S., Khan, F. R., Nickson, J. J.: Mediastinoscopy for assessing mediastinal spread in clinical staging of carcinoma of the lung. Cancer **25**, 347—353 (1970).
Goldman, K. P.: Prognoses of coal-miners with cancer of the lung. Thorax **20**, 170—174 (1965a).
Goldman, K. P.: Histology of lung cancer in relation to prognoses. Thorax **20**, 298—302 (1965b).
Guttmann, R. J.: Effectiveness of radiotherapy in explored inoperable carcinoma of the lung. Bull. N.Y. Acad. Med. **45**, 657—664 (1969).
Hinds, J. R., Hitchcock: Adenocarcinoma of the lung. Thorax **24**, 10—17 (1969).
Hinson, K. F. W., Kuper, S. W. A.: The diagnosis of lung cancer by examination of sputum. Thorax **18**, 350—353 (1963).
Holsti, L. R.: Clinical experience with split-course radiotherapy. Radiology **92**, 591—596 (1969).
Kreyberg, L., Liebow, A. A., Uehlinger, E. A.: International Histological Classification of Tumours No. 1. Histological Typing of Lung Tumors. Geneva: WHO 1967.
Limas, C., Japaze, H., Garcia Bunuel, R.: Scar carcinoma of the lung. Dis. Chest. **59**, 219—222 (1971).
Madey, Y.: Clinical evaluation of 745 cases of primary lung carcinoma. Pol. med. J. **7**, 917—927 (1968).
Nasiel, M.: Comparative histological and sputum-cytological studies of the bronchial epithelium in inflammatory and neoplastic lung disease. Acta path. microbiol. scand. **72**, 501—518 (1968).
Neyazaki, T., Ikeda, M., Seki, Y., Egawa, N., Suzuki, C.: Bronchial artery infusion therapy for lung cancer. Cancer **24**, 912—922 (1969).
Nohl, H. C.: An investigation into the lymphatic and vascular spread of carcinoma of the bronchus. Thorax **11**, 172—185 (1956).
Pindborg, J., Kramer, I., Torloni, H.: International Histological Classification of Tumours No. 5. Histological Typing of Odontogenic Tumours, Jaw Cysts and Allied Lesions. Geneva: WHO 1971.
Rasmussen, P. S.: The incidence of local recurrence and distant metastases in surgically treated cases of lung cancer. Acta path. microbiol. scand. **62**, 145—150 (1964).
Razzuk, M. A., Race, G. J., Lynn, J. A., Martin, J. A., Urschel, H. C., Paulson, D. L.: Observations on ultrastructural morphology of bronchogenic carcinoma. J. thorac. cardiovasc. Surg. **59**, 581—587 (1970).
Roswit, B., Patno, M. E., Rapp, R., Veinbergs, A., Feder, B., Stuhlbarg, J., Reid, C. B.: The survival of patients with inoperable lung cancer: A large-scale randomized study of radiation therapy versus placebo. Radiology **90**, 688—697 (1968).
Saccomanno, G., Archer, V. E., Auerbach, O., Kuschner, M., Saunders, R. P., Klein, M. G.: Histologic types of lung cancer among uranium miners. Cancer **27**, 515—523 (1971).

SCARFF, R. W., TORLONI, H.: International Histological Classification of Tumours No. 2. Histological Typing of Breast Tumours. Geneva: WHO 1968.
SELLORS, T. H.: Results of surgical treatment of carcinoma of the lung. Brit. med. J. **1**, 445—448 (1955).
SENSENIG, D. M., ROSSI, N. P., EHRENHAFT, J. L.: Results of the surgical treatment of bronchogenic carcinoma. Surg. Gynec. Obstet. **116**, 279—284 (1963).
SHIMIZU, K.: Epidemiological study on lung cancer among A-bombs survivors in Hiroshima. Hiroshima J. med. Sc. **16**, 241—253 (1967).
SIMECEK, C.: Cytological investigation of intrathoracic lymph nodes in carcinoma of the lung. Thorax **21**, 369—371 (1966).
SMITH, L., PARNSINGHA, T.: Post-irradiation surgery for bronchogenic carcinoma. Thorax **24**, 457—460 (1969).
SNIDER, G. L., PLACIK, B.: The relationship between pulmonary tuberculosis and bronchogenic carcinoma. Amer. Rev. resp. Dis. **99**, 229—236 (1969).
SOBIN, L. H.: The World Health Organization's programme for the histopathological definition and classification of tumors. Meth. Inf. Med. **10**, 120—122 (1971).
STEENSBERG, J.: Survival in males with surgically treated localized cancer of the lung. Cancer **22**, 1—7 (1968).
THORARINSSON, H., HALLGRIMSSON, J., BJARNASON, O., PETERSEN, G.: Carcinoma of the lung in Iceland. Dis. Chest. **52**, 754—759 (1967).
UYS, C. J.: Bronchial carcinoma in the population groups of Cape Town. A histological survey. S. Afr. Cancer Bull. **14**, 8—14 (1970).
WAHI, P. N., COHEN, B., LUTHRA, U. K., TORLONI, H.: International Histological Classification of Tumours No. 4. Histological Typing of Oral and Oropharyngeal Tumours. Geneva: WHO 1971.
WANEBO, C. K., JOHNSON, K. G., SATO, K., THORSLUND, T. W.: Lung cancer following atomic radiation. Amer. Rev. resp. Dis. **98**, 778—787 (1968).
WARREN, S., GATES, O.: Lung cancer and metastatis. Arch. Path. **78**, 467—474 (1964).
WATSON, W. L.: Ten year survival in lung cancer. Cancer **18**, 133—135 (1965).
WATSON, W. L., SCHOTTENFELD, D.: Survival in cancer of the bronchus and lung. 1949—1962. Comparison of men and women patients. Dis. Chest. **53**, 65—72 (1968).
WEISS, W., BOUCOT, K. R., COOPER, D. A.: The histopathology of bronchogenic carcinoma and its relation to growth rate, metastases and prognosis. Cancer **26**, 965—970 (1970).
WEISS, W., COOPER, D. A., BOUCOT, K. R.: Operative mortality and 5-year survival rates in men with bronchogenic carcinoma. Ann. int. Med. **71**, 59—65 (1969).
World Health Organization: International classification of diseases. Manual of the international statistical classification of diseases, injuries and causes of death. 8th revision. Geneva: WHO 1967.
YESNER, R., FEINSTEIN, A., GELFMAN, N. A.: Relation of lung cancer histopathology to cigarette smoking. Amer. J. Path. **59**, 92 (1970).
YESNER, R., GERSTL, B., AUERBACH, O.: Application of the WHO classification of lung cancer to biopsy material. Ann. Thorac. Surg. **1**, 33—49 (1965).

# The Significance of Asbestos in Tissue

J. C. WAGNER [1]

Medical Research Council's Pneumoconiosis Unit, Llandough Hospital, Penarth, Glamorgan, Wales, Great Britain

In Muenster in 1957 [1], I presented a paper entitled "A preliminary experimental assessment of the significance of asbestos bodies". I stated in the paper that following FAHR's [2] first observation of peculiar bodies in sections from the lung of a patient dying of asbestosis, there had been considerable controversy concerning the composition of these bodies and the role that they play in the pathogenesis of the disease.

At that stage the following facts had been generally accepted. STEWART [3] showed that the bodies were formed as a result of the inhalation of asbestos dust. GLOYNE [4] demonstrated that the bodies were formed from asbestos fibres and are not present in asbestos dust. GARDNER [5] and VORWALD [6] showed that intratracheal injection of these bodies did not cause pulmonary fibrosis. In addition, if the bodies were injected subcutaneously there was no granulomatous reaction. The experimental and human evidence in my paper [1] indicated that all three major types of asbestos—chrysotile, crocidolite and amosite—when inhaled, could produce both asbestos bodies and fibrosis. There seemed to be three major problems which required further investigation. These were:

1. Whether all types of asbestos were equally dangerous.
2. The size of the toxic asbestos particles.
3. The mechanism of the inhalation of the various types of asbestos.

During the intervening fifteen years we have studied these problems. The following paper is a summary of our investigations and the conclusions we have reached.

There are several types of asbestos. All are fibrous silicates and have similar properties. They are used mainly to produce fireproof insulation or as a matrix for cement or plastics in building materials. Asbestos has hundreds of other uses and is essential in our industrial society. For example, the brakes of automobiles depend on the abrasive nature and heat resistance of asbestos. The inhalation of asbestos dusts can lead to pulmonary fibrosis and carcinoma of the lung or to the development

1 The following team members were responsible for these studies: Dr. J. C. GILSON (Director), J. C. WAGNER, C. GOLD, D. E. MUNDAY, W. H. ROBERTS (Pathology); G. BERRY (Statistics); V. TIMBRELL, J. W. SKIDMORE, M. GRIFFITHS (Physics); T. G. MORRIS (Chemistry) from MRC Pneumoconiosis Unit; B. COMMINS (MRC Air Pollution Unit); A. MORGAN and A. HOLMES (A.E.R.E. Harwell); and F. D. POOLEY (Department of Mineral Exploitation, University College, Cardiff).

of diffuse mesotheliomas of the pleura and peritoneum. The problem has been to discover which type or types of asbestos are responsible for the development of the tumours; if a specific variety could be incriminated, then its use could be discouraged and that of the less harmful varieties recommended.

Three types of asbestos are important commercially: chrysotile (white), most abundant and accounting for about 95% of the total; amosite (brown) and crocidolite (blue). A small amount of anthophyllite, a talclike fibre, is produced in Finland. Chrysotile is widely distributed in the main mining areas of Canada, Russia, Southern Africa, and Cyprus. Crocidolite is found in Cape Province and Transvaal in South Africa, and until recently was produced in Western Australia; a deposit is being developed in Bolivia. Amosite is mined only in the Transvaal in South Africa, but a large deposit of similar fibre has just been discovered in India.

The physical nature of the chrysotile fibre from different deposits varies considerably, as do the associated minerals found in the ore. However, after the fibre has been separated from the ore and processed in the mills, all chrysotile fibres consist of bundles of very fine fibrils and have a soft wavy appearance. In contrast, the crocidolite and amosite fibres are much more rigid and straight, and have larger diameters than the unit fibrils of chrysotile. They are also more resistant to acids and alkalis. From 1900, crocidolite was in demand in the shipbuilding industry because chrysotile was not a good insulating material when exposed to sea water. Crocidolite is now used mainly to form a matrix in chrysotile asbestos cement products, pressure piping, and automobile battery boxes. Amosite bonds well with plastics and is used in the manufacture of floor tiles and in decorative insulations to replace timber in passenger ships. The use of asbestos has increased tremendously in the last twenty years and the current annual consumption is over four million tons.

Asbestosis, the fibrosis of the lung caused by inhalation of asbestos, was first detected at the turn of the century in France and Britain, but it was not until the early 1930's that it was shown to be a major occupational hazard in the asbestos textile industry [7]. The first suggestion that there might be an association between asbestosis and bronchial carcinoma came from pathologists in Britain and the United States in 1935. This was supported in Britain by the Inspector of Factories, who reported that in 1947 [8] 15% of all death certificates for males, on which asbestosis was mentioned, stated that death was due to carcinoma of the lung. This excessive risk was confirmed in 1955 by Doll [9] who showed that those first employed before 1930 in "scheduled" occupations in an asbestos textile factory had a death rate from lung cancer ten times greater than that of the general population. Later studies on the same population confirmed that with improvement in factory conditions the incidence of carcinoma dropped substantially. This suggested that carcinoma of the lung was associated with the incidence of severe pulmonary fibrosis due to heavy asbestos exposure [10]. In 1960, the situation was further complicated by our demonstration of the association between exposure to asbestos dust and the development of diffuse mesotheliomas of the pleura and peritoneum [11]. This has several intriguing features:

1. These rare tumours were associated only with exposure to the crocidolite (blue) asbestos mined in the North West Cape Province, and not to the chrysotile and amosite mining areas of Southern Africa or to the crocidolite deposit adjoining the amosite area.

2. The association was with exposure to asbestos dust and not necessarily with the pulmonary fibrosis of asbestosis; a number of the cases were environmental rather than occupational exposures.

3. The average latent period between initial exposure to asbestos dust and development of the tumour was over forty years.

This was the first indication that the different types of asbestos varied in their biological effect.

Crocidolite has been used in Britain since 1900, but by 1962 the Inspectorate of Factories' records of 130 cancers of the lung in asbestos workers contained no cases of mesothelioma [12]. A search was therefore made in the departments of pathology and surgery, and cases were referred to a panel of pathologists formed to establish criteria for the diagnoses of these previously rare tumours [13—15].

By 1964 it was clear that mesotheliomas had occurred and were increasing in number [16], but as most British asbestos workers had been exposed to more than one type of fibre, it was impossible to implicate a single type. More than 600 mesotheliomas are now recorded in the United Kingdom—the majority associated with exposure to asbestos [17].

To study the effect of exposure to one type of fibre, epidemiological studies were required in the mining areas. A comparison of the South African crocidolite mines with the chrysotile mines in Canada was needed. International co-ordination for this was possible through a UICC Working Group which, in 1964, reviewed the problem of asbestos and cancer and recommended lines for further work. A committee to implement these proposals was formed [18]. In this way it was possible to initiate international epidemiological surveys, develop a new radiological classification [19], organise international and national pathology panels, and prepare, characterize and distribute reference samples of asbestos dust for experimental work [20]. The working party will reconvene in October 1972 to consider how successfully the recommendations have been implemented and to report on the information that has been obtained concerning "Asbestos and Health".

Meanwhile, preliminary information is available on several aspects of the problem. A survey of Quebec asbestos miners has been undertaken by epidemiologists of McGill University with support of the Quebec Asbestos Mining Association. They conducted a remarkably complete follow-up of about 12,000 workers and showed a slight excess of lung cancer in the most heavily exposed group. Despite the heavy general air pollution by chrysotile dust over many years, the crude death rates for lung cancer in the population of the mining towns are less than the death rate for the Province of Quebec [21]. No mesotheliomas were recorded in the mining population. On the whole, the situation was entirely different from that in the asbestos fields in the North West Cape.

In the United States, prospective mortality studies, with the use of social security records, showed an excess risk of bronchial cancer in those working in an asbestos-textile factory just before the Second World War [22]. In New York insulation workers, death rates from lung cancer were also about seven times those expected [23]. Mesotheliomas of the peritoneum were observed among those on the union books in 1942, but more recently employees show an increased incidence of pleural tumours. Carcinoma of the lung was particularly prevalent among heavy cigarette smokers, and the effect appears to be multiplicative [24], but there was no correlation between cigarette smoking and the development of the mesotheliomas. Information about the type of asbestos used in the past by these workers is incomplete, but crocidolite, if used at all, was present in very small amounts compared to chrysotile and amosite.

The Soviet Union is second only to Canada in chrysotile production. At a meeting in Dresden in 1968, Professor Kogan indicated an increased incidence of carcinoma of the lung in the asbestos area near Svedlovsk. Professor J. C. McDonald, who was in charge of the survey in Quebec, has recently discussed results with Kogan, and the situations in the Ural and Quebec asbestos fields are similar, with slight increase in carcinoma of the lung among heavily exposed workers, and with no mesotheliomas. Similar results have been obtained in Finland among the anthophyllite miners.

In contrast, mesotheliomas have been reported from shipbuilding ports, particularly in dockyards in Britain, the United States, Germany, and Holland. The whole situation was considered in Britain by a panel of experts under the chairmanship of the Chief Medical Inspector of Factories. Their report, "Problems Arising from the Use of Asbestos" [25], concluded there was sufficient evidence to suggest "other types of fibre should be substituted for crocidolite wherever possible". The law concerning the use of asbestos has been changed, and since 1970 the use of crocidolite has been restricted in Britain. It is disquieting to realise that, while the use of crocidolite has dropped rapidly during recent years in Britain, there has been a steady increase of the importation into the United States, Germany, and Japan.

It was shown that pleural mesotheliomas, histologically similar to those seen in man, could be induced in rats by intrapleural inoculation of asbestos [26]. Hence animal experiments may help in identifying factors influencing the occurrence of the tumours. The results of two experiments, one with specific pathogen free (SPF) rats, the other with Standard rats, have been reported [27]. The two experiments gave similar results; chrysotile and crocidolite produced mesotheliomas in over 60% of the animals and amosite in 35%. It was shown that the main difference between the types of asbestos was that, after adjustment for natural mortality the distribution of mesothelioma occurrence was about 200 days later for amosite than the other two dusts. The crocidolite was also used after oil-extraction and gave similar results to the sample used in natural form.

## Recent Experiments

All the experiments used SPF rats of the Wistar strain bred at the MRC/PU from stock given to us by Imperial Chemical Industries, Pharmaceutical Division. Each rat was allowed to live until it died or appeared to be distressed and a necropsy examination was carried out on each animal.

### Experiment A — Varying Dose Experiment

Samples of chrysotile and crocidolite, each at 5 doses, 0.5, 1, 2, 4 and 8 mg were inoculated intrapleurally. There were 12 rats per dose per dust and inoculation was during March 1965.

### Experiment B — Canadian Chrysotile Inoculation

Samples of chrysotile from seven Canadian mines (an eighth was not available in time), the same superfine grade chrysotile (SFA) as in Experiment A and a saline control were the treatments. A dose of 20 mg was inoculated intrapleurally and there were 16 rats per Canadian chrysotile and double this number of the SFA chrysotile and controls. Inoculation was during December 1966.

### Experiment C — Asbestos Dust Inoculation

The dusts used were the UICC reference samples of amosite, anthophyllite, chrysotile A, chrysotile B, and crocidolite, all in natural form and after the oils had been removed by Dr. B. Commins, samples from eight Canadian chrysotile mines, brucite, barium sulphate, and saline controls. The dose was 20 mg inoculated intrapleurally with 24 rats for each Canadian chrysotile and 32 for the other treatments. Inoculation took place between November 1967 and February 1968.

### Experiment D — Asbestos Dust Inhalation

Rats were exposed in the cabinets described by Timbrell [28] to a dust cloud of concentration of approximately 12 mg/m$^3$ 'respirable' dust as measured by the MRE size selective sampler. The five UICC reference samples were used and there were two lengths of exposure, 1 day (7 hrs) and 3 months (450 hrs). Each cabinet holds about 50 rats but after killing to determine the retention of the dust, about 37 remained for each dust after long exposure, and 45 for short exposure. Exposure was between May and August, 1967.

## Results

### Experiment A

The results of this experiment were reported at the Johannesburg 1969 Conference [29]. It was shown that the risk of developing a mesothelioma at a given time after inoculation could be taken as proportional to the dose, although with such a small experiment this point could not be checked very rigorously.

### Experiments B and C

In experiment B, 69% of the rats inoculated with the SFA chrysotile developed mesotheliomas and between 25 and 62% for the Canadian samples. In experiment C some animals in all except the control groups, have developed mesotheliomas, and over all asbestos samples 41% of rats had a mesothelioma. The results have been analysed using the method shown to be applicable to experiments of this type [30]. The risk of developing a mesothelioma at time t after inoculation is $3c(t-w)^2$ where c and w are constants. The constant w has been taken as 250 days for all dusts; this may not be the optimum value for all the dusts but enables comparisons to be made in terms of c, which is then proportional to the mesothelioma rate. The method of estimation makes the necessary allowance for natural mortality.

The comparison between Canadian chrysotiles is given in Table 1. In neither experiment are differences between the effects of the eight samples significant but sample C from a mine in Western Canada (the remaining samples were from mines in a relatively small area of Eastern Canada) gave the lowest value in both experiments. At the Johannesburg 1969 Conference when preliminary results were given for experiment B the correlations between c and the cobalt, chromium, iron, nickel, and scandium contents were considered. Only chromium showed anything of interest but this result must be discounted since the chromium content of sample C is now known to be 1200 ppm and not 120 ppm as reported. Two other comparisons of interest are shown in Table 1; the SFA chrysotile used in experiment B was from

Table 1. Experiments B and C — values of c for canadian chrysotiles

| Sample | $c \times 10^9$ | |
|---|---|---|
| | Expt. B | Expt. C |
| A | 5.4 | 5.0 |
| B | 9.2 | 4.8 |
| C | 2.9 | 2.9 |
| D | 9.4 | 5.2 |
| E | 7.6 | 4.0 |
| F | 7.9 | 5.8 |
| G | — | 8.4 |
| H | 4.3 | 7.4 |
| SFA chrysotile | 17.7 | — |
| UICC chrysotile B | — | 2.2 |

Table 2. Experiment C — values of c for UICC samples

| | $c \times 10^9$ | |
|---|---|---|
| | Natural | Oil-extracted |
| Amosite | 2.9 | 2.8 |
| Anthophyllite | 1.5 | 3.3 |
| Chrysotile A | 1.9 | 1.3 |
| Chrysotile B | 2.2 | 1.8 |
| Crocidolite | 6.0 | 7.7 |

mine D but the c value of $17.7 \times 10^{-9}$ (which fits in with experiment A) is double that of the D sample. However, the former is a superfine grade more finely ground than the D sample which also differed in that it was obtained several years later, In experiment C the UICC chrysotile B sample is a mixture of the eight Canadian samples but has a c value less than all the separate samples. The explanation is probably that the Canadian samples were ground more finely than the UICC samples before experimental use.

We now turn to the UICC samples. The values of c are given in Table 2. In two out of five samples the oil-extracted gave the higher values of c, producing 58 mesotheliomas compared with 56 for the natural samples. The crocidolite has a much larger mesothelioma rate than the other four samples which gave similar values. This contrasts with the early experiments in which chrysotile and crocidolite gave similar results.

## Experiment D

In Table 3 are shown the cumulative dosage for each dust and each length of exposure. There is little variation between the five dusts for the long exposure but more for the short exposure since there was insufficient time for any irregularities to be evened out. Also shown is the amount of dust retained in the lungs at the end

Table 3. Experiment D — Dose and retention of asbestos

| Dust | Total dosage (mg/m³ hours) | | Weight of dust (mg) in lungs at end of long exposure |
|---|---|---|---|
| | Short exposure | Long exposure | |
| Amosite | 99 | 5004 | 3.6 |
| Anthophyllite | 103 | 5243 | 3.6 |
| Chrysotile A | 68 | 5068 | 0.7 |
| Chrysotile B | 90 | 4928 | 0.6 |
| Crocidolite | 88 | 5033 | 3.0 |

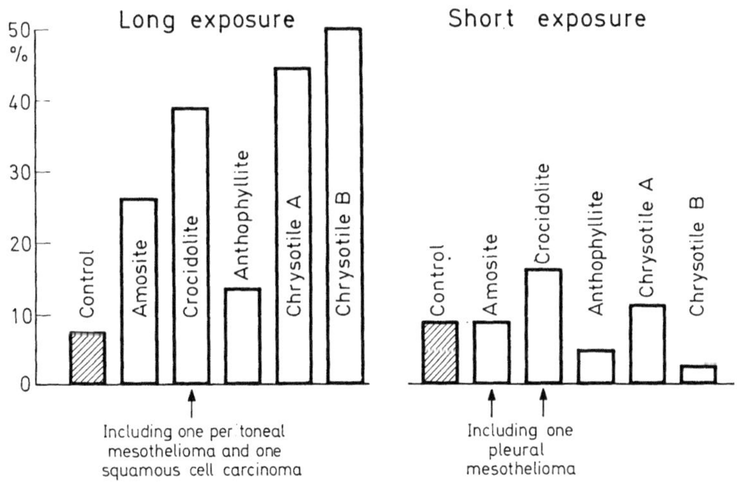


Fig. 1. Inhalation of UICC asbestos reference samples by SPF rats
Percentage with "Pulmonary Adenomas"

of the long exposure, determined by reference to the silica content from six rats per dust. The chrysotile samples gave values about a sixth of the other samples. TIMBRELL [20] has shown how differential deposition of this order can occur due to the curliness of the chrysotile fibres. After one day's exposure the amount of dust retained would be too small for determination but on the basis of the results in Table 3 it can be calculated that the amount retained would be about 0.06 mg for the amphiboles and 0.01 mg for the chrysotiles.

Only three mesotheliomas occurred; two of these were after short exposure, one to amosite the other to crocidolite: the third which was a peritoneal tumour, was after long exposure to crocidolite. There was also a squamous cell carcinoma of the lung after long exposure to crocidolite. Lung adenomas were observed with all dusts and controls but for long exposure there was significant excess for all dusts except anthophyllite (Fig. 1). For the short exposure there was little evidence of an excess of lung adenomas.

## Conclusions on Asbestos Experiments

All samples of asbestos tried produced mesotheliomas after intrapleural inoculation. Since Harington [31] reported the presence of oils in asbestos samples it has been suspected that the oils might be responsible for causing the mesotheliomas. However, it has again been demonstrated that removal of the oils, which was this time by repeated extractions with boiling benzene for 64 hours, does not remove the components producing mesotheliomas. The more finely ground samples produced more mesotheliomas but this could be due to factors besides particle size; for example, different mills were used to grind the samples.

Thus there was a big difference between the effects of inoculation and inhalation; the former caused a high incidence of mesotheliomas whilst the latter produced an excess of lung adenomas and only three mesotheliomas, two, surprisingly, after short exposure. The difference is probably due to inhaled dust not penetrating as far as the mesothelial surface.

## Physical Aspects

The physicists have considered the aerodynamics of the different types of asbestos in relation to inhalation. To a first approximation, the rate of fall of an asbestos fibre depends on its diameter, not its length, so that when asbestos fibres are inhaled, deposition due to sedimentation is almost independent of length [32]. This explains why long fibres (up to about 200 $\mu$) can penetrate to the alveolar regions if they are thin enough ($< 3\ \mu$ diameter). On the other hand, interception on the walls, a deposition mechanism which is important in narrow airways, depends almost entirely on fibre length. Chrysotile fibres, resembling stretched coils, are readily deposited by interception, especially at bifurcations, since the curvature gives them large collision cross-section areas. Amphibole fibres, which are straight, are less readily deposited by interception, since they tend to turn into the direction of the stream-lines in the airflow and thus have small collision cross-sections. In experiment D in which rats were exposed by inhalation to dust clouds generated from the UICC reference samples, the retention of amphiboles was six times greater than for chrysotile [33, 34]. A similar result was obtained when asbestos aerosols were sucked through hollow lung casts in which the airways were left open at the respiratory bronchioles [35]. This ratio for the different types of fibre may be substantially higher in industry. Many chrysotile mining areas are characterized by dense clouds of dust, but a substantial proportion of particles are in the form of large flocks which settle quickly and are available for inhalation for a limited period. Even in chrysotile mills, enough fibre may reach the bronchus to cause asbestosis and carcinoma of the lungs but, in general, exposure to the amphiboles is more likely to produce these diseases. But chrysotile is seldom likely to be associated with mesothelioma of the pleura since its curly nature allows it to reach this region only in minute amounts. The distribution of different types of fibre within the lungs after inhalation needs further study.

By using the electron microscope for measurement, the physicists have shown that the fibres of crocidolite mined in the North West Cape and Australia are much thinner and shorter than those of the crocidolite and amosite mined in the Transvaal and consequently have a much greater chance of reaching the pleura. This hypothesis could account for the high rate of pleural mesotheliomas in the North West Cape, and their presence in Australia compared to only one case in the Transvaal.

Carcinomas of the lung are associated with the moderate-to-severe fibrosis of asbestosis, but there is no evidence as yet to implicate a particular type of asbestos or to measure the relative risks for exposure to only one type of fibre. It would seem that excessive exposure to all types of fibre could be responsible. There is evidence to support the contention that the incidence of carcinoma can be greatly reduced by good industrial hygiene. Mesotheliomas appear to occur after slight exposures to crocidolite; the use of this type of fibre should therefore be restricted if not essential. The position of amosite is not yet clear, so that a high standard of dust control is required when it is used. The use of chrysotile carries only a small risk when the dust control is at a level which is now practical and economic. However, there is a considerable difference between the chrysotile from various deposits, and results of current intrapleural experiments [36] suggest that chrysotile from certain individual mines are more reactive than others. Thus the need is still urgent for further studies on the biological effects of the various types of asbestos to find a relatively inert fibre for industry. Further work on the effect of crocidolite on the mesothelial cells may provide useful information in the study of carcinogenesis.

## References

1. Wagner, J. C.: In: Jotten, K. W. and Klosterkötter, W. (ed.). Die Staublungenerkrankungen **3.** Bericht über die 3. Internationale Staublungen-Tagung, Münster, 29—31 Oktober 1957. Wiss. Forschber. **66**, 566 (1958). Darmstadt: Steinkopff 1958.
2. Fahr, T.: Münch. med. Wschr. **61**, 625 (1914).
3. Stewart, M.: Brit. med. J. **11**, 581 (1929).
4. Gloyne, S. R.: Lancet **1**, 1351 (1932).
5. Gardner, L. U.: Amer. Rev. Tuberc. **45**, 762 (1942).
6. Vorwald, A. J., Durkan, T. M., Pratt, P. C.: A. M. A. Arch. industr. Hyg. **3**, 42 (1951).
7. Merewether, E. R., Price, C. W.: Report on Effects of Asbestos Dust on the Lungs and Dust Suppression in the Asbestos Industry. London HMSO (1930).
8. Minister of Labour and National Service. Annual Report of the Chief Inspector of Factories for the Year 1947. (Cmd. 7621) London HMSO (1949).
9. Doll, R.: Brit. J. industr. Med. **12**, 81 (1955).
10. Knox, J. F., Holmes, S., Doll, R., Hill, I. D.: Brit. J. industr. Med. **25**, 293 (1968).
11. Wagner, J. C., Sleggs, C. A., Marchand, P.: Brit. J. industr. Med. **17**, 260 (1960).
12. Buchanan, W. D.: Ann. N. Y. Acad. Sci. **132**, 507 (1965).
13. Elmes, P. C., McCaughey, W. T., Wade, O. L.: Brit. med. J. 1, 350 (1965).
14. Hourihane, D. O.: Thorax **19**, 268 (1964).
15. Owen, W. G.: Ann. N. Y. Acad. Sci. **132**, 674 (1965).
16. Gilson, J. C.: Trans. Soc. Occup. Med. **16**, 62 (1966).
17. Wagner, J. C., Gilson, J. C., Berry, G., Timbrell, V.: Brit. med. Bull. **27**, 71 (1971).
18. International Union Against Cancer. Brit. J. industr. Med. **22**, 165 (1965).

19. UICC Committee. Chest. **58**, 57 (1970).
20. TIMBRELL, V.: In: SHAPIRO, H. A. (ed.). Pneumoconiosis: Proceedings of the International Conference, Johannesburg, 23 April—2 May 1969, p. 28. Cape Town: Oxford University Press 1970.
21. MCDONALD, J. C., MCDONALD, A. D., GIBBS, G. W., SIEMIATYCKI, J., ROSSITER, C. E.: Arch. environm. Hlth **22**, 677 (1971).
22. MANCUSO, T. F., EL-ATTAR, A. A.: J. occup. Med. **9**, 147 (1967).
23. SELIKOFF, I. J., HAMMOND, E. C., CHURG, J.: In: SHAPIRO, H. A. (ed.). Pneumoconiosis: Proceedings of the International Conference, Johannesburg, 23 April—2 May 1969, p. 180. Cape Town: Oxford University Press 1970.
24. DOLL, R.: J. Roy. Statist. Soc. **134**, 133 (1971).
25. Ministry of Labour: Problems Arising from the Use of Asbestos. London HMSO: 1967.
26. WAGNER, J. C.: Nature (Lond.) **196**, 180 (1962).
27. WAGNER, J. C., BERRY, G.: Brit. J. Cancer **23**, 567 (1969).
28. TIMBRELL, V., SKIDMORE, J. W., HYETT, F., WAGNER, J. C.: J. Aerosol Sci. **1**, 215 (1970).
29. WAGNER, J. C., BERRY, G., TIMBRELL, V.: In: SHAPIRO, H. A. (ed.). Pneumoconiosis: Proceedings of the International Conference, Johannesburg, 23 April—2 May, 1969, p. 216. Cape Town: Oxford University Press 1970.
30. BERRY, G., WAGNER, J. C.: Brit. J. Cancer **23**, 582 (1969).
31. HARINGTON, J. S.: Nature (Lond.) **193**, 43 (1962).
32. TIMBRELL, V.: Ann. N. Y. Acad. Sci. **132**, 255 (1965).
33. TIMBRELL, V., POOLEY, F., WAGNER, J. C.: In: SHAPIRO, H. A. (ed.). Pneumoconiosis: Proceedings of the International Conference, Johannesburg, 23 April—2 May, 1969, p. 120. Cape Town: Oxford University Press 1970.
34. TIMBRELL, V. In: Mercer, T. T., Morrow, P. E., and Stöber, W. (ed). Assessment of Airborne Particles. Proceedings of the Third Rochester International Conference on Environmental Toxicity, Rochester, June 18—20, 1970, p. 429. Springfield, Illinois: Charles C Thomas 1972.
35. TIMBRELL, V.: In: SHAPIRO, H. A. (ed.). Pneumoconiosis: Proceedings of the International Conference, Johannesburg, 23 April—2 May, 1969, p. 3. Cape Town: Oxford University Press 1970.
36. WAGNER, J. C.: In: NETTESHEIM, P., HANNA, M. G., Jr., DEATHERAGE, J. W., Jr. (ed.). Morphology of Experimental Respiratory Carcinogenesis. Proceedings of a Conference, Gatlinburg 13—16 May, 1970, p. 347. U.S. Atomic Energy Commission. Symposium Series No. 21, 1970.

# *Thyroid Gland*

# Histologic Classification as a Problem in the Epidemiology of Thyroid Cancer

K. Franssila and E. Saxén

Finnish Cancer Registry and the Third Department of Pathology, University of Helsinki, Helsinki, Finland

In the International Classification of Diseases all malignant tumours of a specific site are usually classified into one group using one code number. This is generally done also in epidemiologic studies. It has been found, however, that the malignant tumours of most organs do not form a homogeneous group but are composed of many individual types which differ in their clinical course and epidemiology. For example, in the nodular sclerosing type of Hodgkin's disease the age and sex distribution and the course of the disease are very different from those of the other histologic types of Hodgkin's disease (Lukes et al., 1966, Franssila et al., 1967). This concurs with the hypothesis based on epidemiologic studies that Hodgkin's disease is actually composed of two different diseases (e.g. MacMahon, 1966). It is also well known that adenocarcinoma of the lung does not show the same sex difference or the same correlation with smoking as epidermoid carcinoma.

Thus, it is apparent that much information is lost if all malignant tumours of a single organ are placed in one group. The special characteristics of one type of cancer may be hidden under the features of the other types. Therefore, the specific histologic types of one organ should be studied separately, epidemiologically also, instead of grouping all cancers together.

We have chosen thyroid cancer as an example to show the correlation between the histology, epidemiology and biologic behaviour of different tumours of the same organ. All cases of thyroid cancer diagnosed in Finland during a five-year period were histologically re-examined and re-typed. In addition, Cancer Registry reports were explored for their suitability for studies of the incidence of different histologic types.

## Materials and Methods

The Cancer Registry has existed in Finland since 1953 and covers the whole country. All hospitals, pathological laboratories, and practicing physicians are requested to report to the Registry all cases of malignant tumours coming to their attention. The number of non-reported cases is kept to a minimum by obtaining the listings of all deaths in Finland, which are then checked against the files of the Registry. This also allows a complete follow-up until death of all patients. Only three per cent of the cancer cases in the incidence statistics are included on the basis of death certificates only.

The present material comprised all the cases (391) of thyroid cancer diagnosed in Finland in the five-year period 1958—1962. The diagnosis had been histologically confirmed in 88 per cent of the cases. The histologic re-examination and re-classification were done without knowledge of any clinical data, and succeeded in 97 per cent of the cases.

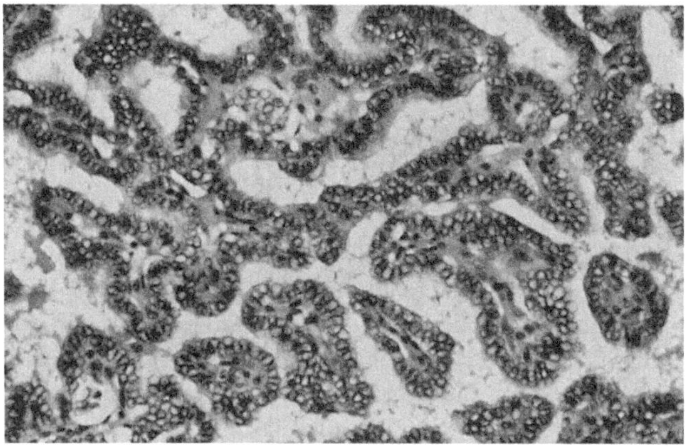

Fig. 1. Papillary carcinoma. Papillary structures with ground glass type of nuclei (H and E, × 300)

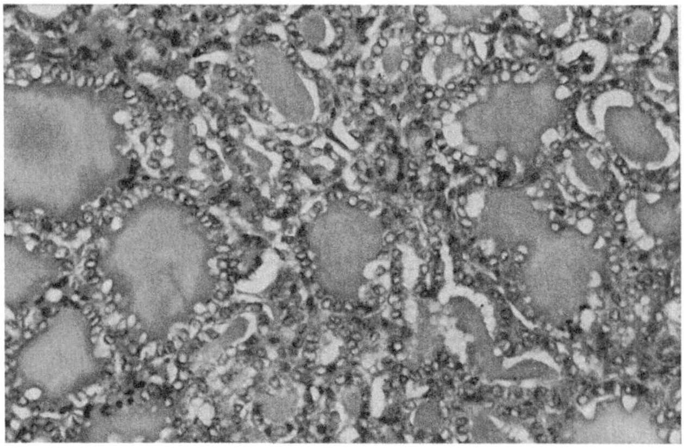

Fig. 2. Papillary carcinoma. Same tumour as in Fig. 1. Follicular pattern with abundant colloid production. Nuclei are of the ground glass type (H and E, ×300)

The observed survival rates were calculated by the actuarial method (BERKSON and GAGE, 1950) and the relative survival rates according to the method proposed by EDERER et al. (1961). The common closing date was December 31, 1968. The longest follow-up time was 11 years.

Thyroid carcinoma was classified into four histologic types (papillary, follicular, medullary and anaplastic) according to the following criteria:

In papillary carcinoma were included all the carcinomas in which neoplastic papillae were seen, regardless of the presence of follicular or solid areas (Fig. 1). The tumours in which either of the last mentioned structures were encountered without papillae were also regarded as papillary carcinomas if the nucleus was of ground-glass type (large, pale, with little chromatin) and the mode of growth was typical of papillary carcinoma, that is, heavily infiltrating (Fig. 2). All papillary neoplasms were considered to be malignant.

In follicular carcinoma were included the cases in which no neoplastic papillae were demonstrated, but which displayed follicular solid and/or trabecular structures

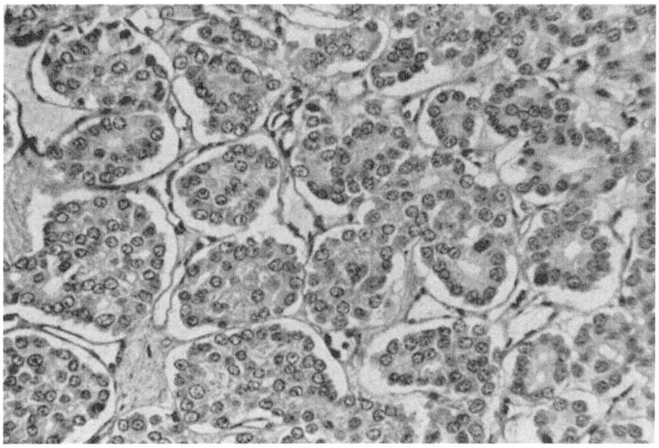

Fig. 3. Follicular carcinoma. Follicular and trabecular structures. The nuclei are not of the ground glass type (H and E, × 300)

and in which the nucleus was not of ground glass type (Fig. 3). All follicular tumours in which tissue or vascular invasion was seen were regarded as malignant. Encapsulated tumours in which the infiltration beyond the capsule was slight or absent were called encapsulated carcinomas (malignant adenoma).

In medullary carcinoma were included carcinomas in which amyloid was seen.

In anaplastic carcinoma were included tumours in which no differentiation was demonstrated. Tumours composed of both differentiated and undifferentiated areas were also regarded as anaplastic.

## Results

*Incidence of thyroid cancer and distribution by histologic type before and after the re-examination.* At re-examination 231 tumours (69 per cent of re-examined cases) were regarded as thyroid cancer, and 16 as suspected carcinoma. On the assumption that also 69 per cent of the tumours which were not examined histologically or re-examined were thyroid cancer, we obtain an annual incidence of $1.22/10^5$. This is markedly lower than the 1.76 incidence based on the original Cancer Registry material before re-examination.

The distribution of the cases into histologic types before and after re-examination is shown in Table 1. There were in the original material many unspecific histologic

Table 1. Number and percentual distribution of cases by histologic type before and after the re-examination

| Histologic type | Before re-examination | | After re-examination | |
|---|---|---|---|---|
| | No. | % of specific diagnoses | No. | % of specific diagnoses |
| Papillary carcinoma | 62 | 27.8 | 100 | 43.7 |
| Follicular carcinoma | 89 | 39.9 | 60 | 26.2 |
| malignant adenoma | 35 | | 9 | |
| Medullary carcinoma | — | — | 10 | 4.4 |
| Anaplastic carcinoma | 51 | 22.9 | 58 | 25.3 |
| Other cancer | 21 | 9.4 | 1 | 0.4 |
| Total specific diagnoses | 223 | 100.0 | 229 | 100.0 |
| Adenocarcinoma | 37 | | — | |
| Malignant tumour | 35 | | 2 | |
| Suspicion of carcinoma | 40 | | 16 | |
| Benign tumour or malignant tumour not of thyroid origin | — | | 88 | |
| Total | 335 | | 335 | |

diagnoses like adenocarcinoma and carcinoma. If we take only specific diagnoses into consideration, the distribution of tumours into histologic types is quite different before and after the re-examination. Follicular carcinoma was the most common histologic type before re-examination, largely because of the big proportion of so-called malignant adenomas. Papillary carcinoma was the most common type after re-examination, and the proportion of follicular carcinoma was markedly smaller.

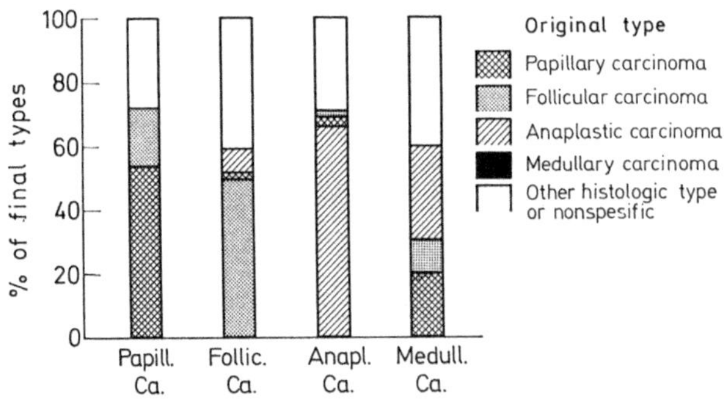


Fig. 4. Percentual distribution of cases by original histologic diagnosis in four final histologic types

Fig. 4 presents the original (before re-examination) histologic diagnoses for each of the final (after re-examination) histologic types and Fig. 5 the final histologic diagnoses for each of the original histologic types. It will be observed that only in one-half of the tumours interpreted at re-examination as papillary or follicular carcinomas was the diagnosis the same as the original diagnosis. On the other hand,

87 per cent of the cases originally diagnosed as papillary carcinoma were still classified as such at re-examination, but only 34 per cent of those originally diagnosed as follicular carcinoma. Forty four per cent of the latter were assessed as benign at the re-examination. The original diagnosis was malignant adenoma in almost all (87%) of these cases.

*Age and sex*. The age-adjusted incidences for both sexes are shown in Fig. 6. The difference between the sexes is great in papillary carcinoma, while in follicular

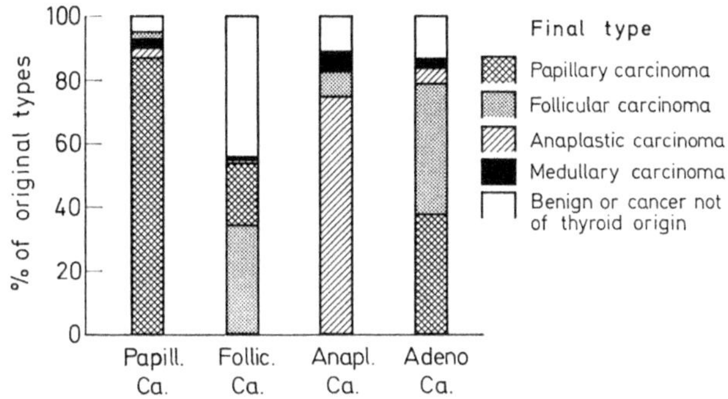


Fig. 5. Percentual distribution of cases by final histologic diagnosis in four original histologic types

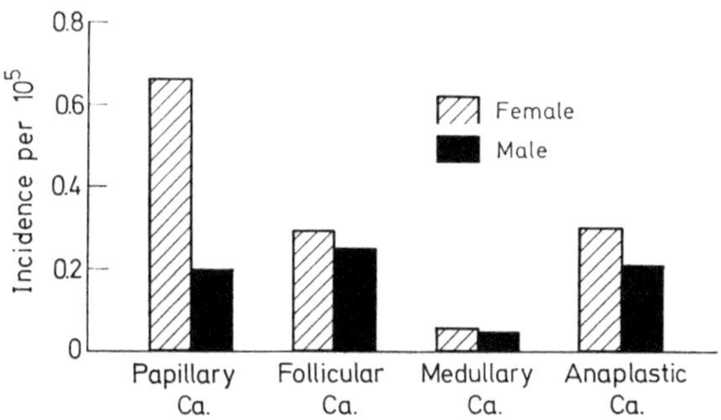


Fig. 6. Age-adjusted incidence rates (total Finnish population as the standard) by sex and histologic type

and medullary carcinoma it is small. In the total series the rate for females is about twice that for men.

Fig. 7 shows the age-specific incidences for both sexes. There are marked differences between the histologic types in the age of occurrence. Anaplastic carcinoma occurs almost solely in old age, while papillary carcinoma occurs in all age groups, and follicular carcinoma in middle and old age.

*Course of the disease*. Table 2 shows the frequency of inoperable tumours and of regional and distant metastases in the different histologic types. There were marked differences between the histologic types in these respects. The primary tumour was inoperable in half of the anaplastic carcinomas, rarely in other histologic types. Regional lymph node metastases were common in papillary and medullary carcinoma, whereas they were detected in only one patient with follicular carcinoma. Distant

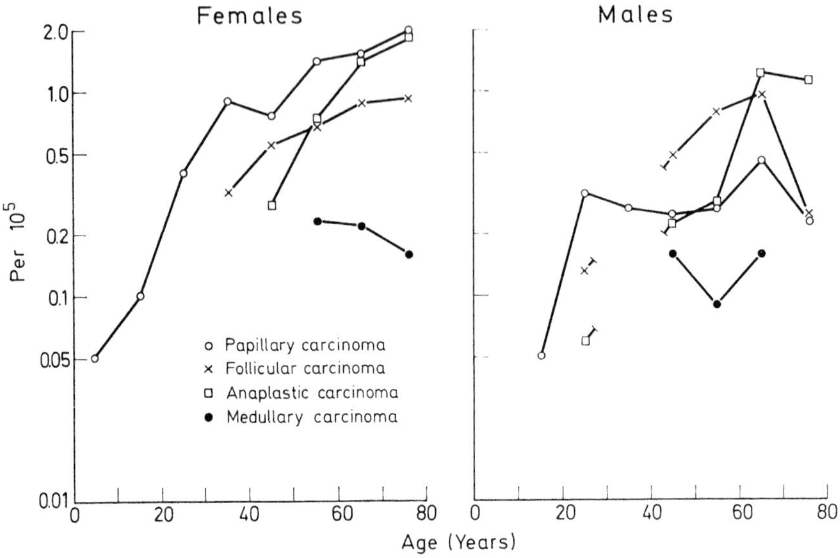


Fig. 7. Age-specific incidence rates for four histologic types of thyroid carcinoma

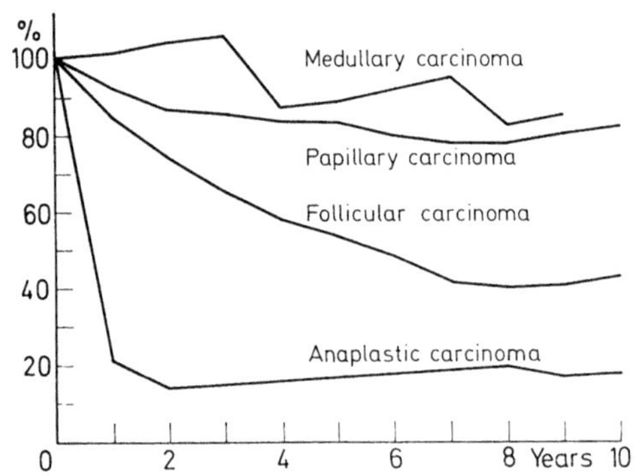


Fig. 8. Relative survival curves for four histologic types of thyroid carcinoma

Table 2. Frequency of inoperable tumours and of metastases by histologic type

| Histologic type | No. of cases | Inoperable tumours | Metastases during the follow-up period | |
|---|---|---|---|---|
| | | | Regional | Distant |
| | | (%) | (%) | (%) |
| Papillary carcinoma | 100 | 8 | 42 | 13 |
| Follicular carcinoma | 60 | 6 | 2 | 70 |
| Medullary carcinoma | 10 | — | 70 | 10 |
| Anaplastic carcinoma | 58 | 47 | 28 | 45 |
| Others | 3 | — | 33 | 67 |
| All cases | 231 | 17 | 29 | 36 |

metastases, on the other hand, were common in follicular carcinoma and rare in the medullary and papillary types. Anaplastic carcinoma was in its mode of metastasising an intermediate form between papillary and follicular carcinoma.

*Survival.* The relative survival curves for the individual histologic types are shown in Fig. 8. The curves for papillary, follicular and anaplastic carcinomas differ from each other significantly ($p < 0.001$) when tested by Mantel-Haenszel method (MANTEL, 1963).

## Discussion

Differential diagnosis between benign and malignant thyroid tumours is difficult. The main problem lies in distinguishing between encapsulated follicular carcinomas (malignant adenomas) and benign atypical adenomas and thyroid nodules. The criteria of malignancy vary largely in this respect. Some authors consider remarkable cellular atypia to suffice for diagnosis of carcinoma, some regard only tumours showing vascular or capsular invasion as malignant. In the present series, only 40 per cent of the tumours originally diagnosed as malignant adenomas were regarded as malignant after the re-examination. The differences between the histologic criteria may partly explain the differences in incidences between different areas. It is possible that the high incidence of follicular carcinoma in endemic goitre areas is due to over-diagnosis: atypical nodules and adenomas, which occur in abundance in such areas are sometimes misdiagnosed as follicular carcinomas of malignant adenoma type (SAXÉN et al., 1969).

The difficulties of differential diagnosis between benign and malignant thyroid tumours are well reflected in our study. The number of cases originally diagnosed as cancer or suspicion of cancer declined by 26 per cent after the re-examination. Thus, the incidences based on Cancer Registry reports seem to be rather unreliable and too high.

There are many different histologic classifications of thyroid cancer. The number of histologic types and the nomenclature vary, as well as the histologic criteria for different types. Most of the classifications have in common the separation of anaplastic carcinoma as a histologic type of its own. In contrast, there are marked differences in the classification of differentiated carcinomas. Opinions differ especially about the necessity to distinguish between papillary and follicular carcinomas, and if they are separated, about the criteria for differential diagnosis. Some authors regard tumours composed mainly of papillae as papillary and those composed mainly of follicles as follicular carcinoma (MEISSNER and WARREN, 1969); others distinguish a separate type of carcinoma containing both papillae and follicles and call it mixed papillary and follicular carcinoma (RUSSELL et al., 1969). However, it has been found that tumours containing follicular and solid structures in addition to papillae behave like purely papillary tumours and differently from follicular carcinoma (FRANSSILA, 1971).

We classified these mixed types as papillary carcinoma and found marked differences between papillary and follicular carcinoma: The age and sex distribution, mode of spread and survival rates of papillary carcinoma were different from those of follicular carcinoma. It has been suggested that the incidence of follicular carcinoma is higher in endemic goitre areas than elsewhere (SAXÉN, 1950), and that this tumour is associated more often than expected with non-neoplastic goitre

(CUELLO et al., 1969). But no difference has been found in the incidence of papillary carcinoma between endemic and non-endemic goitre areas (SAXÉN, 1950). Irradiation is obviously an etiologic agent in some papillary carcinomas, especially in those of children (WINSHIP and ROSVOLL, 1961), but apparently not in follicular carcinoma. Papillary and follicular carcinoma thus differ from each other in many respects. It is obvious that they are two biologically different tumours, which ought to be distinguished between.

In anaplastic carcinoma both the histologic features and the course of disease are so different from those of differentiated carcinoma that its separation into a type of its own is generally accepted. RUSSELL et al., (1969) found a differentiated component, either papillary or follicular, in all the anaplastic carcinomas they studied with subserial sections. Consequently, it is possible that anaplastic carcinoma derives from either papillary or follicular carcinoma, and should perhaps be classified into the histologic type from which it derives. However, differentiated carcinoma is seen in only 9—18 per cent of routine biopsies from anaplastic carcinoma (SMEDAL and MEISSNER, 1961; WOOLNER et al., 1961). In addition, anaplastic carcinoma behaves differently from differentiated carcinomas. Therefore, its separation as a histologic entity may be regarded as justified.

Medullary carcinoma differs histogenetically from all other thyroid carcinomas by probably arising from parafollicular cells (WILLIAMS, 1966), while other thyroid carcinomas are considered to derive from follicular epithelial cells. It is, therefore, most clearly a pathologic entity among all carcinomas of the thyroid gland.

In addition to these four histologic types, Hürthle and clear cell carcinomas are often classified separately. It has been found, however, that they behave according to their main structural pattern. They are therefore generally classified into one of the previous histologic types.

Encapsulated follicular carcinoma (malignant adenoma) is usually included in follicular carcinomas. This is apparently justified as the course of the disease and histology are qualitatively similar although the infiltrating type behaves more malignantly and shows histologically more pronounced infiltration. However, there is good reason to distinguish between encapsulated carcinoma and other follicular carcinomas in epidemiologic studies, as regional differences between the incidence of follicular carcinoma may largely depend on the lack of consistency in the pathologist's differential diagnosis between encapsulated carcinoma and benign atypical adenoma.

Sarcomas were earlier quite common in series from Central Europe where they have formed even 28—50 per cent of all thyroid cancers (THALMAN, 1954; KIND, 1966). On the other hand, the American literature has only isolated reports of thyroid sarcoma. The great differences are mainly due to the different criteria applied. When the Swiss material published by KIND (1966) was histologically reexamined according to recent interpretations the proportion of sarcomas declined from 20 to 0.6 per cent (HEDINGER, 1969).

It appears from the foregoing that it is possible to divide thyroid cancers into histologic types that differ from each other so clearly that they should be regarded as different diseases also in epidemiologic studies. Cancer Registry materials are not yet suitable for this kind of study as they are based on diagnoses made by pathologists applying different criteria. To make the histologic diagnoses as comparable as possible, we require a uniformly accepted classification. For the present, comparable results are possible only if the same pathologist studies the slides of the materials compared. This is valid also for many other organs.

In conclusion, we may say that much information is lost if malignant tumours of one specific site are treated as a single group in epidemiologic studies. This is shown clearly by the present study as far as thyroid cancer is concerned.

## References


BERKSON, J., GAGE, R. P.: Calculation of survival rates for cancer. Proc. Mayo Clin. **25**, 270—286 (1950).

CUELLO, L., CORREA, P., EISENBERG, H.: Geographic pathology of thyroid carcinoma. Cancer (Philad.) **23**, 230—239 (1969).

EDERER, F., AXTELL, L. M., CUTLER, S. J.: The relative survival rate: a statistical methodology. In: End results and mortality trends in cancer. Nat. Cancer Inst. Monogr. No. 6, 1961, p. 101—121.

FRANSSILA, K. O., KALIMA, T. V., VOUTILAINEN, A.: Histologic classification of Hodgkin's disease. Cancer (Philad.) **20**, 1594—1601 (1967).

FRANSSILA, K.: Value of histologic classification of thyroid cancer. Acta path. microbiol. scand. Sect. A, suppl. 225, 1971.

HEDINGER, C. E.: Sarcomas of the thyroid gland. In: HEDINGER, C. E. (ed.): Thyroid Cancer. UICC Monograph series, vol. 12. Berlin-Heidelberg-New York: Springer 1969, p. 47—52.

KIND, H. P.: Die Häufigkeit der Struma maligna im Sections- und Operationsgut des Pathologischen Instituts der Universität Zürich von 1900 bis Mitte 1964. Schweiz. med. Wschr. **96**, 560—568 (1966).

LUKES, R. J., BUTLER, J. J., HICKS, E. B.: Natural history of Hodgkin's disease as related to its pathologic picture. Cancer (Philad.) **19**, 317—344 (1966).

MACMAHON, B.: Epidemiology of Hodgkin's disease. Cancer Res. **26**, 1189—1200 (1966).

MANTEL, N.: Chi-square tests with one degree of freedom; extensions of the Mantel-Haenszel procedure. J. Amer. stat. Ass. **58**, 690—700 (1963).

MEISSNER, W. A., WARREN, S.: Tumors of the thyroid gland. Atlas of Tumor Pathology. Second series. Fascicle 4. Armed Forces Institute of Pathology: Washington 1969.

RUSSELL, W. O., IBANEZ, M. L., CLARK, R. L., HILL, C. S., Jr., WHITE, E. C.: Follicular (organoid) carcinoma of the thyroid gland. Report of 84 cases. In: HEDINGER, C. E. (ed.): Thyroid Cancer. UICC Monograph series, vol. 12. Berlin-Heidelberg-New York: Springer 1969, p. 14—25.

SAXÉN, E.: Carcinoma thyreoideae and its incidence in Finland. Acta chir. scand., suppl. 156, 1950.

SAXÉN, E. A., FRANSSILA, K., HAKAMA, M.: Effect of histological typing of registry material on the results on epidemiolgcal comparisons in thyroid cancer, In: HEDINGER, C. E. (ed). Thyroid Cancer. UICC Monograph Series vol. 12. Berlin—Heidelberg—New York: Springer 1969, p. 98—103.

SMEDAL, M. L., MEISSNER, W. A.: The results of X-ray treatment in undifferentiated carcinoma of the thyroid. Radiology **76**, 927—935 (1961).

THALMANN, A.: Die Häufigkeit der Struma maligna am Berner Pathologischen Institut von 1910 bis 1950 und ihre Beziehung zur Jodprophylaxe des endemischen Kropfes. Schweiz. med. Wschr. **84**, 473—478 (1954).

WILLIAMS, E. D.: Histogenesis of medullary carcinoma of the thyroid. J. clin. Path. **19**, 114—118 (1966).

WINSHIP, T., ROSVOLL, R. V.: Childhood thyroid carcinoma. Cancer (Philad.) **14**, 734—743 (1961).

WOOLNER, L. B., BEAHRS, O. H., BLACK, B. M., MCCONAHEY, W. M., KEATING, F. R., Jr.: Classification and prognosis of thyroid carcinoma: A study of 885 cases observed in a thirty-year period. Amer. J. Surg. **102**, 354—387 (1961).

# Leukemia and Thyroid Carcinoma Found among A-Bomb Survivors in Hiroshima

Susumu Watanabe and Yukio Shimosato
National Cancer Center Research Institute, Tokyo, Japan

Takeshi Ohkita, Haruo Ezaki, Takao Shigemitsu, and Nanao Kamata
Research Institute for Nuclear Medicine and Biology, Hiroshima University, Hiroshima, Japan

## Introduction

It is a well-known fact that various neoplasms can be induced by ionizing radiation. In humans, leukemia, and carcinomas of the skin, lung, thyroid gland, etc., have been reported among persons exposed to either total body or local irradiation, mostly for diagnostic and therapeutic purposes with X-rays. On the other hand, the final conclusion has not been reached yet, whether certain types of neoplasm were induced significantly by the atomic bomb explosions at Hiroshima and Nagasaki. But at present it is considered to be almost certain that leukemia and thyroid carcinoma were induced in high incidences by atomic bomb radiation. Induction of malignant lymphoma and carcinomas of the breast, ovary and lungs by atomic bomb irradiation is inconclusive and accepted by some and denied by others. For these reasons, presentation of data and discussion on this occasion will be limited to leukemia and thyroid carcinoma.

Although there is a difference opinion among the investigators on classification of leukemias, the overall incidence is known by the death statistics, because leukemia is almost 100% fatal. On the other hand, statistical assessments of thyroid carcinoma vary greatly, since many of the thyroid carcinomas, especially occult carcinoma, are not lethal, and since criteria not only for each histologic type but also for malignity of the thyroid lesions vary among the pathologists.

The diagnostic criteria employed by us were very similar to those of Hazard. We tried to use the general tendency of thyroid carcinoma in Japan as control for the study at Hiroshima, and cases experienced in the National Cancer Center in Tokyo were also studied.

## A. Leukemia

### I. Incidence of Leukemia among Hiroshima Survivors

The annual change in the total and exposed populations in Hiroshima city during the period of 1946 to 1970 is shown in Table 1. The numbers in this table are based on the national and local censuses. The exposed population has gradually decreased, however, there are about 79,000 survivors still living in the city. The number of deaths and death rate of leukemia per 100,000 in Hiroshima in each year during the past 25 years are indicated in Table 2 and Fig. 1. In 1970, the total number of deaths from leukemia among the population who were born before atomic bomb detonation

Table 1. Change in population of Hiroshima (1946—1970)

| Year | Population[a] estimated | Exposed population estimated | Non-exposed population estimated |
|---|---|---|---|
| 1946 | 183.535 | 102.036 | 81.499 |
| 1947 | 220.551 | 101.052 | 119.499 |
| 1948 | 234.126 | 100.069 | 134.057 |
| 1949 | 246.463 | 99.085 | 147.378 |
| 1950 | 252.643[b] | 98.102[b] | 154.541 |
| 1951 | 258.654 | 97.119 | 161.535 |
| 1952 | 265.198 | 96.135 | 169.063 |
| 1953 | 271.730 | 95.152 | 176.578 |
| 1954 | 278.899 | 94.168 | 184.731 |
| 1955 | 287.140 | 93.185 | 193.955 |
| 1956 | 292.207 | 92.201 | 200.006 |
| 1957 | 297.784 | 91.218 | 206.566 |
| 1958 | 305.738 | 90.234 | 215.504 |
| 1959 | 311.074 | 89.251 | 221.823 |
| 1960 | 318.896 | 88.267 | 230.629 |
| 1961 | 321.747 | 87.284 | 234.463 |
| 1962 | 324.623 | 86.300 | 238.323 |
| 1963 | 327.503 | 85.317 | 242.186 |
| 1964 | 330.372 | 84.336 | 246.036 |
| 1965 | 333.257[c] | 83.350[c] | 249.907 |
| 1966 | 334.503 | 82.367 | 252.136 |
| 1967 | 335.114 | 81.383 | 253.731 |
| 1968 | 342.141 | 80.400 | 261.741 |
| 1969 | 345.802 | 79.416 | 266.386 |
| 1970 | 349.740 | 78.433 | 271.307 |

[a] Population born before Aug. 6, 1945.
[b] Figures from census on Oct. 1, 1950.
[c] Figures from census on Nov. 1, 1965.

was 11, of which only two were from the exposed cases. The death rates per 100,000 were 3.15 and 2.55, respectively, and it is clear from the table that in these three years, the death rates of leukemia of the exposed population are almost equal to or a little less than that of all Japan. Fig. 2 illustrates the death rate of leukemia per successive three years from 1946 through 1969. It is obvious that the high mortality of the exposed population is mostly due to the death rate of the proximally exposed survivors. In 1970, no deaths were found from the people exposed within 2,000 m. The number of leukemia cases that developed and the incidence of leukemia during the same period is shown in Table 3. In recent years, the sudden rise of the incidence of the disease was noted in both 1966 and 1967: nevertheless, none of the cases was found among the survivors in 1969. It is noteworthy that the latter is the first phenomenon since 1947. The general trends of the incidence of leukemia among

Table 2. Death-rate of leukemia in Hiroshima citizens (1946—1970)

| Year of onset | Total cases[a] | | Exposed cases (within 5 km) | | Death-rate of all Japan |
|---|---|---|---|---|---|
| | Number of cases | Death-rate/ 100,000 | Number of cases | Death-rate/ 100,000 | |
| 1946 | 1 | 0.54 | 0 | — | — |
| 1947 | 3 | 1.36 | 2 | 1.98 | 1.07 |
| 1948 | 7 | 2.99 | 3 | 3.00 | 1.19 |
| 1949 | 7 | 2.84 | 3 | 3.03 | 1.37 |
| 1950 | 8 | 3.17 | 6 | 6.12 | 1.47 |
| 1951 | 13 | 5.03 | 10 | 10.30 | 1.58 |
| 1952 | 17 | 6.41 | 10 | 10.40 | 1.67 |
| 1953 | 22 | 8.10 | 13 | 13.66 | 1.91 |
| 1954 | 7 | 2.51 | 4 | 4.25 | 2.12 |
| 1955 | 12 | 4.18 | 8 | 8.59 | 2.28 |
| 1956 | 19 | 6.50 | 12 | 13.02 | 2.41 |
| 1957 | 17 | 5.71 | 11 | 12.06 | 2.44 |
| 1958 | 16 | 5.23 | 8 | 8.87 | 2.65 |
| 1959 | 19 | 6.11 | 12 | 13.45 | 2.67 |
| 1960 | 12 | 3.76 | 4 | 4.53 | 2.81 |
| 1961 | 18 | 5.59 | 7 | 8.02 | 2.89 |
| 1962 | 13 | 4.00 | 7 | 8.11 | 3.06 |
| 1963 | 9 | 2.75 | 6 | 7.03 | 3.07 |
| 1964 | 8 | 2.42 | 3 | 3.56 | 3.19 |
| 1965 | 11 | 3.30 | 5 | 6.00 | 3.21 |
| 1966 | 10 | 2.99 | 6 | 7.28 | 3.30 |
| 1967 | 16 | 4.77 | 10 | 12.29 | 3.30 |
| 1968 | 4 | 1.17 | 3 | 3.73 | — |
| 1969 | 7 | 2.02 | 2 | 2.52 | — |
| 1970 | 11 | 3.15 | 2 | 2.55 | — |

[a] Cases born before Aug. 6, 1945.

survivors is visualized in Fig. 3. Even in the proximally exposed population, the incidence has also markedly decreased in the last three years. In 1970, the incidence per single year was higher than the average of all Japan: however, it might be said that the peak of the prevalence of leukemia among the survivors has already passed.

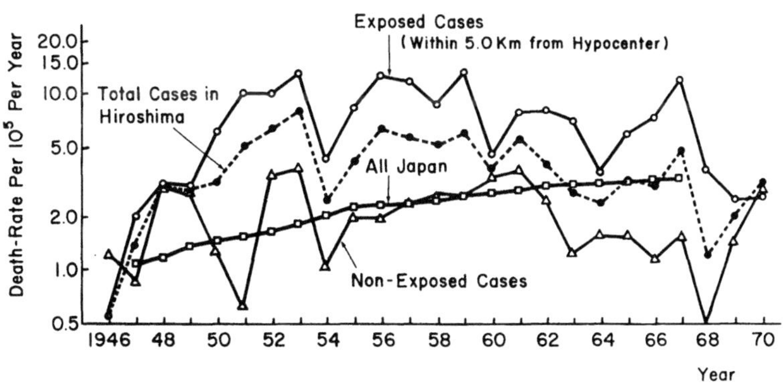


Fig. 1. Death-rate of leukemia in Hiroshima citizens (1946—1970)

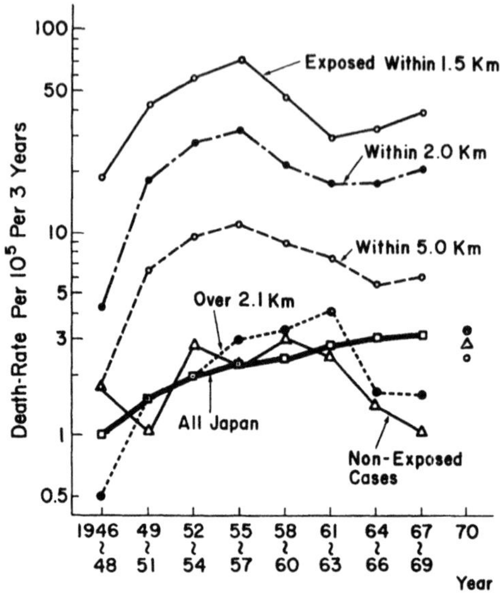


Fig. 2. Death-rate of leukemia in Hiroshima citizens (1946—1970)

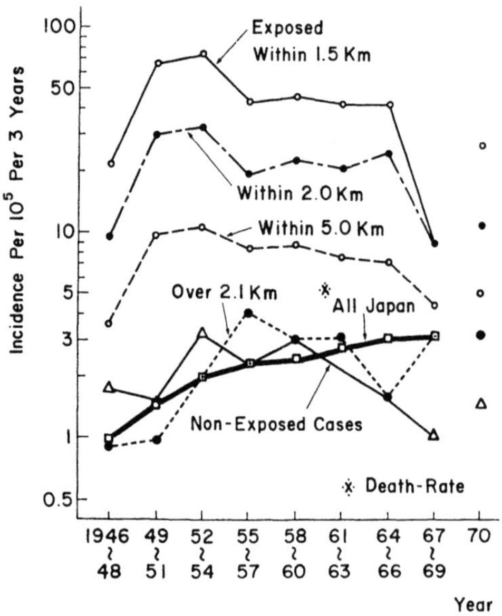


Fig. 3. Incidence of leukemia in Hiroshima citizens (1946—1970)

These observations are summarized in Table 4. During the past 25 years, 300 cases of leukemia occurred in Hiroshima citizens: 170 of these cases were derived from people exposed to the atomic bomb within 5,000 meters from the hypocenter. Thus, the total incidence of leukemia per 100,000 per year during the period was 4.07, whereas that of exposed persons was 7.54. The total number of deaths from leukemia was 287, of which 157 were in the exposed group. The total death rate

Table 3. Incidence of leukemia in Hiroshima citizens (1946—1970)

| Year of onset | Total cases[a] | | Exposed cases (within 5 km) | |
|---|---|---|---|---|
| | Number of cases | Incidence/ 100,000 | Number of cases | Incidence/ 100,000 |
| 1946 | 1 | 0.54 | 0 | — |
| 1947 | 5 | 2.27 | 4 | 3.96 |
| 1948 | 11 | 4.70 | 7 | 7.00 |
| 1949 | 9 | 3.65 | 6 | 6.06 |
| 1950 | 11 | 4.35 | 8 | 8.15 |
| 1951 | 18 | 6.96 | 14 | 14.42 |
| 1952 | 19 | 7.16 | 11 | 11.44 |
| 1953 | 19 | 6.99 | 12 | 12.61 |
| 1954 | 13 | 4.66 | 8 | 8.50 |
| 1955 | 12 | 4.18 | 7 | 7.51 |
| 1956 | 14 | 4.79 | 5 | 5.42 |
| 1957 | 16 | 5.37 | 11 | 12.06 |
| 1958 | 18 | 5.89 | 9 | 9.97 |
| 1959 | 19 | 6.11 | 12 | 13.44 |
| 1960 | 11 | 3.45 | 3 | 3.40 |
| 1961 | 17 | 5.28 | 7 | 8.02 |
| 1962 | 10 | 3.08 | 7 | 8.11 |
| 1963 | 11 | 3.36 | 6 | 7.03 |
| 1964 | 11 | 3.33 | 5 | 5.93 |
| 1965 | 9 | 2.70 | 3 | 3.60 |
| 1966 | 17 | 5.08 | 10 | 12.14 |
| 1967 | 13 | 3.88 | 8 | 9.83 |
| 1968 | 4 | 1.17 | 3 | 3.75 |
| 1969 | 4 | 1.16 | 0 | — |
| 1970 | 8 | 2.29 | 4 | 5.10 |

[a] Cases born before Aug. 6, 1945.

from leukemia per 100,000 per year during this period was 3.89, while that of exposed cases was 6.96. The mean value of the death rate from leukemia in all Japan within the same period was 2.36: in Hiroshima and in exposed cases it was, respectively, about 1.6 and 2.9 times higher than that of all Japan.

The type of leukemia observed among the survivors in Hiroshima and the rate of acute and chronic leukemia in relation to the onset of the disease is shown in

Table 4. Incidence and mortality of leukemia in Hiroshima citizens (1946—1970)

| | | Exposed cases (within 5,000 m) | Non-exposed cases[a] | All Japan |
|---|---|---|---|---|
| No. of cases | 300 | 170 | 108 | |
| Incidence per 100,000 per year | 4.07 | 7.54 | 2.11 | |
| No. of deaths | 287 | 157 | 106 | |
| Death-rate per 100,000 per year | 3.89 | 6.96 | 2.07 | 2.36[b] |

[a] Cases born after Aug. 6, 1945 and early entrants are excluded. [b] 1947—1967.

Table 5. There were 101 cases of acute form and the majority of them belonged to the myeloid type. Similar trends were also apparent in cases of chronic forms: only three of lymphoid type. Furthermore, the majority of cases developing in the early period after the bombing belonged to the chronic type. Therefore, if the cases are grouped into 5-year periods, a gradual switch from the acute type to chronic type is noted. The type of leukemia developed in Hiroshima survivors in relation to the

Table 5. Rate of acute and chronic leukemia in Hiroshima survivors by period of onset

| Period of onset | Acute form | Chronic form | Ratio of acute/chronic |
|---|---|---|---|
| 1946—1950 | 12 | 13 | 0.92 |
| 1951—1955 | 24 | 28 | 0.86 |
| 1956—1960 | 29 | 11 | 2.64 |
| 1961—1965 | 19 | 9 | 2.11 |
| 1966—1970 | 17 | 8 | 2.13 |
| All exposed cases | 101 | 69 | 1.46 |
| Mean of all Japan | | | 5.00—5.88 |

exposure distance was also studied and a significant observation has been made, as shown in Table 6. Among cases exposed within 2,000 meters from the hypocenter, there was an increase in the chronic form as compared with the exposed beyond 2,000 meters or nonexposed cases. The ratio of the acute and chronic forms among cases exposed within 2,000 meters was about 1.15. In contrast, in the cases beyond 2,000 meters, the ratio rises as the exposure distance increases, approaching

Table 6. Rate of acute and chronic leukemia in Hiroshima survivors by exposure distance (within 5,000 m) (1946—1970)

| Distance from hypocenter (m) | Acute form | Chronic form | Ratio of acute/chronic |
|---|---|---|---|
| Within 2,000 | 70 | 61 | 1.15 |
| 2,001—3,000 | 15 | 4 | 3.75 |
| 3,001—5,000 | 16 | 4 | 4.00 |
| Non-exposed | 86 | 20 | 4.30 |
| Mean of all Japan | | | 5.00—5.88 |

the value of 4.30 seen in nonexposed cases. Although no data are available on the accurate ratio of these two forms of leukemia in all Japan, it could be set somewhere between 5.00 and 5.88, judging by the statistics made by the leading clinics in Japan.

In analyzing these findings, there is no doubt about the causative role of the atomic radiation in induction of leukemia among the Hiroshima survivors. Moreover, it appears to be true that an increase in the incidence of chronic myeloid type is the most characteristic among leukemias developed in the Hiroshima survivors.

## II. Incidence of Leukemia among the "Early Entrants"

In Hiroshima, shortly after the detonation thousands of people went into the city where the disasters were heaviest, and they stayed there for rescue work, ground cleaning, or to search for their relatives. Of course, estimation of radiation doses received by these people is almost impossible, and there is tendency to ignore the existence of appreciable residual radioactivity in the city. There are various possible modes of radioactivity being given to the human body and in cases of B, D, F, and G, as indicated in Table 7, radiation injury might have occurred not only to

Table 7. Procedures of the actions of the radiations from the atomic bomb explosions to the organism[a]

| | External irradiation | Internal irradiation |
|---|---|---|
| 1. Gamma irradiation | A. $\gamma \rightarrow$ External irradiation<br>B. $\gamma \rightarrow$ Elements in the surrounding sphere<br>↓<br>Formation of radioisotopes<br>↓<br>External irradiation | |
| 2. Neutron irradiation | C. N → External irradiation | E. N → Bone<br>↓<br>Mobilization of $P^{32}$ (AMANO, 1953) |
| | D. N → Elements in the surrounding sphere<br>↓<br>Formation of radioactive isotopes<br>↓<br>External irradiation | F. N → Elements in the surrounding sphere<br>↓<br>Formation of radioactive isotopes<br>↓<br>Inhalation, ingestion, absorption<br>↓<br>Deposition in the tissues, especially in the bone (WATANABE, 1953) |
| 3. Irradiation from the fission products | | G. Fission products<br>↓<br>Inhalation, ingestion, absorption<br>↓<br>Deposition in the tissues |

[a] From WATANABE (1955).

exposed people but also to early entrants. Concerning the modes of irradiation which possibly give late effects to early entrants, we have emphasized the importance of factor F in the paragraph of the introduction of this section. In fact, it has been noted that some of the early entrants showed various acute radiation syndromes such as hemorrhagic diathesis and epilation. Therefore, the incidence of leukemia among these early entrants has been investigated by us as well. According to our survey, no leukemia had developed among these people until 1950. Ever since then, however, leukemia began to appear sporadically among those living in and out of the city, and no clear peak of the incidence has been observed. In order to carry out an accurate survey of the incidence of leukemia in early entrants, it was essential to ascertain their exact number, which was very difficult. However, a dependable figure was provided by a survey concurrent with the general census taken by the Hiroshima city officials in 1960, shown in Table 8. Of a total of 75 cases, 71 cases were derived from those entering the city within 2 weeks of the detonation. Fifty-eight of these cases were from those who entered the city within 3 days after the explosion. Since the number of people who entered the city within 3 days following the atomic bomb detonation was estimated as 25,799, the incidence of leukemia per

Table 8. Incidence of leukemia among the early entrants into Hiroshima after A-bomb detonation (1946—1970)

| | Cases entered within 3 days | Cases entered between 4—7 days | Cases entered between 8—14 days |
|---|---|---|---|
| Population[a] | 25,799 | 11,001 | 7,326 |
| Number of Cases | 58 | 9 | 4 |
| Incidence per 100,000/year | 8.99 | 3.27 | 2.18 |

[a] From census on Oct. 1, 1960.

Table 9. Type of leukemia among the early entrants into Hiroshima after A-bomb detonation (1946—1970)

| | Acute | Chronic myeloid | Chronic lymphoid | Total |
|---|---|---|---|---|
| Male | 27 | 17 | 5 | 49 |
| Female | 15 | 10 | 1 | 26 |
| Total | 42 | 27 | 6 | 75 |
| No. of cases entered within 7 days | 36 | 26 | 5 | 67 |
| No. of cases entered within 3 days | 31 | 22 | 5 | 58 |

100,000 early entrants per year comes to 8.99, which is much higher than that of the nonexposed and of all Japan. These leukemia cases are classified by type of the disease as shown in Table 9. There were 42 cases of acute type against 33 cases of chronic type. Although we cannot explain the high incidence of the chronic form, especially chronic myeloid leukemia in these cases, it may be recalled that the same trend has been obseved in cases exposed within 2,000 meters from the hypocenter. If we take the ratio of the acute and chronic types among cases that entered the city within 3 days following the explosion, the ratio is 1.41. Therefore, leukemias occurring among the early entrants could be considered as possessing the same characteristics as those occurring among the heavily irradiated survivors. In an attempt to demonstrate the possible role of internal irradiation of leukemia among the early entrants, we performed a series of experiments in which small doses of diverse radioactive isotopes such as $P^{32}$, $Sr^{89}$, $Sr^{90}$, or $Ce^{144}$ were administered to mice. As expected, leukemia developed in some of the experimental animals after a latent period. Among these, the incidence was highest in $Sr^{90}$ treated mice.

## III. Correlation of the Type of Radiation Exposure and the Type of Leukemia Induced

Correlation of the high incidence of leukemia and exposure to ionizing radiation in human beings has been definitely established. The relevant findings from the available data on the type of leukemia developed among irradiated persons are summarized in Table 10. It is obvious from these data that the majority of leukemias induced in persons who had received multiple irradiations to confined areas of the body for therapeutic purposes, were of the acute form, and the ratio of acute to chronic myeloid was around 3.7. In contrast, most cases exposed to occupational irradiation, such as multiple total body irradiation with small doses over a long period of time, were of the chronic myeloid type. Therefore, the ratio of acute to chronic myeloid leukemia was much less in this group. Moreover, chronic lymphoid

Table 10. Type of leukemia among radiation exposed persons

| Categories | | Authors | Acute | Chronic Myeloid | Chronic Lymphoid | AL/CML |
|---|---|---|---|---|---|---|
| Therapeutic | | Court-Brown and Doll | 33 | 9 | 1 | 3.7 |
| | | Moloney | 63 | 17 | 1 | 3.7 |
| | | Wakisaka and Miyata | 42 | 11 | 0 | 3.8 |
| Occupational | | Moloney | 5 | 5 | 2 | 1.0 |
| | | Wakisaka and Miyata | 22 | 20 | 1 | 1.1 |
| A-bomb | within | Hiroshima | 70 | 59 | 2 | 1.2 |
| survivors | 2000 m | Nagasaki | 45 | 17 | 0 | 2.6 |
| | over | Hiroshima[a] | 31 | 7 | 1 | 4.4 |
| | 2001 m | Nagasaki | 74 | 9 | 3 | 8.2 |

[a] Within 5000 m from hypocenter.

leukemia, in general, very rarely developed among the radiation exposed persons. According to the atomic bomb survivors, chronic myeloid leukemia was also predominant in the proximally exposed and early entrants, as mentioned before. In this group, the radiation received was quite different because of the individual situations at the time of exposure: such as total body exposure, partial body exposure, selective partial body exposure with scattered irradiations, as directly exposed with or without shielding, and prolonged internal total body irradiation with deposited radioactive elements, as supposed in the early entrants. The mechanism involved in radiation leukemogenesis is extremely complicated. However, based on these findings, together with some histological evidence, we may speculate that the chronic form of radiation-induced leukemia might develop multicentrically from hyperplastic or "maturation-arrested" marrow after irradiation, whereas the acute form might originate unicentrically in intensely irradiated, hypoplastic marrow, with abrupt onset and rapid invasion.

## IV. Cytogenetic Studies on Atomic Bomb Survivors

Chromosome abnormalities seem to be one of the most apparent residual abnormalities recognizable in radiation exposed persons for many years after the exposure. The biological significance of these abnormalities seems to be necessary for the understanding of the effect of radiation to human beings, especially in relation to eventuality of the late effects of radiation. We have been investigating chromosome aberrations in atomic bomb survivors from three points of view. The first study is chromosome aberrations in peripheral blood from physically normal survivors. The second is that of bone marrow cells from physically normal individuals who were exposed to the atomic bomb at proximal distances from the hypocenter. The third is a chromosome study of leukemia patients among atomic bomb survivors. A number of reports of cytogenetic studies on the atomic bomb survivors have been published. According to these reports, the presence of cells with abnormal chromosomes is low in frequency. However, even more than 20 years after

Table 11. Chromosome aberrations in peripheral blood from physically normal survivors[a]

| | Under 30 years of age | | Over 30 years of age at time of bombing | |
|---|---|---|---|---|
| | control | exposed | control | exposed |
| No. of survivors examined | 94 | 94 | 80 | 77 |
| % of aberration | 0.01 | 0.6 | 0.3 | 1.5 |
| Survivors with chromosome aberrations | 1.1% | 34% | 16% | 61% |

[a] Exposed survivors were within 1400 m of the hypocenter, and received an estimated 200 rad or more. Controls were 3000—3999 m from the hypocenter, and received an estimated dose of less than 1 rad.

the bombing, abnormal chromosomes are still present. Chromosome aberrations in peripheral blood of atomic bomb survivors are shown in Table 11. Exposed survivors were within 1,400 meters of the hypocenter and received an estimated dose of 200 rad or more. Controls were 3,000 to 3,999 meters from the hypocenter, and received an estimated air dose of less than 1 rad. Survivors were divided into two groups, under 30 years and over 30 years at the time of bombing. For each exposed person control of the same sex and the same age was selected. Preparations were scrutinized without knowledge of the patient's exposure status. As indicated in this table, percentage of chromosome aberrations in the younger age group was 0.01% in the controls and 0.6% in the exposed. We found 50 exchange types of chromosome aberrations in the exposed group, including translocation, dicentrics, rings and fragments. Thirty-three of 94 exposed survivors had one or more exchange type of aber-

Table 12. Chromosome aberrations in bone marrow cells of atomic bomb survivors

| Distance from hypocenter | No. examined | Total cells observed | Mean modality % | No. of chromosome abnormalities | No. of subjects with chromosome aberrations |
|---|---|---|---|---|---|
| 0—1000 m | 14 | 495 | 94.5 | 20 | 5 (35%) |
| 1001—1500 | 18 | 545 | 93.7 | 0 | 0 |
| 1501—2000 | 23 | 728 | 96.1 | 0 | 0 |
| 2001—3000 | 20 | 591 | 94.7 | 0 | 0 |
| Control | 17 | 624 | 95.5 | 0 | 0 |

rations. In the higher age groups, 61% of the survivors had one or more exchange type of chromosome aberrations.

Table 12 indicates the study on bone marrow chromosomes of the physically normal survivors. Bone marrow direct method was used for chromosome analysis and specimens were obtained from 75 survivors, of whom 14 were exposed to the bomb within 1,000 meters. All the 17 cases in the control group had modal number of 46 with mean modality percentage of 95.5. Chromosome analysis of the 14 cases exposed within 1,000 meters showed 46 modal numbers of chromosomes in all cases with modality percentage ranging from 84% to 100%. There was no significant statistical difference in modality percentage between the control and exposed. However, five of 14 survivors exposed within 1,000 meters had structurally abnormal chromosomes in their bone marrow cells. The history at the time of bombing and clinical remarks of these five patients with chromosome abnormalities are also tabulated in Table 13. All of them had some acute radiation symptoms such as epilation, burns and diarrhea at the time of disaster. None had hematological disorders at time of examination except for one case with slight grade of bleeding tendency of vascular type. Case No. 2 had 13 abnormal cells in 76 examined cells, of which eight karyotypes were identical in abnormality. She seemed to have an abnormal clone in the bone marrow. One and a half years later from the first examination, the clone increased in percentage. Case No. 3 had another type of abnormal chromosome. The patient's estimated dose was 639 rad. Fig. 4 illustrates the karyotype from case No. 2, representing Ph1-like chromosomes considered to be an abnormal clone, and Fig. 5 from case No. 3, another patient who had an abnormal clone. Judging from our findings together with those of other investigators studying bone marrow chro-

Table 13. Chromosome aberrations in bone marrow and history of A-bomb exposure in patients without hematological disorders

| Case | Sex | Age[a] | Distance from Hypocenter (m) | Acute Rad. Epilation | Symptoms Burn | Diarrhea | No. of Cells with Abnorm. Chromosomes | Karyotype of Abnorm. Cells | Clinical remarks |
|---|---|---|---|---|---|---|---|---|---|
| 1 | M | 17 | 500 | + | + | | 1/31 | 46, XY, Dq+ | Nil |
| 2 | F | 15 | 500 | + | + | + | 13/76 | 46, XX, t(Dp+; E 18q-), Gq-[b]<br>46, XX, t(Alq+; Bq-), Gq- | Nil |
| 3 | M | 37 | 800 | + | + | + | 12/63 | 46, XY, Gq-[b]<br>46, XY, Dq+ | Hypertension<br>Cholecystopathia |
| 4 | F | 34 | 900 | + | | | 1/50 | 46, XX, Cq- | Hypertension |
| 5 | M | 44 | 1000 | + | + | | 2/48 | 46, XY, inv(Ap-; q+) | ASHD[c]<br>Cataracta radiatica |

[a] Age at the time of atomic bombing. [b] Clone formation. [c] Arteriosclerotic heart diesase.

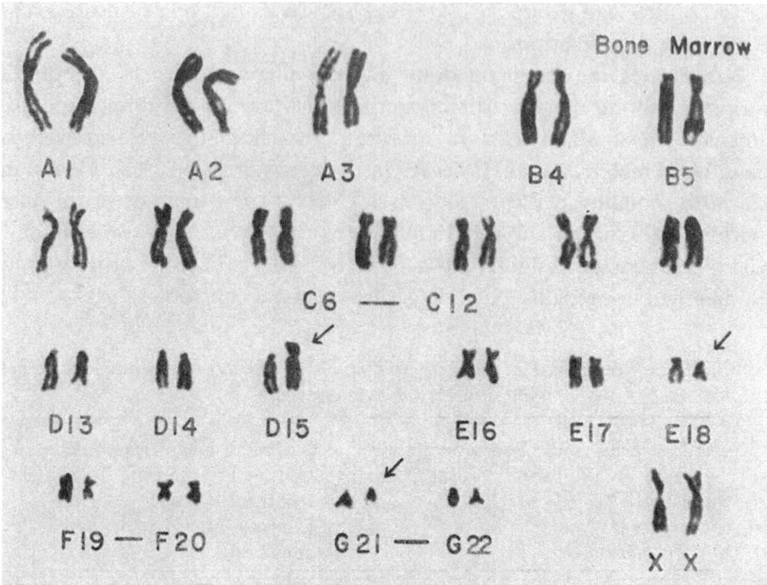


Fig. 4. Bone marrow karyotype with Ph¹-like and other abnormal chromosomes (case No. 2 in Table 13)

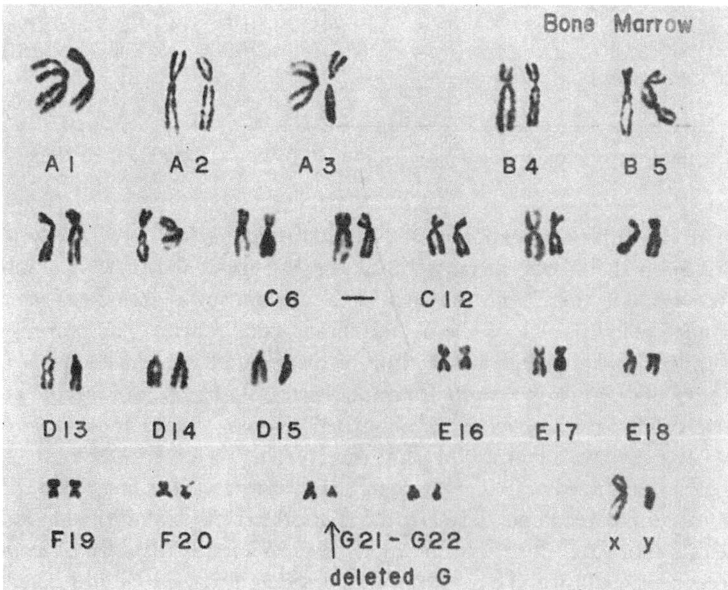


Fig. 5. Bone marrow karyotype with Ph¹-like chromosome deletion (case No. 3 in Table 13)

mosome aberration in irradiated individuals who did not have leukemia or other hematological disorders, it can be concluded that there are no unique abnormalities specific to atomic bomb survivors. However, the presence of clone of cells with abnormal chromosome such as smaller G in hematologically normal exposed persons, may give some clue to the problems of leukemogenesis following radiation exposure.

As regards the leukemia patients, a total of 147 cases with various types of the disease have been examined cytogenetically. Of 79 acute cases, 20 were exposed to the atomic bomb. Of 52 chronic myeloid leukemia cases, involving 15 blastic crisis, 19 were exposed cases. In chronic myeloid leukemia patients all had $Ph^1$ chromosome in high percentage and had low neutrophilic alkaline phosphatase activity. There were no findings to indicate that the tendency to aneuploidy and pseudodiploidy was high in chronic myeloid leukemia of the exposed. In acute leukemia, chromosome abnormalities common to all exposed cases were not noted. Moreover, there were no cytogenetic differences between the group with and without the history of atomic bomb exposure.

## B. Thyroid Carcinoma

### I. Incidence of Thyroid Carcinoma among Hiroshima Survivors and "Early Entrants"

Since Duffy and Fitzgerald (1950) suggested the possibility that carcinoma of the thyroid gland would be induced by ionizing radiation in man, cases were reported by Simpson et al. (1955). Clark (1959) and Rooney Powell (1959). In experimental animals many radiation-induced thyroid carcinomas were reported after similar suggestions were made by Goldberg et al. (1950, 1952).

Among persons exposed to atomic bomb explosion at Hiroshima, Kaneko (1957) first reported a case of 12 year-old girl, who had been exposed at 800 m from the hypocenter, and developed acute leukemia and papillary adenocarcinoma of the thyroid gland 9 years later. Fujimoto et al. (1959) reported 3 cases of thyroid carcinoma among Hiroshima survivors including a case reported by Kaneko. The second case was a 23 year-old female who had been at a place 800 m from the hypocenter and developed chronic myelogenous leukemia and papillary adenocarcinoma of the thyroid gland about 6 years later. The third case was a 61 year-old female who had been 1100 m away from the hypocenter and developed about 8 years later acute myelogenous leukemia and papillary adenocarcinoma of the thyroid gland. These three are considered to have been induced thyroid carcinoma with the intervals of 6 to 9 years after atomic bomb exposure.

It is noteworthy that for some time thereafter no cases with thyroid carcinoma have been reported among leukemic patients at Hiroshima. After a survey of cases with thyroid carcinoma among Hiroshima and Nagasaki survivors during a period of 16 months in 1958 and 1959, Hollingworth et al. (1963) pointed out that the incidence of thyroid carcinoma tended to increase among persons exposed to the atomic bomb at places relatively close to the hypocenter. Harano et al. (1961) reported that they experienced 18 cases of thyroid carcinoma among Nagasaki survivors between 1946 and 1961. Wood et al. (1968) also reported the results on thyroid carcinoma, chiefly clinically manifested, in Hiroshima and Nagasaki. They found

39 cases of thyroid carcinomas among 13,000 persons examined in both cities. At Hiroshima, 4 male patients among 2431 exposed and 18 female patients among 4436 exposed were found, the rate being 320 patients per 100,000 exposed. Twelve cases were exposed within 1400 m from the hypocenter, 4 cases between 1400 and 2000 m and 3 cases between 3000 and 3500 m. When 2 male and 7 female patients who were not examined by them were added to make total of 31 patients, incidence was as high as 466 per 100,000. The incidence of the thyroid carcinoma was high among the proximately exposed and significantly high in persons who received larger estimated radiation doses.

SHIGEMITSU (1965) conducted a survey on thyroid carcinoma among patients examined at the Surgical Department of Hiroshima University Hospital in 12 years from 1951 through 1963. Total number of patients examined were 14,720, among whom 1509 (10.3%) were exposed to the atomic bomb explosion. Of total cases, 1972 cases were found to have thyroid disorders, of which 136 (7.1%) were carcinoma. The number of cases and incidences of thyroid carcinoma among the exposed and non-exposed were listed in Table 14. In order to see the incidence of thyroid carcinoma in Hiroshima City, survey was conducted with people insured by National Health Insurance including healthy persons, and the results were shown in Table 15.

A similar study was carried out by EZAKI (1970) and his results are shown in Tables 16 and 17. In his study, it is noted that the incidence of thyroid carcinoma among persons seen at the Surgical Department was similar to the previous study but it increased more in the exposed among the health insured group.

Table 18 includes the cases studied by SHIGEMITSU and EZAKI (1965, 1966). As to the histological types of the thyroid carcinoma, the incidence of follicular carcinoma appears to be relatively high among the exposed, but conclusive statement can not be made since histological criteria used in these 2 studies were dissimilar.

The incidences of thyroid carcinoma among the exposed at varying ranges from the hypocenter were shown in Table 19. It was quite high among persons exposed within 1500 m from the hypocenter. It decreased to one half among those exposed at 1500 to 3000 m and further decreased to two thirds of this among the exposed at 3000 to 5000 m. This study clearly indicates the relationship between radiation dose and development of thyroid carcinoma.

On the whole, the incidence of thyroid carcinoma among the exposed is 66.37 per 100,000. According to the data presented in Tables 14 through 17, that among the non-exposed was 4.3 to 7.0 per 100,000. Therefore, the incidence is about 10 times higher among the exposed than that among the non-exposed. Of course, this does not include all the cases with thyroid carcinoma at Hiroshima in these periods of time, because these cases were chiefly found among persons examined at the Surgical Department of Hiroshima University Hospital and included a few cases found elsewhere, for which sufficient information was obtained.

According to the report of SHIGEMITSU (1965), among the proximately exposed, that is, persons exposed within 1000 m from the hypocenter, thyroid carcinomas were found in 6 cases, the incidence being 15.8%, whereas other thyroid disorders were found in only 7 cases (3.2%). The difference was significant statistically. EZAKI (1966) also stated that almost no difference in the incidences of hyperthyroidism was noted among the exposed and non-exposed as shown in Table 20.

Table 14. Incidence of thyroid carcinoma among patients examined at surgical clinic of Hiroshima University Hospital (1951—1963)

| | A-bomb exposed | Non-exposed |
|---|---|---|
| Number of patients with thyroid carcinoma | 34 | 58 |
| Number of patients examined | 1509 | 13.211 |
| Incidence per $10^2$ patients | 22.5 | 4.4 |
| (SHIGEMITSU, 1965) | $P < 0.01$ | |

Table 15. Incidence of thyroid carcinoma in National Health Insurance Cases in Hiroshima City (August 1950 to December 1961)

| | A-bomb exposed | Non-exposed |
|---|---|---|
| Number of patients with thyroid carcinoma | 6 | 6 |
| Number of insured persons | 22,386 | 114,262 |
| Incidence per $10^5$ | 26.84 | 5.25 |
| (SHIGEMITSU, 1965) | $X^2 = 9.78$ | $P < 0.01$ |

Table 16. Incidence of thyroid carcinoma among patients examined at surgical clinic of Hiroshima University Hospital (1958—1965)

| | A-bomb exposed | Non-exposed |
|---|---|---|
| Number of patients with thyroid carcinoma | 53 | 74 |
| Number of patients examined | 2331 | 16,989 |
| Incidence per $10^2$ patients | 22.7 | 4.3 |
| (EZAKI, 1970) | $X^2 = 106$ | $P < 0.01$ |

Table 17. Incidence of thyroid carcinoma in National Health Insurance Cases in Hiroshima City (August 1960 to December 1962)

| | A-bomb exposed | Non-exposed |
|---|---|---|
| Number of patients with thyroid carcinoma | 9 | 8 |
| Number of insured persons | 24,994 | 114,083 |
| Incidence per $10^5$ | 36.0 | 7.0 |
| (EZAKI, 1970) | $X^2 = 14.1$ | $P < 0.01$ |

Table 18. Histological types of thyroid carcinoma among A-bomb survivors in Hiroshima (H.U.H. Surgical Clinic) (1951—1968)

| | Exposed | Non exposed |
|---|---|---|
| Papillary carcinoma | 35 (67.3%) | 46 (82.2%) |
| Papillary carcinoma with follicular differentiation | 3 (5.76%) | 3 (5.4%) |
| Follicular carcinoma | 12 (23.08%) | 7 (12.4%) |
| Undifferentiated carcinoma | 1 (0.9%) | |
| Unknown | 1 (1.9%) | |
| Total | 52 | 56 |

Table 19. Incidence of thyroid carcinoma among A-bomb survivors in Hiroshima (H. U. H. Surgical Dept.) (1951—1968)

| Distance from Hypocenter [m] | ♂ | ♀ | Total | Incidence per $10^5$ exposed population | | |
|---|---|---|---|---|---|---|
| 0—500 | 0 | 0 | 0 | 0 | 308.95 | 109.07 |
| 501—1000 | 2 | 8 | 10 | 336.0 | | |
| 1001—1500 | 0 | 9 | 9 | 63.35 | 51.11 | 57.82 |
| 1501—2000 | 1 | 7 | 8 | 41.99 | | |
| 2001—2500 | 0 | 8 | 8 | 65.64 | 70.23 | |
| 2501—3000 | 4 | 5 | 9 | 74.82 | | |
| 3001—5000 | 1 | 3 | 4 | 29.08 | | 29.08 |
| Unknown | 1 | 3 | 4 | | | |
| Total | 9 | 44 | 53 | | 66.37 | |

Table 20. Incidence of hyperthyroidism (H.U.H. Surgical Clinic) (1958—1965)

| | Exposed | Non-exposed |
|---|---|---|
| Number of patients with hyperthyroidism | 77 | 491 |
| Total number of patients | 2331 | 16,989 |
| Incidence per $10^5$ patients | 3303 | 2890 |

(EZAKI, 1970)

Table 21. Correlation between exposure doses and latency of thyroid carcinoma among A-bomb survivors in Hiroshima (1951—1963)

| Interval (years) | 0—5 | 6—10 | 11—15 | 15 < | Total |
|---|---|---|---|---|---|
| <10 (Rad) | 2 | 5 | 7 | 4 | 18 |
| $10$—$10^2$ | 0 | 1 | 4 | 2 | 7 |
| $10^2$—$10^3$ | 1 | 1 | 3 | 3 | 8 |
| $10^3$—$10^4$< | 0 | 1 | 1 | 2 | 4 |
| Total | 3 | 8 | 15 | 11 | 37 |

(SHIGEMITSU, 1965)

Table 22. Interval between exposure and onset of initial symptom of thyroid carcinoma among A-bomb survivors in Hiroshima (1958—1965)

| Interval (years) | 0—5 | 5—10 | 11—15 | 16—20 | Total |
|---|---|---|---|---|---|
| Number | 5 | 11 | 17 | 23 | 56 |

(EZAKI, 1970)

The intervals between the time of the atomic bomb exposure and the time of detection of thyroid carcinoma were shown in Tables 21 and 22.

These studies included overlapped cases. The first case of thyroid carcinoma was detected 5 years after the exposure, and thereafter the number of cases gradually increased. Interestingly the highest incidence was noted 16 to 20 years after the exposure. The peak was delayed as compared with that of leukemia. This result coincided with the general assumption. According to SHIGEMITSU, incidence of thyroid carcinoma within 10 years after exposure was higher among persons exposed to lower doses of irradiation, but it tended to increase after 10 years even among persons exposed to higher doses.

The age at the time of diagnosis of thyroid carcinoma was studied by EZAKI (1970) (Fig. 6). Among the exposed, the peak of the incidence was between 30 and

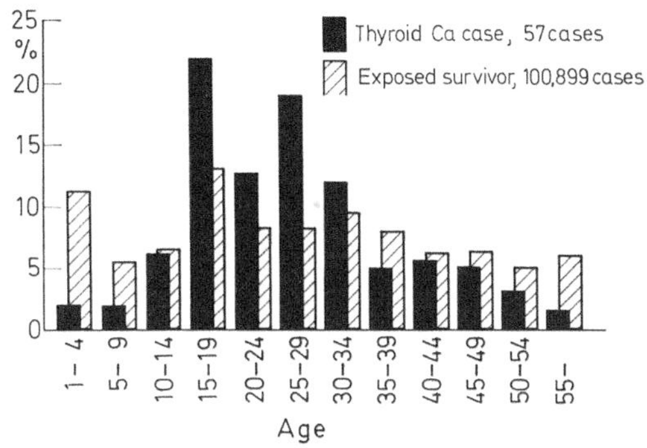


Fig. 6. Thyroid Ca cases by age at time of A-bomb exposure

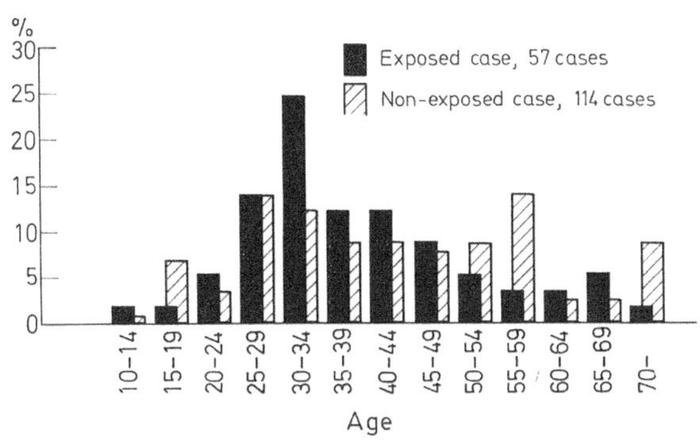


Fig. 7. Onset of initial symptom of thyroid Ca by age

34 years of age and it gradually decreased with aging. The incidence among the non-exposed, however, showed almost no difference between the age of 20 and 50, without a peak at early thirties, but with a peak at the age between 55 and 59. The age of the patients with thyroid carcinoma at the time of exposure was reviewed (Fig. 7). The highest incidence was noted among persons exposed at the age between 15 and 19. And the comparative value though slightly lower was also obtained among persons exposed at the age of 25 to 29. The population by age group at the time of atomic bomb explosion at Hiroshima does not agree with that of patients with thyroid carcinoma, indicating that two peaks in the incidence at the age 15 to 19 and 25 to 29 are probably due specific to the effect of atomic bomb exposure. Thyroid carcinoma developed more frequently among persons exposed to radiation

when they were relatively young. And the high incidence was not noted among persons who were elderly at the time of the exposure, indicating that ionizing radiation of the atomic bomb explosion has not promoted induction of thyroid carcinoma in an age group with involuted thyroid function. However, in children with developing thyroid function, carcinogenesis may in some degree be promoted by ionizing radiation.

As stated already, leukemia was also seen among entrants into Hiroshima City immediately after the explosion. And its incidence was highest among those entering the city within 3 days of the explosion, with a gradual decrease with the lapse of time. In case of thyroid carcinoma also, there have been 10 reported cases among entrants. Six patients entered the city within 3 days of the explosion, 3 within 1 week and in one date of entrance was unknown (Table 23).

Table 23. Incidence of thyroid carcinoma among the early entrants into Hiroshima City after A-bomb detonation (H. U. H. Surgical Dept.) (1951—1968)

| | Cases entered within 3 days | Cases entered between 4—7 days | Cases entered between 8—14 days |
|---|---|---|---|
| Number of cases | 6 | 3 | 0 |
| | 9 | | |
| Population of entrants | 25.798 | 11.001 | 7.327 |
| Incidence per $10^5$ entrants | 23.2 | 27.11 | |
| | 24.45 | | |

The incidence of thyroid carcinoma among the directly exposed was between 22.5 and 36.0 per 100,000. That among the entrants immediately after the explosion was notably as high as 23.2 to 27.11 per 100,000 entrants, which was about equal to the former, and an increase in the thyroid carcinoma has not been observed among those entering the city a week or more after the explosion.

It is known that Marshallese people also developed thyroid carcinoma where test explosions of hydrogen bombs were carried out. This is probably due to the fall-out of the radioactive substances. However, not only the effects of external irradiation but also of internal irradiation should be considered. As in the case of leukemia, we have found for the first time in this study such a fact that all the patients who developed thyroid carcinoma entered the city within 1 week of explosion, and two thirds did so within 3 days.

## II. Thyroid Carcinomas at the National Cancer Center

We reported above the development of thyroid carcinoma at Hiroshima City, particularly placing emphasis on that among persons exposed to the atomic bomb explosion. We now proceed to the status of thyroid carcinoma in Japan in general, which is based on the experience at the National Cancer Center in Tokyo.

The number of thyroid carcinomas at National Cancer Center Hospital was 40 among 2398 autopsies, which was 1.7% of all malignant neoplasms (Table 24). Of these, 24 cases were clinically manifested thyroid carcinomas, and remaining 16 cases were of incidentally found thyroid carcinoma, indicating relative infrequency of this tumor in Japan. Among the clinically manifested thyroid carcinomas, one half were papillary carcinoma and follicular carcinoma made up 16.7% of all. Frequency of undifferentiated carcinomas was 25%. Among the latent thyroid carcinomas, the majority were papillary adenocarcinomas which were followed by follicular carcinoma. Other types were very rare.

Table 24. Histological type of thyroid carcinoma (autopsy cases, NCC) (1963.6—1970.12)

| | Number | Incidence (%) |
|---|---|---|
| Manifest: (24 cases: 1% of total autopsy cases) | | |
| Papillary | 12 | 50 |
| Follicular | 4 | 16.7 |
| Poorly differentiated adenocarcinoma | 2 | 8.3 |
| Undifferentiated (includes one case of probable medullary carcinoma) | 6 | 25 |
| Latent: (16 cases: 0.7% of total autopsy cases) | | |
| Papillary (2—18 mm) | 13 | 81.3 |
| Follicular (3—15 mm) | 2 | 12.5 |
| Medullary (4 mm) | 1 | |
| Total | 40 | |
| Total autopsy cases | 2398 | 1.7 |

As to the surgical materials in the period from 1964 through 1970, 82.3% of 158 thyroid carcinomas were of papillary type and 16.5% follicular (Table 25), probably representing a tendency in Japan. Beside these, 4 malignant lymphoma, 8 metastatic carcinomas, 119 follicular adenomas and solitary colloid nodules, 45 nodular and diffuse goiters, 24 Hashimoto's strumas, 5 subacute thyroiditis and 16 with no localized lesions were resected during the same period, totalling 209 benign lesions.

Table 25. Histological type of thyroid carcinoma (surgical materials, NCC) (1964.7—1970.12)

| | Number | Incidence [%] |
|---|---|---|
| Papillary | 130 | 82.3 |
| Follicular | 26 | 16.5 |
| Undifferentiated | 2 | 1.3 |
| Total | 158 | |

Malignant lymphoma 4; metastatic carcinoma 8

Upon comparison of autopsy and surgical materials, frequency of each histologic type is very close in surgically resected thyroid carcinomas and latent thyroid carcinomas found at the time of autopsy. This is due in part to the detailed examination of the surgically resected specimens disclosing latent foci of carcinoma.

In regard to the size of the latent carcinoma found at autopsy, 9 tumors were smaller than 5 mm in diameter of which 7 were papillary carcinomas. Tumors 6 to

10 mm in diameter were none. Those 11 to 15 mm were 6, of which 4 were of papillary type. And those larger than 16 mm were 2, both of which were papillary carcinomas (Table 26). Data on surgical materials are summarized in Table 27; they are divided into 2 groups, that is, preoperative diagnosis of non-carcinoma group and of carcinoma group. Many of the carcinomas which were not diagnosed as malignant preoperatively were smaller than 10 mm in diameter, and a few cases with carcinomas larger than 11 mm in diameter have been diagnosed incorrectly. On the whole, there were 15 cases of papillary carcinoma, 2 cases of follicular carcinoma and 2 cases with independent foci of a papillary carcinoma and a follicular carcinoma. Many of the tumors diagnosed preoperatively as malignant were larger

Table 26. Size of latent thyroid carcinoma (autopsy, NCC) (1963—1970)

| | | | | |
|---|---|---|---|---|
| Papillary | —5 mm | 6—10 mm | 11—15 mm | 16—20 mm |
| | 7 | 0 | 4 | 2 |
| Follicular | 3 mm | 15 mm | | |
| | 1 | 2 | | |
| Medullary | 4 mm | | | |
| | 1 | | | |

Table 27. Size of thyroid carcinoma (surgical materials, NCC) (1963.6—1970.12)

| | —5 mm | 6—10 mm | 11—15 mm | 16— mm |
|---|---|---|---|---|
| Cases with preoperative diagnosis of non-carcinoma | 5 ((1)) | 9 (1) | 2 (1) | 3 ((1)) |
| Cases with preoperative diagnosis of carcinoma | 2 | 6 | 13 ((1)) | 18 (2) ((1)) |
| Total | 7 ((1)) | 15 (1) | 15 (1) ((1)) | 21 (2) ((2)) |
| Incidence in 158 cases Examined (%) | 4.43 | 9.45 | 9.49 | 13.29 |
| | 13.42 (—5 mm + 6—10 mm) | | | |
| | 23.42 (—5 mm to 11—15 mm) | | | |

( ) Number of follicular carcinoma; (( )) Number of follicular + papillary carcinoma.
Single primary carcinomas larger than 16 mm are excluded

than 11 mm in diameter, but there were 8 tumors of less than 10 mm which were correctly diagnosed preoperatively. Thirty five of these 39 cases were of papillary type. Two were follicular and 2 cases contained independent foci of a papillary carcinoma and a follicular carcinoma.

On the whole 22 cases of 158 (13.4%) surgically resected thyroid carcinomas were smaller than 10 mm in diameter. Tumors of less than 15 mm in diameter were 37 (23.4%). In general, it can be said that thyroid carcinomas smaller than 5 mm were latent carcinoma, those of 6 to 10 mm were either latent or clinically manifested carcinomas and those of larger than 11 mm were clinically manifested carcinomas.

Occult carcinoma is defined by some as carcinomas smaller than 15 mm in diameter which are clinically not detected. In autopsy materials, most of latent carcinomas were less than 5 mm in diameter and in surgical materials less than 10 mm in diameter. In spite of the definition, thyroid carcinomas of less than 15 mm, even smaller than 5 mm were not infrequently correctly diagnosed as carcinoma before surgery.

Table 28. Cases of thyroid carcinoma with history of previous radiation exposure (NCC: 1963—1970)

| Age | Sex | Previous history | Age at exposure | Radiotherapy | Age at time of diagnosis of carcinoma | Histological diagnosis |
|---|---|---|---|---|---|---|
| *Autopsy cases* | | | | | | |
| 31 | ♀ | L. colli tbc | 19 | 6 months | 22 | Pap. ca. and squam. ca. |
| 42 | ♀ | Struma (ca. ?) | 29 | X-ray 2×/W. for mo. | 37 | Pap. ca. and squam. ca. |
| 63 | ♀ | Thyroid Tumor (ca. ?) | 52 | X-ray 1000 rad. | 62 | Poorly diff. adeno ca. |
| 61[a] | ♀ | L. colli tbc | 26 | X-ray 10× | 55 | Pap. ca. |
| *Surgical cases* | | | | | | |
| 43[a] | ♀ | Struma (foll. Adenoma ?) | ca. 10 | X-ray | 43 | Foll. ca. (deriv. from adenoma) |
| 42[a] | ♂ | L. colli tbc | 17 | X-ray 3—4 weeks | 41 | Pap. ca. |
| 48[a] | ♀ | Struma | 18 | X-ray 3—4× | 48 | Pap. ca. |
| 59[a] | ♂ | X-ray tube manufacturing | 20—35 | (small dose 15 years) | 57? | Pap. ca. |
| 67[a] | ♀ | Struma | 27 | X-ray 3× | 37 | Foll. ca. and sclerosing tumors |
| ?[a] | ♀ | L. colli tbc | ca. 15 | X-ray? | | |
| 56[a] | ♀ | Struma | 16 | X-ray | | Foll. ca. |
| 50 | ♀ | Struma | 30 | X-ray 3× | 42 | |

[a] Cases with possible radiation induced carcinoma.

Table 29. Cases of thyroid carcinoma with history of previous radiation exposure (autopsy and surgical materials, NCC) (1963—1970)

| | Number of cases exposed | Total number of cases | Incidence [%] |
|---|---|---|---|
| Autopsy | 4 (1) | 40 | 10 (2.5) |
| Surgical | 8 (7) | 158 | 5.1 (4.4) |
| Total | 12 (8) | 198 | 6 (4.5) |

( ) Cases with possible radiation induced carcinoma.

Four autopsied cases with thyroid carcinoma had previous history of radiation therapy to the neck (Table 28). Two cases were irradiated for a thyroid tumor and "struma", both of which could have been carcinoma already at the time of irradiation. One case was irradiated for tuberculous lymphadenitis but diagnosis of thyroid carcinoma was established 3 years later, which should also be excluded from cases of

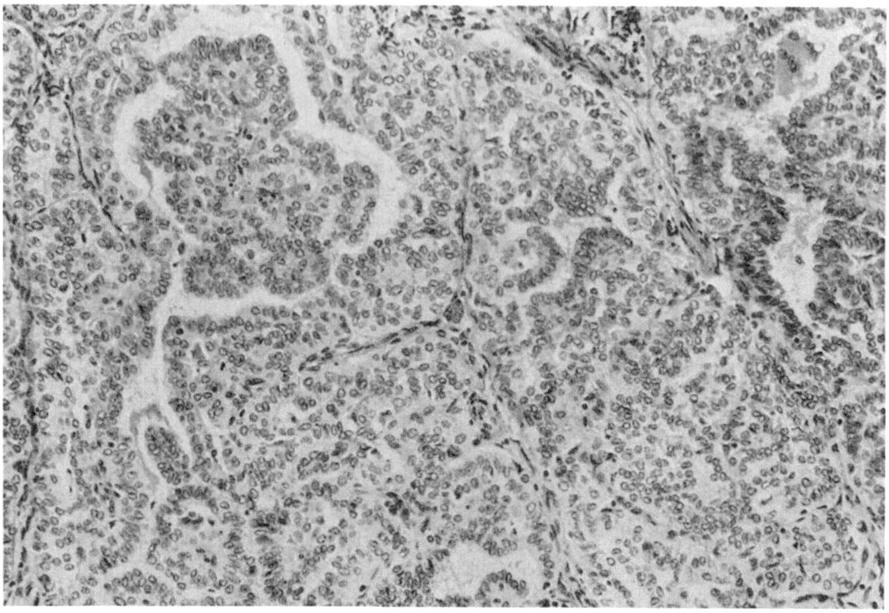

Fig. 8. Papillary carcinoma of the thyroid gland (61 year old female) after radiotherapy of the neck

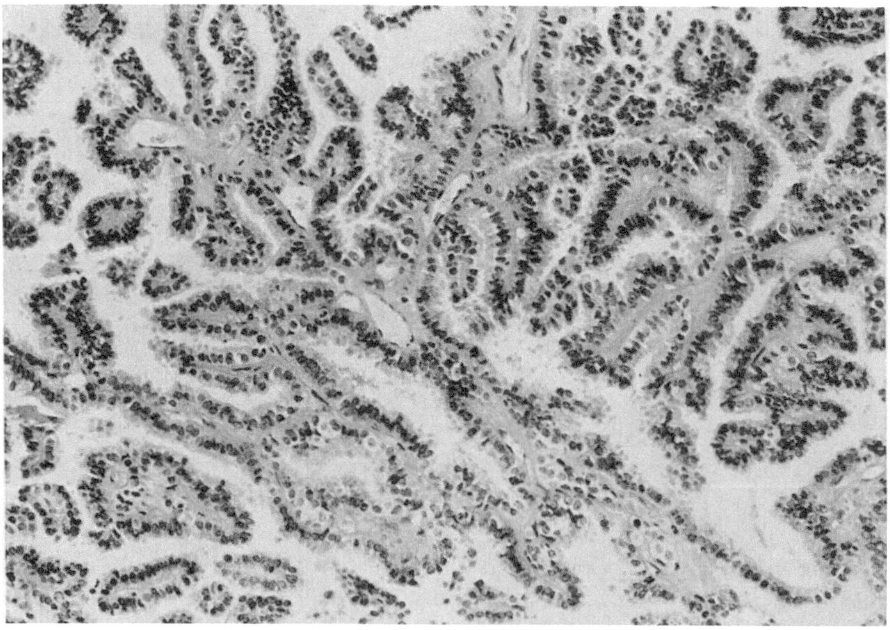

Fig. 9. Papillary adenocarcinoma of the thyroid gland (59 year old man) after small dose X-ray exposure between the age of 20 and 35

radiation induced carcinoma. Only 1 patient, a 61 year-old female, is probably placed in the category of radiation induced thyroid carcinoma, in whom radiotherapy was repeated 10 times for tuberculous lymphadenitis of the neck at the age of 26 and diagnosis of papillary carcinoma of the thyroid gland (Fig. 8) (S-78-69) was established at the age of 55.

Among the surgical materials, eight cases had past history of radiotherapy to the neck. All but one case may be radiation induced carcinoma, which was a 50 year-old female treated with X-ray three times for "struma" at 30 years of age and diagnosed as carcinoma at age of 42. Those cases were briefly summarized in Table 15. One case was illustrative, which was a 59 year-old man manufacturing X-ray tubes, had been exposed to small dose of X-ray between the age of 20 and 35, and developed papillary adenocarcinoma of the thyroid gland (Fig. 9) and basal cell carcinoma of the facial skin (Fig. 10) at the age of 57. Among these 7 cases, 3 cases each were papillary and follicular carcinoma, and histology of 1 case was not known. Here too, follicular carcinoma appears to be relatively frequent among persons exposed to ionizing radiation but of course no conclusion was reached.

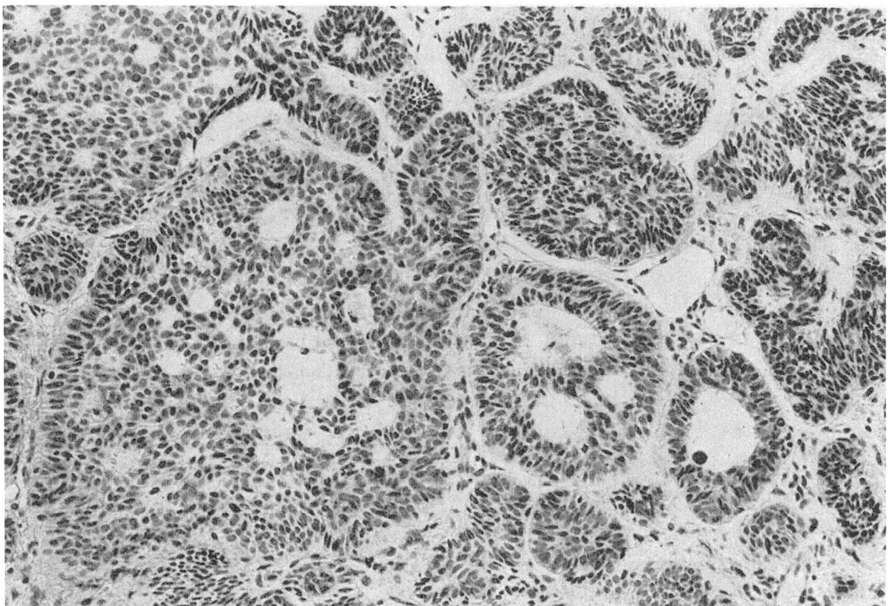

Fig. 10. Basal cell carcinoma of the facial skin at the age of 57 (same patient as Fig. 9)

Cases with past history of radiation exposure were found in 10% of autopsy materials and 5.1% of surgical (as a whole about 6%). However, incidences of possible radiation induced carcinoma were 2.5 and 4.4%, respectively (Table 29). Among 12 cases with past history of radiation exposure, there were 8 cases with possible radiation induced carcinoma. All but one were clinically manifested carcinoma. But precise incidence of radiation induced thyroid carcinoma in Japan is unknown, because clinical records were often insufficient and no detailed studies have been performed yet.

## III. Small Thyroid Carcinomas at Hiroshima and Nagasaki

SAMPSON and KEY at Hiroshima ABCC jointly with IIJIMA at Hiroshima University, found 536 cases of primary carcinoma of the thyroid gland in 3067 autopsies (2327 autopsies performed at Hiroshima ABCC during the period from January 1957 through February 1968, and 740 autopsies performed at Nagasaki ABCC during the period from January 1951 through September 1967). Of these, 525 (98%) were papillary adenocarcinoma, and 518 (97%) were smaller than 1.5 cm in the greatest dimension, being occult carcinomas which had not been suspected clinically. Incidences of thyroid carcinoma were 18.1% (137/740) at Nagasaki and 17.3% (402/2327) at Hiroshima; 15.7% (254/1614) in male and 19.4% (282/1453) in female, slightly more frequent in female. Age distribution disclosed that in male it was most frequent at the age 35 to 44, gradually decreasing with aging, and in female frequency was about the same between the age 25 and 64, being reduced after the age of 70. Two thirds of papillary carcinomas of male and one half of female were smaller than 0.2 cm in diameter. Eleven non-papillary carcinoma included 8 follicular carcinoma, 2 anaplastic carcinoma, and 1 medullary carcinoma. Two of follicular carcinomas were 5.5 cm and 2.2 cm in diameter, remaining 6 were smaller than 1 cm.

The size of primary tumors of 5 patients who died of thyroid carcinoma were 1.5 cm, 1.8 cm, 3 cm, and larger. Relative risk for thyroid carcinoma of persons exposed to more than 50 rads was 1.41 times that of the non-exposed, which was significantly high.

In another report, they divided microcarcinoma of the thyroid gland into the "circumscribed" and "invasive". The incidence of invasive microcarcinoma was not different between a group exposed to 50 rads or more and groups exposed to less than 50 rad, or of the nonexposed, whereas the incidence of circumscribed carcinoma increased in a group exposed to 50 rads or more. However, circumscribed carcinoma is more frequent than invasive carcinoma among persons exposed to less than 50 rads and the non-exposed. The invasive carcinoma was larger in size than the circumscribed, the mean value of tumors of less than 0.1 cm being 0.7 mm and 0.4 mm respectively. And the invasive carcinomas of less than 0.05 cm were found to be 8%, whereas the circumscribed were 68%. From these findings, they consider that the circumscribed carcinoma lacks evidence of growth, and in these lesions carcinomatous changes were initiated in the thyroid gland but not promoted by ionizing radiation. On the other hand, in the invasive carcinoma evidence of growth was present, in which the promoting factor participated more, thyroid stimulating hormone being considered to be a probable promoting factor.

The number of tumors less than 0.1 cm in diameter were 141: 86 circumscribed and 55 invasive. It is of great interest that their emphasis was placed on the occult carcinomas and induction of carcinoma by atomic bomb radiation particularly in the circumscribed type. However, in spite of their meticulous studies, we still have some doubts on their view. The occult invasive carcinoma is probably accepted as carcinoma, but the circumscribed type might be questioned by some pathologists whether they are truly carcinoma or not, since their histological diagnosis was entirely based on the cytological features and therefore insufficient. The cell aggregates without proliferation will certainly give rise to discussion. Although they stated the frequency of these 2 types in microcarcinoma of less than 0.1 cm in diameter, they did not show their frequency in tumors larger than 0.1 cm. If the circumscribed carcinomas were more frequent than the invasive ones in tumors larger than 0.1 cm in diameter, subsequently a different view may be introduced whether they are truly carcinoma or not.

There were no descriptions in the report of WOOD *et al.* (1968) as to the size o tumors but they included 6 female cases of occult sclerosing carcinoma. They consisted of 12 papillary and 13 follicular carcinomas. If occult sclerosing type is included which is presumed to be a papillary type, papillary-follicular ratio will be 18 to 13. From these figures, the incidence of follicular carcinomas would be higher as compared to that in the non-exposed. This fact was not stated by the authors.

# Conclusion

Our analysis of the data given above shows that there is no doubt about the role of atomic bomb irradiation in the induction of leukemia among A-bomb survivors in Hiroshima. Furthermore, it appears to be true that the increase in the incidence of the chronic myeloid type is the most striking.

In addition to the prevalence of leukemia in the survivors, it has become evident since 1950 that the incidence of leukemia was increased also among the early entrants who had entered Hiroshima city shortly after the bombing.

We may speculate that the chronic form of radiation-induced leukemia might develop multicentrically from hyperplastic bone marrow after irradiation, whereas the acute form with abrupt onset and rapid invasion might originate unicentrically in intensely irradiated, hypoplastic marrow.

One-third to two-thirds of the atomic bomb survivors had one or more chromosome aberrations in their peripheral blood. Radiation-induced chronic myeloid leukemia showed typical $Ph^1$ chromosome. There was no tendency to aneuploidy and pseudo-diploidy in chronic myeloid leukemia of the exposed, and no cytogenetic difference was found between the exposed and non-exposed leukemia patients.

The incidence of thyroid carcinoma apparently increased among persons exposed to atomic bomb explosion, and it seems to require a relatively long period of time such as 15 to 20 years before carcinoma develops. This finding is of interest as compared to the incidence of leukemia among the exposed which is presently declining towards that in the non-exposed population. The thyroid carcinoma is more prevalent in females among both exposed and non-exposed persons. It developed more frequently in persons exposed to atomic bomb explosion at the age of 15 to 19 and 25 to 29, and much less frequently in persons exposed in old age. This fact suggests that decrease in the thyroid function is not necessarily a contributing factor to the thyroid carcinogenesis. On the contrary carcinogenic action of radiation is apt to work efficiently in the age group with active thyroid function.

It is noteworthy that thyroid carcinoma was seen in high incidence among the entrants into Hiroshima within 1 week after atomic bomb detonation. In these instances, $^{131}I$ and other radioactive substances might have played a role in induction of carcinoma. Besides, the incidence of follicular carcinoma appears to have increased among the exposed, although histological criteria at present and a decade ago for each type of thyroid carcinomas are somewhat different. Follicular carcinoma appears to be relatively more frequent also among persons with past history of radiotherapy to the neck region.

Lastly, the incidence of thyroid carcinoma fluctuates greatly by the detection rate or confirmation rate of occult or latent carcinomas. Therefore, great care is needed in the evaluation of the incidence in variable samples.

## References

### *A. Leukemia*


BLOOM, A. D., AWA, A. A., NERIISHI, S., HONDA, T., ARCHER, P. G.: Chromosome aberrations in leukocytes of older survivors of the atomic bombing of Hiroshima and Nagasaki. Lancet II, 802—805 (1967).

BLOOM, A. D., NERIISHI, S., KAMADA, N., ISEKI, T., KEEHN, R. J.: Cytogenetic investigation of survivors of the atomic bombings of Hirsohima and Nagasaki. Lancet II, 672—674 (1966).

COURT-BROWN, W. M., DOLL, R.: Leukemia and aplastic anemia in patients irradiated for ankylosing spondylitis. Medical Research Council Special Report No. 295. London: H. M. Stationery Office 1957.

GOH, K.: Smaller G chromosome in irradiated man. Lancet I, 659—660 (1966).

HIROSE, F.: Leukemia in atomic bomb survivors, Hiroshima, 1946—1967. Acta haemat. jap. **31**, 765—771 (1968).

ISHIHARA, T., KUMATORI, T.: Cytogenetic studies on fisherman exposed to fallout radiation in 1954. Jap. J. Genet. **44**, Suppl. **1**, 242—251 (1969).

ITO, T.: Leukemogenic effect of radiostrontium ($^{90}$Sr) in mice: A comparative study of leukemogenicity of $^{90}$Sr and X-rays. I. Incidence and characteristics of $^{90}$Sr-induced and X-ray-induced leukemias. Acta haemat. jap. **33**, 415—431 (1970).
II. Transmissibility of the induced leukemia, alkaline phosphatase activity and cytogenetic changes of leukemic cells. ibid. **33**, 432—448 (1970).

ITO, T., YOKORO, K., ITO, A., NISHIHARA, E.: A comparative study of the leukemogenic effects of strontium-90 and X-rays in mice. Proc. Soc. exp. Biol. (N.Y.) **130**, 345—350 (1969).

KAMADA, N.: The effects of radiation on chromosomes of bone marrow cells. II. Studies on bone marrow chromosomes of atomic bomb survivors in Hiroshima. Acta haemat. jap. **32**, 236—248 (1969).

KAMADA, N.: The effects of radiation on chromosomes of bone marrow cells. III. Cytogenetic studies on leukemia in atomic bomb survivors. Acta haemat. jap. **32**, 249—274 (1969).

KAMADA, N., TSUCHIMOTO, T., UCHINO, H.: Smaller G chromosomes in the bone marrow cells of heavily irradiated atomic-bomb survivors. Lancet II, 880—881 (1970).

MIYATA, H., ENOMOTO, H., MAEDA, K.: Statistical survey on leukemia among individuals irradiated occupationally and therapeutically in East Japan. Acta haemat. jap. **31**, 784—791 (1968).

MOLONEY, W. C.: Leukemia and exposure to X-ray. A report of 6 cases. Blood **14**, 1137—1142 (1959).

OHKITA, T.: Recent trends of leukemia in atomic bomb survivors. Hiroshima J. med. Sci. **22**, 383—391 (1969).

TOMONAGA, M., ICHIMARU, M., *et al.*: Leukemia in atomic bomb survivors from 1949 to 1965 and some aspects of epidemiology of leukemia in Japan .J .Kyushu hemat. Soc. 17: 375-396, (1967)

WAKISAKA, G., KARIYONE, S.: Leukemia in radiological workers and in patients treated with ionizing radiation (West Japan). Acta haemat. jap. **31**, 792—804 (1968).

WATANABE, S.: Patho-anatomical studies on the development of leukemia, with special references to experimental studies with some radioisotopes. Tr. Soc. path. Jap. **46**, 183—239 (1957).

WATANABE, S., HIROSE, F., MATSUBAYASHI, Y.: The incidence of leukemia in Hiroshima during the years from 1946 to 1960. Proc. Second Congr. Asian and Pacific Soc. Hematol. **1961**, 81—90.

WATANABE, S.: Late hematological effects following the exposure of atomic bomb in Hiroshima with particular considerations on leukemia. Proc. VIIIth Congr. Int. Soc. heamat. **1**, 19—29 (1962).

WATANABE, S.: Nuclear hematology: Based on experience with atomic explosions. In Nuclear Hematology, ed. by SZIRMAI, E., pp. 485—537. New York and London: Academic Press 1965.

YOKORO, K.: Patho-anatomical and hematological studies on the effects of internal irradiation with radioactive-strontium ($^{89}Sr$) in mice. Acta haemat. jap. **21**, 817—841 (1958).

*B. Thyroid Carcinoma*

CLARK, D. E.: Association of irradiation with cancer of the thyroid in children and adolescents. JAMA **159**, 1007—1009 (1959).

CONARD, R. A., DOBYNS, B. B., SUTOW, W. W.: Thyroid neoplasia as late effect of exposure to radioactive iodine in fallout. JAMA **214**, 316—324 (1970).

DUFFY, B. J., Jr., FITZGERALD, P. J.: Thyroid cancer in childhood and adolescence a report on 28 cases. Cancer **3**, 1018—1032 (1955).

EZAKI, H., SHIGEMITSU, T.: Studies on thyroid cancer induced by A-bomb exposure. Proc. Hiroshima Univ. RINMB **11**, 166—168 (1970).

YUKIO, FUJIMOTO, *et al.*: Three autopsy cases of myeloid leukemia associated with thyroid carcinoma (Japanese) Hiroshima J. med. Sci. **12**, 1059—1065 (1959).

HARANO, A., *et al.*: Thyroid disease found among A-bomb survivors in Nagasaki, especially on thyroid carcinoma (Japanese). Report of symposium on A-bomb late effect study, 201—204 (1961).

HAZARD, J. B.: Nomenclature of thyroid Tumors, In Thyroid Neoplasia ed YOUNG, S., and INMAN, D. R. New York: Academic Press 1968, p. 3—37.

HAZARD, J. B., SMITH, D. E.: The Thyroid IAP Monograph. Baltimore: Williams-Wilkins 1964.

HOLLINGWORTH, D. R., *et al.*: Thyroid disease. A study in Hiroshima. Jap. med. J. **42**, 47—71 (1963).

KANEKO, N., *et al.*: An autopsy case of leukemia associated with thyroid carcinoma found at an A-bomb exposed infant in Hiroshima (Japanese). Shonika-Shinryo **20**, 478 (1957).

ROONEY, D. R., POWELL, R. W.: Carcinoma of the thyroid in children after X-ray therapy in early childhood JAMA **169**, 1—4, (1959).

SAMPSON, R. J., KEY, C. R., BUNCHER, C. R., IIJIMA, S.: Thyroid carcinoma in Hiroshima and Nagasaki. JAMA **209**, 65—70 (1969).

SAMPSON, R. J., KEY, C. R., BUNCHER, C. R., IIJIMA, S.: Smallest forms of papillary carcinoma of the thyroid. A study of 141 micro carcinomas less than 0.1 cm in greatest dimension. Arch. Path. **91**, 334—339 (1971).

SHIGEMITSU, T.: Studies on thyroid cancer induced by A-bomb exposure and its clinical characteristics (Japanese). Hiroshima J. med. Sci. **13**, 665—692 (1965).

SIMPSON, C. L., HEMPELMANN, L. H., *et al.*: Neoplasia in children treated with X-ray in infancy for thymic enlargement. Radiology **64**, 840—845 (1955).

WOOD, J. W., TAMAGAKI, H., *et al.*: Thyroid carcinoma in atomic bomb survivors. ABCC Technical Report: **4**-68, 1—17 (1968).

# Migrant Studies in Alimentary Tract Cancer

Jerzy Staszewski

Institute of Oncology, Gliwice, Poland

Migrant studies are an effective, but largely unexploited tool for studying cancer epidemiology and etiopathogenesis. I shall not discuss the strategy, merits and limitations of the studies of migrant populations, as this was the subject of several recent publications. For example, a part of the papers presented on the symposium on cancer in migratory populations was published in a special issue of the Journal of Chronic Diseases (Volume 23, Number 5/6, November 1970), and the proceedings were summarized by Haenszel [1].

A comparative study on cancer patterns in Poland and in the United States of America, and on shifts in cancer risks of Polish migrants as related to their home and host country, is conducted as a co-operative project of the American National Cancer Institute and the Polish Institute of Oncology. Presently available for comparison are mortality data, but soon it will be possible to compare also the incidence data from cancer registration in Poland with the data on Polish-born and native Americans, ascertained by a survey conducted 1969—1971 in the United States.

My presentation, limited to gastro-intestinal cancer, is based mainly on the mortality data from the study mentioned. Additionally, some of the data on Polish migrants to Australia were utilized. The available material consisted of:

1. Polish mortality statistics [1] for the 1959—1969 period, which permit analyses of rates by primary site of cancer, sex, age, urban-rural residence, of time trends and, to some extent, of regional differences inside Poland [2, 3, 4]. Before 1959 these statistics considered cancers of the various parts of the digestive system as one group only, without any subdivision, and thus were of no use for our purpose.

2. American mortality data [1] for Polish-born and native white Americans for 1950 (discussed in a previous paper [5]) and for 1959—1961. Availability of data for these two periods permits studying changes with time of cancer risks of migrants.

3. Australian mortality data [1] for 1962—1966 for Polish migrants to Australia. It should be kept in mind that their mortality rates, based on just over 300000 person-years, are subject to substantial chance variation. These data will be described in more detail in another paper [6].

Besides age-specific, also age-adjusted rates are presented in the present paper. The latter were computed using the "world population" as the standard [7]. Also the age-adjusted indices will be utilized for presentation purposes. These indices, described elsewhere [8], are the components of the all-over age-adjusted rates for the ages below and over 65, and closely correspond to the "truncated rates" [9].

1 See Acknowledgment.

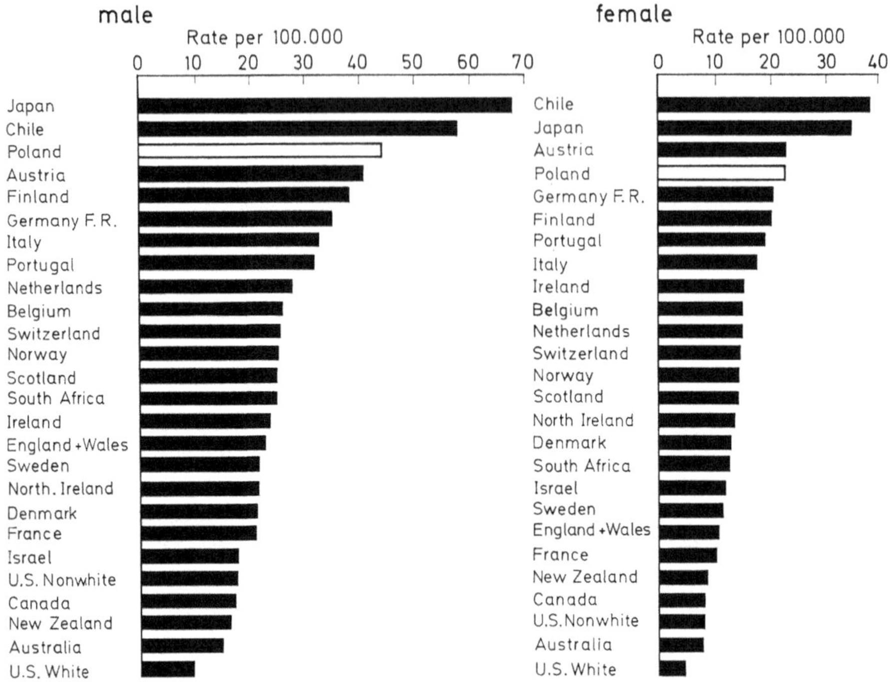


**Fig. 1.** Age-adjusted stomach cancer mortality rates in 1964—1965 in 24 countries [7] and in Poland

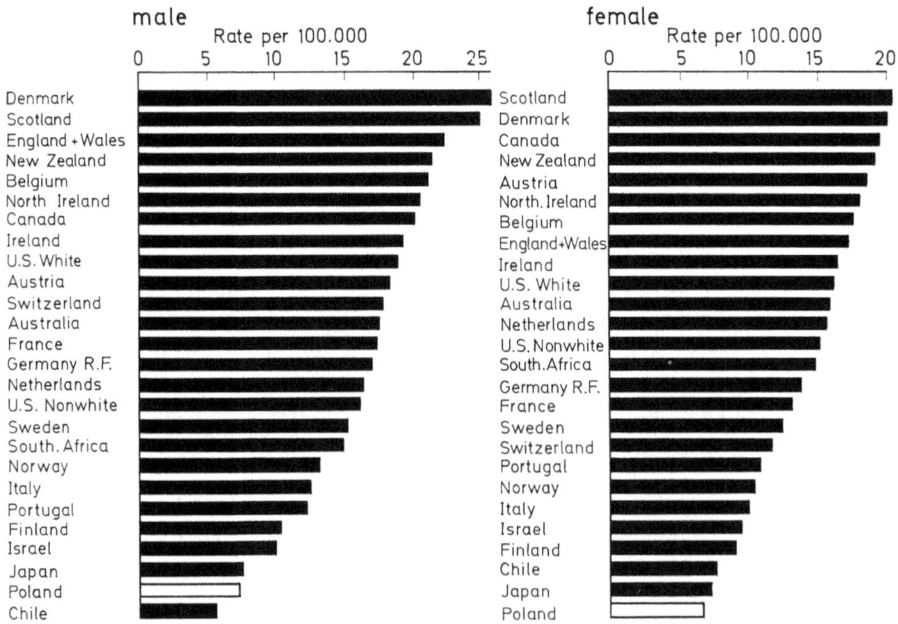


**Fig. 2.** Age-adjusted intestinal tract cancer mortality rates in 1964—1965 in 24 countries [7] and in Poland

Our interest in the experience of Polish-born Americans was aroused by the observation of large differences in the patterns of both stomach and intestinal tract cancer occurrence in Poland and in the United States.

Whereas the United States population experiences a very low stomach cancer risk, as compared to most countries (Fig. 1), Poland belongs to the most unfortunate of high risk countries in respect to this cancer. For intestinal tract cancer the situation is reversed: from the American point of view the risk to this cancer is enviably low in Poland (Fig. 2). In Australia, another host country of Polish migrants, the risk level for both stomach and intestinal tract cancer is much more similar to the one observed in the U.S. than in Poland.

Poland is similar as to the occurrence of both these cancers rather to Japan, Chile, Finland.

I shall begin with considering stomach cancer, and than turn to intestinal tract cancer.

## Stomach Cancer

Stomach cancer displays in Poland further epidemiologic pecularities. Until the very recent years, the decrease of its risk, observed in most countries, was absent in Poland (Fig. 3). Here again a similarity with Japan may be noted. The increase in stomach cancer mortality in Poland, observed up to 1964, was probably spurious, due to the improving diagnosis and death certification, whereas the recent decrease, apparent in urban population and in younger age-groups, reflects probably the

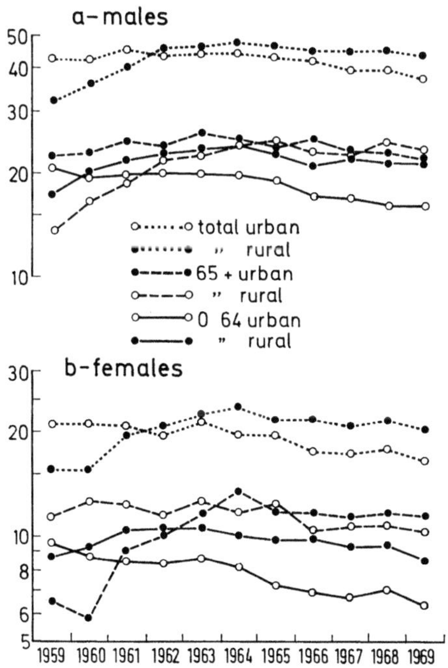


Fig. 3. Time-trends of the age-adjusted stomach cancer mortality rates and "age-adjusted indiees" up to and over 65 of age, in the 1959—1969 period in Poland, by urban-rural residence

begin of a real decrease of stomach cancer risk. (Also in Japan a slight decrease of stomach cancer mortality became apparent, since ca. 1958.)

Furthermore, the available data indicate that in Poland the stomach cancer risk is higher in rural than in urban population—contrary to almost all other cancers. The urban-rural ratio of stomach cancer mortality rates by age is shown in Fig. 4. Also the incidence data from cancer registration in the selected regions of Poland [9] indicate that in Warszawa City the stomach cancer incidence is lower, and in rural areas higher than in regions with a mixed population (Fig. 5).

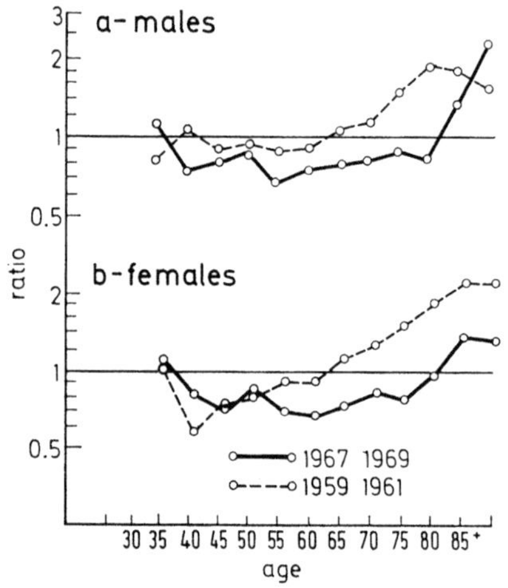


Fig. 4. Urban-rural ratios, U/R, of the stomach cancer mortality rates in 1959—1961 and 1967—1969 in Poland, by age

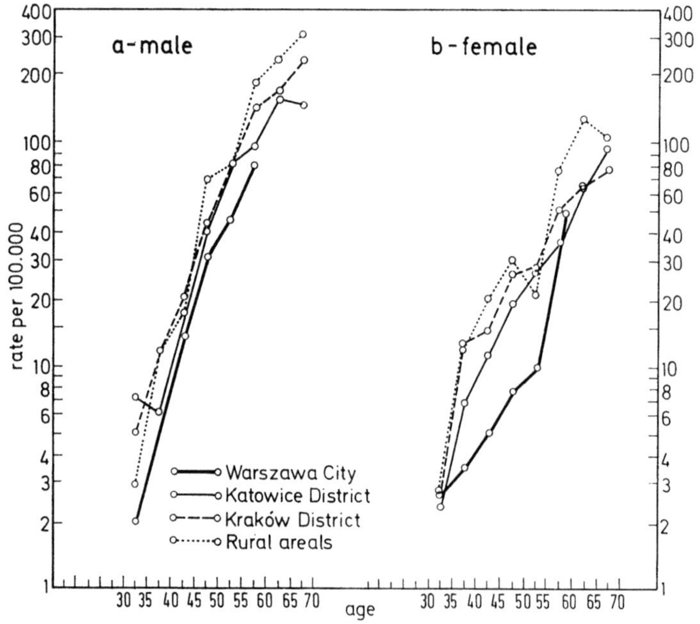


Fig. 5. Age-specific stomach cancer incidence rates in 4 regions of Poland, in 1965—1966

No increased risk was demonstrated in Katowice District, where most of the population is exposed to a heavy air pollution caused by coal mines, foundries, etc.

Turning to Polish migrants and their host country, except for the oldest age-groups, the 1959—1961 stomach cancer mortality in Poland was approximately 4—5 times as high as in native white Americans (Fig. 6). The Polish-born migrants

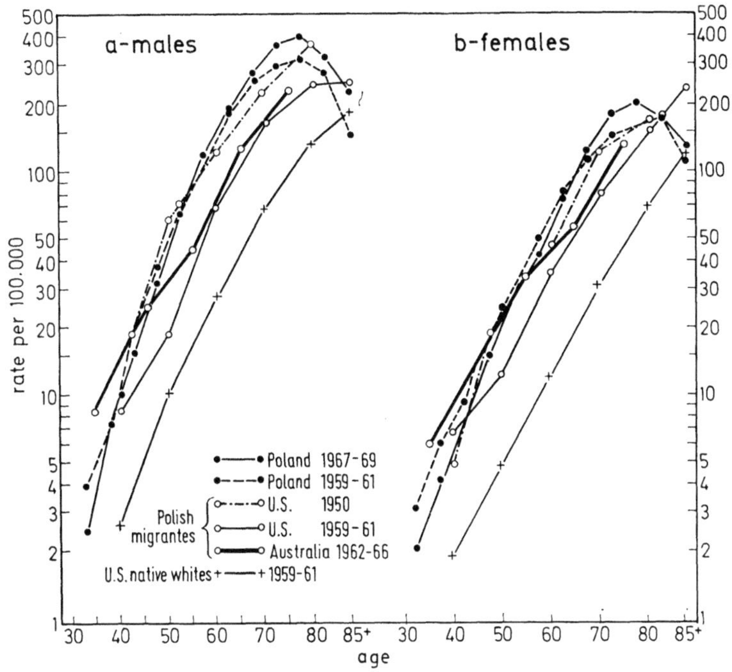


Fig. 6. Age-specific stomach cancer mortality rates in Poland, in Polish migrants to the U.S. and Australia, and in the native white Americans

to the United States experienced in 1950 about the same mortality as prevailed in Poland in 1959—1961, and presumably in 1950, too (judging by the after—1959 trends). Ten years later, however, their mortality rates decreased, becoming intermediate between the rates in their countries of origin and of adoption. In Australia, too, the 1962—1966 mortality of Polish migrants was intermediate, but (despite Australian data being a few years more recent) was more close to the mortality experienced in their country of origin than was the case for the migrants to the United States.

Also in other migrant populations the stomach cancer mortality rates were noted to remain similar as in their country of origin. Around 1950, mortality rates of migrants from other European countries and Japan to the United States were intermediate between the rates prevailing in their respective countries of birth and in their host country, but much closer to the rates in their countries of birth [10, 11]. Ten years later, stomach cancer mortality rates decreased not only in migrants from Poland, but also in Japanese [11], as well as in all foreign born inhabitants of New

York City [12]. Second generation of Japanese migrants to the U.S., Nisei, seems to experience a further decrease of stomach cancer risk, which remains higher, however, than in native whites [11].

## Intestinal Tract Cancer

Cancers of the small intestine and of the colon will be considered combined, because they were not separated in some of the source tabulations. They will be referred to as cancer of the colon, because cancer of the small intestine makes here only a negligible proportion.

Cancer of the rectum is usually classified separately. However, distinction between colon and rectum cancer is not always simple nor uniformly made in both incidence and mortality data; as a substantial part of neoplasms of the intestinal tract is located

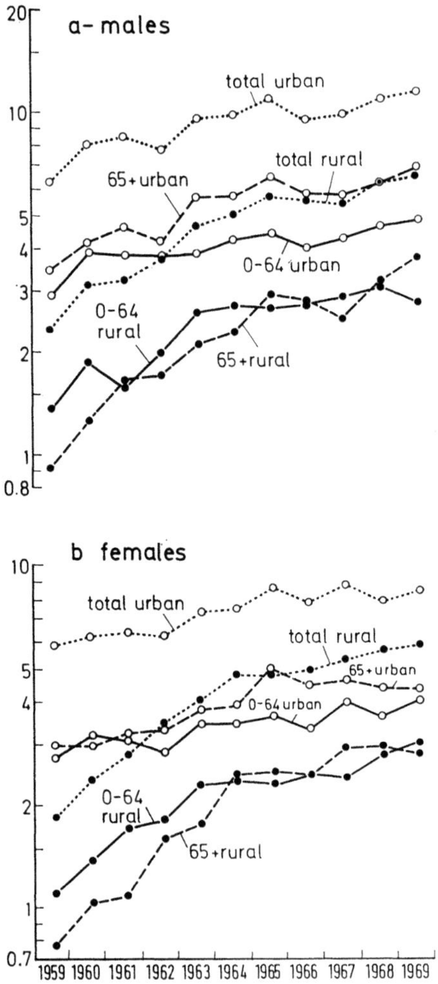


Fig. 7. Time-trends of the age-adjusted intestinal tract cancer mortality rates and "age-adjusted indices" up to and over 65 of age, in the 1959—1969 period in Poland, by urban-rural residence

in sigmoid colon and in rectum, even slight differences in interpretation and application of classification rules may largely influence the results of classification of intestinal tract cancer, and distort comparisons of data from various sources. Hence, colon and rectum cancer will be discussed under the one heading, of intestinal tract cancer, but their separation will be attempted.

Unlike most countries, Poland appears to experience an increase in intestinal tract cancer mortality rates (Fig. 7). This increase, similar for colon and rectum cancers, concerned all ages. It was more marked in the older and in the rural populations (which may, at least partly, be due to an improvement in diagnosis). Despite that increase, the intestinal tract cancer risk in Poland appears to be still low.

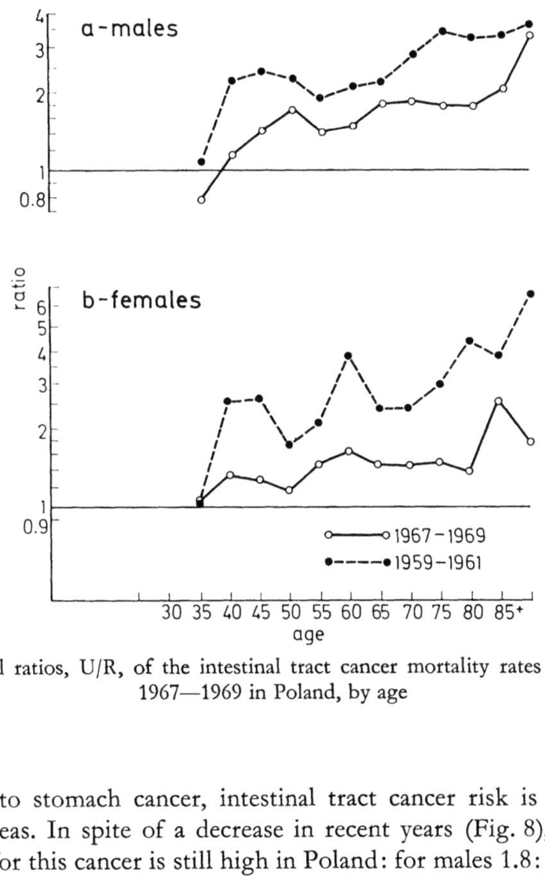


Fig. 8. Urban-rural ratios, U/R, of the intestinal tract cancer mortality rates in 1959—1961 and 1967—1969 in Poland, by age

In contrast to stomach cancer, intestinal tract cancer risk is higher in urban than in rural areas. In spite of a decrease in recent years (Fig. 8), the urban-rural mortality ratio for this cancer is still high in Poland: for males 1.8:1 and for females 1.5:1, as of 1967—1969. Also the incidence data [9] indicate that the intestinal tract cancer incidence is lowest in the rural areas (Fig. 9).

As for Polish migrants, in 1959—1961 the Polish-born Americans experienced a higher colon and rectal cancer mortality than the U.S. native whites (Fig. 10). However, mortality rates of Polish-borns were similar to those of the natives in the northeast and north central states, where those rates are above the U.S. average [10] and where most Polish migrants reside. This finding corraborates the earlier conclusion—based on data for 1950 only—that mortality for these cancers among

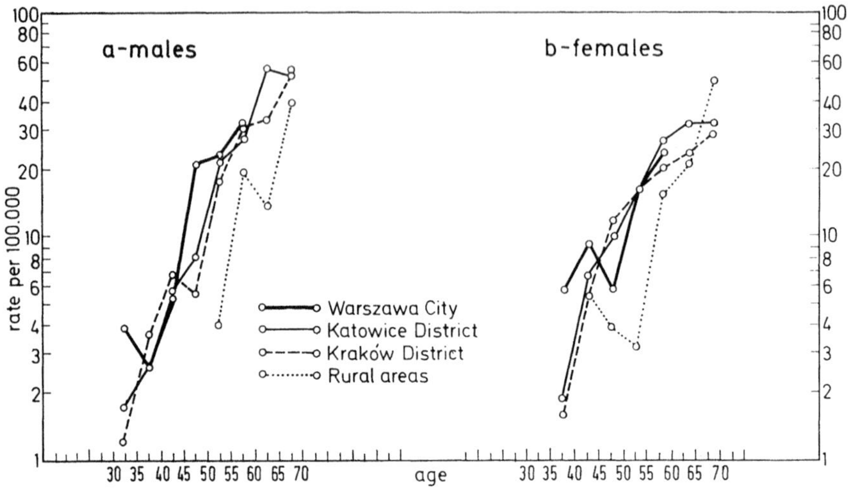


Fig. 9. Age-specific intestinal tract cancer incidence rates in 4 regions of Poland, in 1965—1966

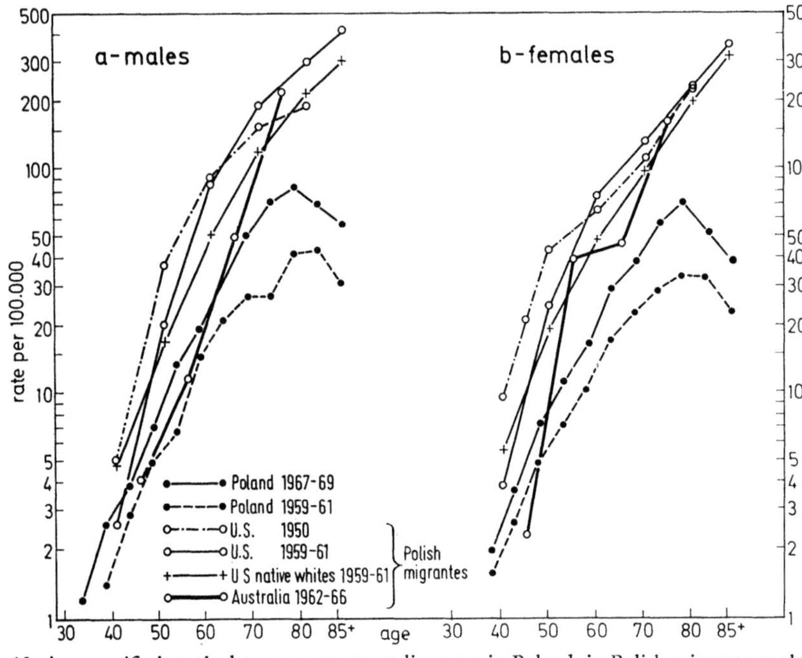


Fig. 10. Age-specific intestinal tract cancer mortality rates in Poland, in Polish migrants to the U.S. and Australia, and in the native white Americans

Polish-born migrants is much higher than in Poland and similar to that in the U.S. native whites [5]. It is worth remembering that Polish migrants to the U.S. were drawn mainly from the farming, rural areas, i.e. those areas where the risk of these cancers was probably even below the low Polish average. The upward displacement of the colorectal cancer risk for those migrants was thus probably even larger than it seems from the rates presented.

A similar increase of the intestinal tract cancer mortality, connected with migration from a low risk to a high risk area for this cancer, was observed in the U.S. in migrants from Norway and Japan [10, 11], as well as from rural to urban areas, whereas mortality decreased in migrants from urban to rural areas [13]. Colorectal cancer risk of migrants is thus similar to the risk prevailing in their last residence area rather than to the risk in their country of birth.

In Polish migrants to Australia a similar increase of the colon and rectal cancer mortality to the high level prevailing in their country of adoption was observed. That increase was only small in males; this deviation may be due to chance variation, the male rates being based on 20 deaths only.

In Polish-born Americans in 1950, the colon-rectum cancer ratio, C/R, was relatively low, 1.6:1. It corroborated the low C/R ratio in Poland (1.4:1) not being due to differences, between the United States and Poland, as to classification of border cases. The C/R ratio in Polish-born Americans in 1959—1961, however, increased to 2.7:1, i.e. to the level prevailing in the United States native whites.

## Comments

Even the limited data presented do permit some conclusions, or at least give some hints, as to the etiopathogenesis of stomach and intestinal tract cancer.

One conclusion is that the shifts in risks to cancers of the stomach and of the intestinal tract, occurring in migrants, are not only going in opposite directions, but that they also are far from synchronous. For intestinal tract cancer the shift from the low risk prevailing in the country of birth to the high risk observed in the host population is completed in one generation, and apparently in less than 30 years: it was complete in 1950 in Polish-born Americans, most of whom came to the United States before 1925. Also migrants inside the United States were found to display risks similar to those prevailing in their last residence [13]. For stomach cancer, on the other hand, the shifts in risks of migrants from the low- to high-risk countries became apparent, if at all, first after over 30 years from the departure from their country of birth, and even then were far from being complete. It appears as if the difference between migrants and the host population did not change but the decreased stomach cancer mortality of migrants were reflecting solely the decreasing trend of rates concerning host and migrant population to the same degree.

The second, perhaps the most important conclusion is that genetic factors do not account for the decreasing frequency of stomach cancer occurrence, observed in most countries. When shifts in cancer risks, observed in migrants, are additionally considered, genetic factors also do not account for the large geographic variations in the occurrence of either stomach or intestinal tract cancer. Much more likely, environmental factors are of primary importance in development of these cancers. Hence, prevention of these cancers may be possible. To this goal, determination of factors, bearing on the risk to these cancers, would be required.

Little is yet known about environmental factors predisposing to stomach or intestinal tract cancer, and the presented data per se offer no information on this subject. However, it may be of interest to examine, how the observed patterns of these cancers in Poland and Polish migrants fit in some of the current hypotheses on their etiopathogenesis.

The belief is widespread that dietary factors are the most important of environmental factors bearing on gastrointestinal tract cancer development.

It was postulated that predisposing to stomach cancer may be alimentary deficiences due to low quality diet—rich in potatoes or rice, and poor in animal proteins and vitamins [14]. The high, but recently decreasing potatoes consumption in Poland (Table 1), corresponding to the high, but recently decreasing stomach cancer risk, fits well in this model. Also the conspicuous negative correlation with socioeconomic class, characteristic for stomach cancer [14], speaks for an association between stomach cancer and dietary deficiences.

Table 1. Average yearly consumption of selected foods in Poland (kilograms per person)

| Item | Year | | | | | | | | | |
|---|---|---|---|---|---|---|---|---|---|---|
| | 1938 | 1946 | 1947 | 1948 | 1949 | 1950 | 1955 | 1960 | 1965 | 1969 |
| Potatoes | 260 | 310 | 305 | 302 | 290 | 270 | 229 | 223 | 215 | 199 |
| Meat | 16.5 | 15.8 | 21.1 | 21.7 | 28.0 | 36.5 | 37.7 | 42.5 | 49.2 | 52.6 |
| Fat | 5.7 | 3.9 | 5.0 | 5.9 | 7.3 | 9.7 | 11.1 | 13.6 | 15.1 | 17.5 |
| Sugar | 9.6 | — | 12.8 | 17.1 | 19.3 | 21.0 | 24.0 | 27.9 | 32.6 | 38.7 |

Source: Rocznik Statystyczny 1970. Warszawa, GUS, 1970.

The higher risk to stomach cancer in the rural than in the urban population of Poland might be related to the low socioeconomic level of the rural population, prevailing up to the last war.

The alimentary deficiences hypothesis is further supported by the finding in Poland of an increased stomach cancer risk among persons eating potatoes at least once daily [15]—which is consistent with the results of a study by GRAHAM *et al.* (conducted in an area with a high proportion of Polish migrants [16]), and with an increased risk of stomach cancer among persons eating much rice, observed in Japan [17].

However, the same observations may be also consistent with another hypothesis: that some food carcinogens, and not dietary deficiences, are of primary importance in stomach cancer development. An association between eating pickled foods and stomach cancer risk was recently observed in Japan and in Japanese migrants [18]. It is possible that microorganisms causing fermentations or accompanying it are producing carcinogens [19]. An increased stomach cancer risk of persons who like sour foods, observed in Poland [15], may perhaps be due to their increased consumption of sauerkraut, sour cucumbers, sour milk, etc. Also the storage of potatoes throughout winter in earth cavities seems to favor their infection by moulds, which in turn might produce carcinogens.

Turning to possible dietary factors which may influence the intestinal tract cancer development, it was postulated that these factors may operate by influencing intestinal bacterial flora and/or peristalsis.

Intestinal bacterial flora is dependent on diet—esp. on relative proportions of fats and carbohydrates [20]. Hence, it can be expected that the possible activation of food carcinogens by intestinal bacterial flora may be also diet dependent.

The low frequency of intestinal tract cancer occurrence in populations with bulky diets [21] is consistent with the hypothesis that the risk of this cancer is decreased by factors which increase peristalsis and thus decrease the contact of intestinal mucosa with carcinogens present in intestinal contents. Such hypothesis would explain the negative correlation of these neoplasms with tobacco smoking, as nicotine increases peristalsis [22, 23].

Evaluation of the relative importance of the postulated ways, in which diet may influence the development of intestinal tract cancer, is made difficult by their interrelations. For example, a diet rich in fats is usually not bulky and thus not much promoting peristalsis; bacterial flora associated with such a diet differs also from the flora connected with a high carbohydrate diet; moreover, fats are increasing bile excretion, and biliary salts may possibly be transformed into carcinogens by the bacterial flora.

The low, but increasing risk of intestinal tract cancer in Poland may depend on the high, but decreasing consumption of potatoes, which are rich in cellulose, provide bulky food and promote peristalsis; it may also depend on the low, but increasing consumption of fats (via effect either on bacterial flora or on supply of material from which carcinogen is made) or of sugar [24]; these changes in consumption are apparent in Table 1.

Bulky, low-fat diet is usually qualitatively poor, low in animal proteins and vitamins. This might account for the negative correlation between cancers of the intestinal tract and of the stomach.

There are indications that nutritional factors may affect the incidence of cancer of the breast, uterine corpus, ovary, and prostate. This is corroborated by a positive correlation between those cancers and intestinal tract cancer—the correlation which may also be noticed in shifts of cancer risks, observed in Polish migrants [25].

This presentation is an interim report on an ongoing study, and not a final report. For the continuation of this study its scope shall be broadened to the following subjects:

1. Incorporation into the study of more detailed information on tumor localisation and histology, on lesions in the adjacent mucosa, etc.

2. Comparative studies of dietary habits, environmental and host characteristics (including the prevalence of cancer precursor lesions) of migrants and of populations in both their country of birth and of adoption.

3. Inclusion, into the study, of Polish migrants to other countries, and also comparisons with other populations.

## Acknowledgments

The Department of Vital Statistics and Demographic Studies of the Central Statistical Office, Warszawa, provided unpublished tabulations of cancer deaths in Poland.

The National Center for Health Statistics, Washington, D.C., provided the unpublished data on cancer mortality among the Polish-born and native white Americans.

Doctors M. G. MCCALL and N. S. STENHOUSE of the University of Western Australia, Perth, provided unpublished data on mortality among Polish migrants to Australia.

The studies described were partly supported by PL 480 Agreement 05-009-01, sponsored by the National Cancer Institute, National Institutes of Health, Bethesda, Md., U.S.A.

The continuous interest and help of Dr. WILLIAM HAENSZEL, without which these studies could not have been carried out, is gratefully acknowledged.

## Summary

Results of the ongoing study of gastrointestinal cancer occurrence in Poland and in Polish migrants to the United States and Australia are described.

In comparison with other countries, Poland is characterized by a high stomach cancer risk (which started to decrease only recently), and by a higher risk in rural than in urban areas. Intestinal tract cancer risk, on the contrary, is relatively low but increasing in Poland, and displays a rather high urban-rural ratio.

The displacements in risks, observed in migrants to the U.S. and Australia, differ for these cancers. Among Polish-born Americans in 1950 the stomach cancer mortality rates appear to have been as high as in their country of birth, and 10 years later (as well as in Australia in 1962—1966) the Polish migrants' mortality rates were still more aligned to the high rates in Poland than to the low rates in natives of the host country. On the contrary, for the intestinal tract cancer a complete transition from the low mortality prevailing in the country of birth to the high rates observed in the country of adoption was observed in those migrants.

The findings are discussed as clues to the etiopathogenesis of gastrointestinal cancer, with a special regard to the role of nutritional factors.

## References

1. HAENSZEL, W.: Report of the working group on studies of cancer and related diseases in migrant populations. Int. J. Cancer **4**, 364 (1970).
2. STASZEWSKI, J.: Cancer in Poland in 1959. Brit. J. Cancer **18**, 1 (1964).
3. STASZEWSKI, J.: Regionalne roznice rejestracji umieralnosci na nowotwory w Polsce w 1961 r. Nowotwory **17**, 297 (1967).
4. STASZEWSKI, J.: Czy czestosc raka zoladka w Polsce rzeczywiscie wzrasta? Nowotwory **19**, 47 (1969).
5. STASZEWSKI, J., HAENSZEL, W.: Cancer mortality among the Polishborn in the United States. J. nat. Cancer Inst. **35**, 291 (1965).
6. STASZEWSKI, J., MCCALL, M., STENHOUSE, N. S.: Cancer mortality in 1962—1966 among Polish migrants to Australia. Brit. J. Cancer **25**, 599 (1971)
7. SEGI, M., KURIHARA, M., MATSUYAMA, T.: Cancer mortality for selected sites in 24 countries. No. 5 (1964—1965). Department of Public Health, Tohoku University School of Medicine, Sendai, 1970.
8. STASZEWSKI, J.: A propos of summarizing indices for comparison of cancer incidence data. Neoplasma (Bratisl.) **16**, 321 (1969).
9. DOLL, R., MUIR, C. S., WATERHOUSE, J. A. H., editors: Cancer incidence in five continents. Vol. II, Geneva: UICC (1970).
10. HAENSZEL, W.: Cancer mortality among the foreign-born in the United States. J. nat. Cancer Inst. **26**, 37 (1961).

11. HAENSZEL, W., KURIHARA, M.: Studies of Japanese migrants. I. Mortality from cancer and other diseases among Japanese in the United States. J. nat. Cancer Inst. **40**, 43 (1968).
12. TERRIS, W., HALL, C. E.: Decline in mortality from gastric cancer in native-born and foreign, born residents of New York City. J. nat. Cancer Inst. **31**, 155 (1963).
13. HAENSZEL, W., DAWSON, E. A.: A note on mortality from cancer of the colon and rectum in the United States. Cancer **18**, 265 (1965).
14. HAENSZEL, W.: Variation in incidence of and mortality from stomach cancer, with particular reference to the United States. J. nat. Cancer Inst. **21**, 213 (1958).
15. STASZEWSKI, J.: Odzywianie a rak zoladka. Nowotwory **21**, 119 (1971).
16. GRAHAM, S., LILIENFELD, A. M., TIDINGS, J. W.: Dietary and purgation factors in the epidemiology of gastric cancer. Cancer **20**, 2224 (1967).
17. SEGI, M., FUKUSHIMA, I., FUJISAKU, S., KURIHARA, H., SAITO, S., ASANO, K., KAMOI, M.: Epidemiological study on cancer in Japan. Gann **48** (Suppl.) (1967).
18. HAENSZEL, W.: personal communication (1971).
19. KINOSITA, R., ISHIKO, T., SUGIYAMA, S., SETO, T., IGARASI, S., GOETZ, J. E.: Mycotoxins in fermented food. Cancer Res. **28**, 2296 (1968).
20. WYNDER, E. L., SHIGEMATSU, T.: Environmental factors of cancer of the colon and rectum. Cancer **20**, 1520 (1967).
21. BREMNER, C. G., ACKERMAN, L. V.: Polyps and carcinoma of the large bowel in the South African Bantu. Cancer **26**, 991 (1970).
22. Smoking and Health: Report of the Advisory Committee to the Surgeon General of the Public Health Service. Public Health Sercive Publication no. 1103, Washington (1964).
23. STASZEWSKI, J.: Smoking and cancer of the alimentary tract in Poland. Brit. J. Cancer **23**, 247 (1969).
24. BURKITT, D. P.: Epidemiology of cancer of the colon and rectum. Cancer **28**, 3 (1971).
25. STASZEWSKI, J.: Cancer epidemiology in Poland and in Polish migrants. Prepared for publication.

# Histological Types of Gastric Cancer and its Relationship with Intestinal Metaplasia

NUBIA MUÑOZ and IVAN MATKO

Unit of Biological Carcinogenesis, International Agency for Research on Cancer, Lyon, France
Gastroenterology Institute, Ljubljana, Yugoslavia

There are two striking features in the epidemiology of gastric cancer. First, the great variation in the incidence of gastric cancer, which has been described from country to country, and also within a given country from one area to another. High rates have been reported for Japan, Finland, Iceland, Poland and mountainous regions of Colombia and Slovenia, and low rates for the Caucasian population of the United States, New Zealand, some African countries and littoral areas of Colombia and Slovenia [1—4]. Second, the persistent decline in gastric cancer rates which has been described in many countries [5—6]. In an attempt to determine if a particular histological type of gastric carcinoma is responsible for these striking features, a modification of the histological classification proposed by LAURÉN [4, 7—8] has been used to classify gastric cancer cases from different geographic areas.

## Material and Methods

Histological sections from surgical specimens or biopsies of gastric cancer cases were used. The modified Laurén's classification has been described in detail elsewhere [8]. Basically, the cases were classified into three groups:

1. *Intestinal type*, characterized by the presence of well defined glandular structures with lumina lined by well polarized cells and/or the tendency of the cells to stick to each other. Variations in this type were recognized according to the size of the glands and the amount of mucinous material (Fig. 1).

2. *Diffuse type*, characterized by the presence of epithelial cells independent from each other, or occasionally forming no well defined glandular structures. Varieties were also recognized in this type according to the amount of signet ring cells and mucinous material (Fig. 2).

3. In this group were classified cases which could not be assigned to either of the two main groups. These included adenoacanthomas, solid carcinomas bearing a resemblance to carcinoids, Brunner cell carcinomas, mixed types (intestinal and diffuse) in which no one type predominated and cases in which the histological sections were not suitable for a diagnosis.

The histological sections were obtained from the departments of pathology of different countries: Colombia [4], Mexico [4], Poland and Yugoslavia.

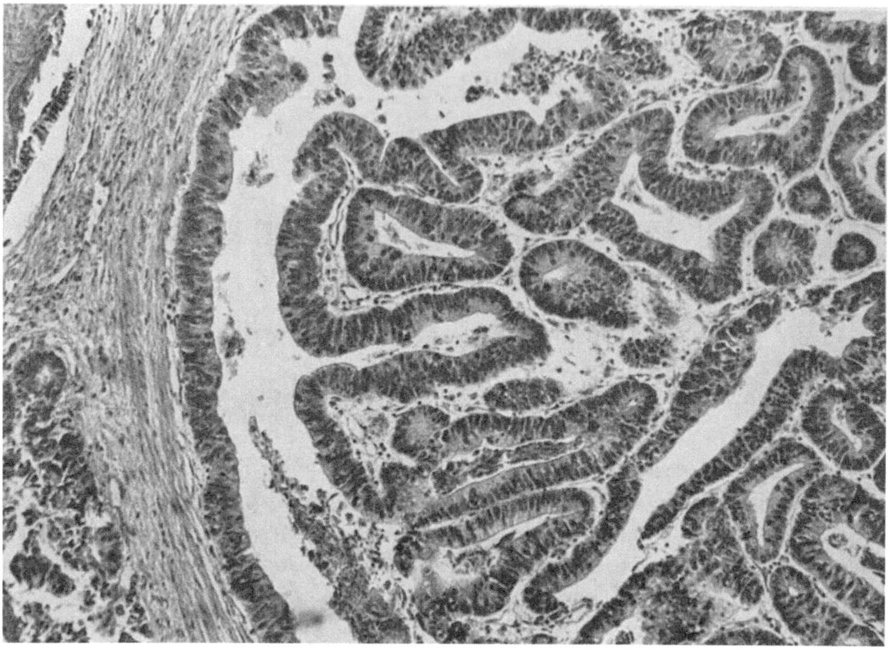

Fig. 1. Intestinal type of gastric cancer with large and well-defined glands formed by large and well-polarized cylindrical cells. Haematoxylin-eosin X100

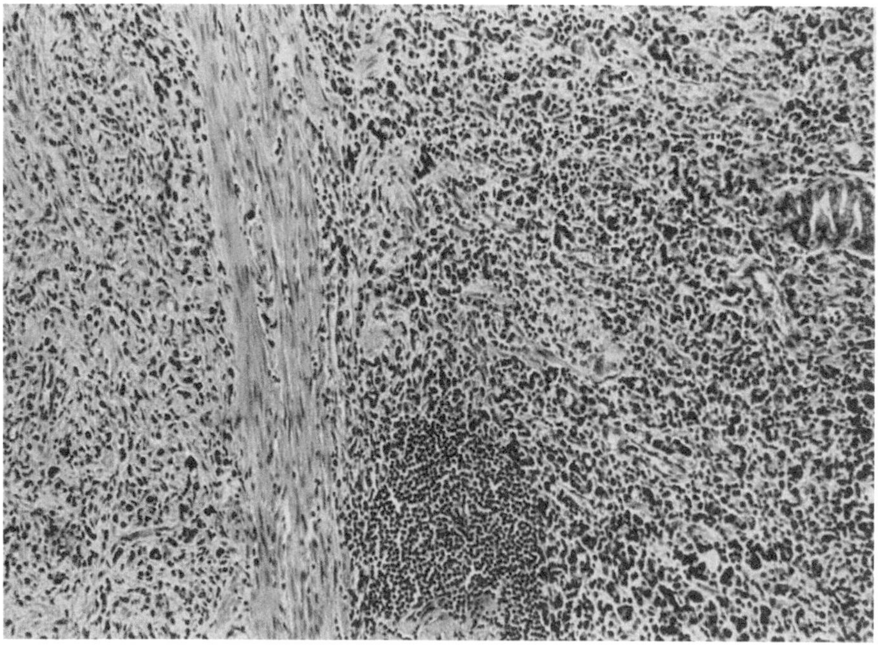

Fig. 2. Diffuse carcinoma with isolate cells spreading diffusely in the mucosa and sub-mucosa. No glandular structures are apparent. Haematoxylin-eosin X100

To study the relationship between gastric cancer and intestinal metaplasia, gastric biopsies performed at the Gastroenterology Institute of Ljubljana were used. Two types of gastric biopsies are usually performed at this Institute: blind biopsies in patients with mild gastrointestinal symptoms and guided biopsies in patients with severe symptoms.

# Results

## Histologic Types

Detailed analysis of part of this material has been published elsewhere [4]. Table 1 gives a summary of the distribution of histologic types of gastric cancer in high- and low-risk areas. The intestinal type was the most frequent type among each of the high-risk areas and the diffuse type in the low-risk areas.

Table 1. Histological types of gastric cancer in high- and low-risk areas

| Geographic areas | Total cases | Histological types (%) | | | Ratio: intestinal/diffuse |
|---|---|---|---|---|---|
| | | Intestinal | Diffuse | Others | |
| High-risk-areas | | | | | |
| Cali-Colombia | 191 | 51.8 | 34.0 | 14.1 | 1.52 |
| Maribor-Yugoslavia | 149 | 51.7 | 34.8 | 13.4 | 1.48 |
| Gliwice-Poland | 94 | 45.7 | 36.2 | 18.1 | 1.26 |
| Total | 434 | 50.5 | 34.8 | 14.7 | 1.45 |
| Low-risk-areas | | | | | |
| Cartagena-Colombia | 38 | 28.9 | 55.3 | 15.8 | 0.52 |
| Barranquilla-Colombia | 13 | 38.5 | 46.1 | 15.4 | 0.83 |
| Mexico City-Mexico | 80 | 38.7 | 46.3 | 15.0 | 0.83 |
| Koper-Yugoslavia | 53 | 39.6 | 50.9 | 9.5 | 0.78 |
| Total | 184 | 37.0 | 49.4 | 13.6 | 0.75 |

## Age and Sex Distribution

Previous studies have also shown that these two types have different sex and age distribution [4, 7—10]. The intestinal type is most frequent in men and in older age groups and the diffuse type does not show a significant difference by sex, but it is more frequent in the younger ages.

## Time Trends

Studies in Norway and the United States have shown that most of the reduction in gastric cancer rates during the last decades can be accounted for by a decrease in the intestinal type since the diffuse and other types have kept their toll fairly constant [8, 10]. In Norway, the decrease in the intestinal type was most marked in females and in the under-49 age group [8].

## Intestinal Metaplasia

It has been defined as "the result of the faulty regeneration of surface epithelium in a mucosa repeatedly damaged by gastritis" [11]. Although there is evidence that suggests an association between intestinal metaplasia and intestinal type of gastric cancer, the nature of this association is not yet clear. In an attempt to clarify this point, the following study is being carried out in the Gastroenterology Institute of Ljubljana.

A total of 2,334 blind gastric biopsies taken from 1962 to 1970 and 437 guided biopsies taken from 1966 to 1970 have been reviewed for the presence of intestinal metaplasia. Table 2 shows the frequency of intestinal metaplasia in these two types of biopsies. The higher frequency among the guided biopsies is not surprising since these biopsies are performed in patients with severe gastrointestinal symptoms. Three hundred and seventy-six patients with intestinal metaplasia and two hundred and ninety-three age- and sex-matched controls with negative biopsies for intestinal metaplasia have been checked in the files of the Cancer Registry of Slovenia for the

Table 2. Frequency of intestinal metaplasia in gastric biopsies Ljubljana/Yugoslavia

| | | |
|---|---|---|
| *Blind biopsies* (1962—1970) | | |
| Total number | —2334 | |
| Number with intestinal metaplasia | — 267 | (11.4%) |
| *Guided biopsies* (1966—1970) | | |
| Total number | — 437 | |
| Number with intestinal metaplasia | — 137 | (30.4%) |

Table 3. Age and sex distribution of intestinal metaplasia cases diagnosed by blind and guided biopsies and of the gastric cancer occurred among them

| | Blind biopsies | | | | Guided biopsies | | | | Total | |
|---|---|---|---|---|---|---|---|---|---|---|
| | Males | Females | Total | Gastric cancer | Males | Females | Total | Gastric cancer | Intest. metapl. | Gastric cancer |
| ≦44 | 58 | 32 | 90 | — | 37 | 10 | 47 | 6 | 137 | 6 |
| 45—54 | 34 | 22 | 56 | 4[a] | 19 | 10 | 29 | 5 | 85 | 9 |
| ≧55 | 50 | 47 | 97 | 3 | 30 | 27 | 57 | 9 | 154 | 12 |
| Total | 132 | 101 | 243 | 7 | 86 | 47 | 133 | 20 | 376 | 27 |

Among 293 age- and sex-matched controls one gastric cancer was found.
[a] Three cases were diagnosed at least one year after the biopsy.

occurrence of gastric cancer. Twenty-seven cases of gastric cancer were found among the 376 patients with intestinal metaplasia and one case among the 293 controls. Table 3 shows the sex and age distribution of the intestinal metaplasia cases and the gastric cancers which occurred among them. As expected, a higher frequency of gastric cancer was found among the guided biopsies, since this is a highly selected group. However, when the clinical records of these 27 cases of gastric cancer were reviewed, it was found that only 3 cases were diagnosed at least one year after the gastric biopsy was taken, and no signs of malignancy were detected at the time of biopsy. These 3 cases were males in the 45—54 age group and belonged to the blind biopsies' group. The other 24 cases which occurred among the intestinal metaplasia patients and the one which occurred among the control group, all were diagnosed at the time of the biopsy or a few months after. Therefore it can be considered that in 3 patients, the intestinal metaplasia preceded the appearance of gastric cancer.

Although this is a very small number, a comparison with the control group and the normal population was attempted (Table 4). The person-years at risk were computed for the cases and controls since they have been followed up for different periods of time. These preliminary results suggest that patients with intestinal metaplasia have a higher risk than the general population of Slovenia and much higher than patients with gastric biopsies negative for intestinal metaplasia.

Table 4. Gastric cancer incidence rate among patients with and without intestinal Metaplasia

| | Person-years at risk | Number of gastric cancer | Annual rate per 100.000 |
|---|---|---|---|
| Cases | 893 | 3 | 330.0 |
| Controls | 859 | 0 | 0.0 |

Truncated standardized incidence rate: (35—64 years) 67.7 per 100.000

## Discussion

There is a considerable evidence to indicate that there are two main types of gastric cancer: intestinal or well-differentiated adenocarcinoma and diffuse or undifferentiated adenocarcinoma. These two types differ not only in morphology, but also in their clinical and epidemiological characteristics. The intestinal type is most frequent in men and in older age group; it has a relatively better prognosis than the diffuse type; it is the predominant type in the high-risk areas for gastric cancer and it is responsible for the decline in gastric cancer rates. The diffuse type does not show a significant difference by sex; it is more frequent in the younger ages; it has a poorer prognosis, a higher relative frequency in low-risk areas for gastric cancer and it does not change significantly in time [4, 7—10].

These observations suggest that these two types of gastric cancer might also have a different aetiology.

There are data that suggest that the intestinal type is more dependent of environmental factors and the diffuse type of genetic factors:

1. When estimates of age-adjusted rates per histologic types are computed for areas with high and low incidence for gastric cancer, it is evident that much of the excess stomach cancer risk in the high-incidence areas could be accounted for by an excess in intestinal type carcinoma. No significant differences are observed in the rates for the diffuse type [4, 8—10].

2. Time trends for these two types of gastric cancer are different. A significant decline in the intestinal type and relatively stable rates for the diffuse types during the last 30 years have been observed in Norway [8].

3. The association with the blood group A is stronger for the diffuse type than for the intestinal type carcinoma [12].

In the search for possible environmental factors associated with the intestinal type carcinoma, the consideration of precancerous lesions becomes very important. Intestinal metaplasia appears to be a good possibility. The evidence for this association has been reviewed recently [13]. In general this evidence is of two types:

*First: Histopathological*

a) Studies in Japan have demonstrated that the histological type in the case of early gastric cancer is basically dependent on the degree of intestinalization of the gastric mucosa. When intestinalization is mild or absent, the cancer arising from this mucosa is usually of diffuse type, but when intestinalization is severe, the resulting gastric cancer is usually of intestinal type [14—15].

b) When intestinal metaplasia is evaluated in the non-cancerous mucosa of gastric cancer specimens, a higher frequency of intestinal metaplasia has been found in the intestinal type carcinomas than in the diffuse type [7—10].

c) A transition from intestinal metaplasia to intestinal type carcinoma is apparent in specimens of early gastric cancer [13, 16], and in experimentally induced gastric cancer in rats [17].

*Second: Epidemiological*

a) A correlation between the prevalence of intestinal metaplasia and the incidence of gastric cancer has been reported in different ethnic groups with different risks of gastric cancer [13, 18—19].

b) The preliminary results of the present study suggest that the patients with intestinal metaplasia have a higher risk of gastric cancer than patients without evidence of intestinal metaplasia or than the normal population.

It is important then, to try to identify the environmental factors associated with intestinal metaplasia. Protein deficiency has been suggested as one of these factors [13]; however, it does not seem to be likely in Norway [8]. A promising approach for the identification of these factors could be the characterization of the diet in areas with high and low prevalence of intestinal metaplasia.

## Summary

Evidence which indicate the existence of two different types of gastric cancer has been reviewed. These two types are: intestinal type or well differentiated adenocarcinoma and diffuse or undifferentiated adenocarcinoma. The fact that these two types differ not only in morphology but also in their clinical and epidemiological characteristics suggests that they also might have a different aetiology. The evidence which suggest an association between intestinal metaplasia and intestinal type of gastric cancer has also been reviewed. Preliminary results of a prospective study which is being done in the Gastroenterology Institute of Ljubljana indicate that patients with intestinal metaplasia have a higher risk of developing gastric cancer than age- and sex-matched controls with biopsies negative for intestinal metaplasia and than the general population.

### Acknowledgement

We thank Dr. J. Staszewski for allowings us to study the material from Poland.

## References

1. Doll, R., Muir, C., Waterhouse, J., eds.: Cancer Incidence in five Continents. In UICC Monograph Series. Berlin: Springer 1970, Vol. II.
2. Kmet, J.: The relationship between diet and stomach cancer in Yugoslavia. Cancro **2**, 163—171 (1966).

3. Correa, P., Llanos, G.: Morbidity and mortality from cancer in Cali/Colombia. J. nat. Cancer Inst. **36**, 717—745 (1966).
4. Muñoz, N., Correa, P., Cuello, C., Duque, E.: Histologic types of gastric carcinoma in high-risk and low-risk areas. Int. J. Cancer **3**, 809—818 (1968).
5. Segi, M., Kurihara, M.: Cancer mortality for selected sites in 24 countries. No. 4, 1962—1963. Department of Public Health, Tohuku University School of Medicine, Sendai, Japan, pp. 271 to 273, 1966.
6. Haenszel, W.: Variations in incidence of and mortality from stomach cancer, with particular reference to the United States. J. nat. Cancer Inst. **21**, 213—262 (1958).
7. Laurén, P.: The two histological main types of gastric carcinoma: diffuse and so-called intestinal type carcinoma. Acta path. microbiol. scand. **64**, 31—49 (1965).
8. Muñoz, N., Asvall, J.: Time trends of intestinal and diffuse types of gastric cancer in Norway. Int. J. Cancer **8**, 144—157 (1971).
9. Muñoz, N., Steinitz, R.: Comparative histology of gastric cancer in migrant groups in Israel. Israel J. Med. Sciences (in press).
10. Muñoz, N., Connelly, R.: Time trends of intestinal and diffuse types of gastric cancer in the United States. Int. J. Cancer, **8**, 158—164 (1971).
11. Magnus, H. A.: Observation on the presence of intestinal epithelium in the gastric mucosa. J. Path. Bact. **44**, 389—398 (1937).
12. Correa, P.: Geographic pathology of cancer in Columbia. Int. Path. **11**, 16—22 (1970).
13. Correa, P., Cuello, C., Duque, E.: Carcinoma and intestinal metaplasia of the stomach in Colombian migrants. J. nat. Cancer Inst. **44**, 297—306 (1970).
14. Nagayo, T., Komagoe, T.: Histological studies of gastric mucosal cancer with special reference to relationship of histological pictures between the mucosal cancer and the cancer-bearing gastric mucosa. Gann **52**, 109—119 (1961).
15. Nagayo, T., Ito, M., Yokohama, H., Komagoe, T.: Early phases of human gastric cancer: morphological study. Gann **56**, 101—120 (1965).
16. Morson, B. C.: Carcinoma arising from areas of intestinal metaplasia in the gastric mucosa. Brit. J. Cancer **9**, 377—385 (1955).
17. Feit, I., Svegda, N., Sochrova, M.: Experimental intestinal metaplasia of rats and its relationship to carcinoma. Neoplasma (Bratisl.) **14**, 285—290 (1967).
18. Imai, T.: Some comments on the geographical pathological aspects of gastric carcinogenesis. Gann Monograph **3**, 123—127 (1968).
19. Bonne, C., Harzt, H., Klerks, I. V., Posthuma, I. H., Radsma, W., Tjorkronegoro, W.: Morphology of the stomach and gastric secretion in Malays and Chinese and the different incidence of gastric ulcer and cancer in these races. Amer. J. Cancer **33**, 265—279 (1938).

# Primary Carcinomas of the Liver in Hong Kong: Some Possible Aetiological Factors

J. B. GIBSON and W. C. CHAN

Department of Pathology, University of Hong Kong, Hong Kong

The incidence of primary liver-cell cancer differs greatly from one part of the world to another. On the basis of the incidence rates published by U.I.C.C. (DOLL, PAYNE and WATERHOUSE, 1966), HUTT (1971) defined three main groups of territories. The first group includes areas in Africa south of the Sahara and in southeast Asia where a rate of 5 or more per 100,000 of the population per year for males was recorded. In the second group, which includes Japan and Denmark, incidence rates from 5 to 3.1 were listed. The third group of low-incidence areas includes northern India, Australia, the Americas and most of Europe for which rates of 3 or less were given. Although strictly comparable rates are not available for Hong Kong, BELAMARIC (1969) worked out a minimum rate of 5.9 there. Primary carcinoma of the liver is also a common tumour in China generally (Chinese Medical Association, 1958). In Chinese in Singapore the incidence rate is 31 per 100,000 per year for males (SIMONS *et al.*, 1971).

Despite striking geographical variations in incidence, *racial factors* are probably of relatively minor importance in determining differences in incidence of primary liver cancer, because such differences may be found between related peoples living in different areas of the same region (ALPERT *et al.*, 1971; SHANK *et al.*, IV) and because the descendants of migrants from Africa to America show a susceptibility to liver cancer which is similar to that of native Americans and not to that of the corresponding populations remaining in Africa (KENNAWAY, 1944; ALPERT and DAVIDSON, 1969). The incidence of the congenital and infantile forms of liver cancer is probably no higher in Asia and Africa than in Europe and America, although that is difficult to establish for these rare forms of liver disease. At all events we are dealing in regions of high incidence almost exclusively with carcinomas that have the appearances of acquired neoplastic disease and with carcinomas occurring in adults and only rarely in older children. Broadly speaking this means liver-cell carcinomas and, in addition in southeast Asia cholangiocarcinomas, like those that occur in Europe and in America.

We have no good reason to suppose that the aetiology of liver cancer is the same throughout the world. Despite its wide distribution, liver cancer may be initiated by a number of different factors in the environment, each of major importance in one high-incidence region and less important or even absent in another region. Individual carcinogenic factors may possibly be combined in synergistic or additive effects in different proportions in different regions. Carcinogens that are effective only after long and continued exposure may be recognizable in the environment on routine surveys of dietary and other environmental conditions. Some carcinogens, however, are capable, in a single dose, of inducing malignancy under experimental conditions in animals. In man a single high-dosage exposure to a carcinogen in the remote past, for instance in childhood, may possibly have similar effects and this may be difficult to detect. The liver cell plays a predominant role in intermediary metabolism

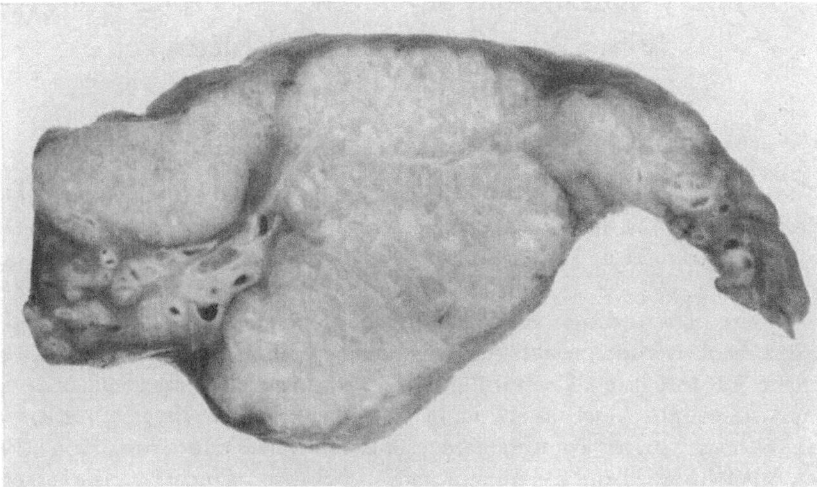

Fig. 1. Surgical left hepatectomy specimen. Mucoid cholangio-carcinoma replaces most of the lobe. In the persisting liver tissue, the bile ducts are grossly thickened by long-standing clonorchiasis; a fluke is seen as a small black fleck (lower left)

and in detoxication and the parenchymal liver cell is exposed to an exceptional extent to the direct carcinogenic effects of many absorbed substances. It is also susceptible to any carcinogenic effects of metabolites of substances which are not in themselves carcinogenic. The search for aetiological agents in the liver-cell form of cancer has accordingly been guided by the results of animal experimentation.

The other form of primary carcinoma of the liver, the *cholangiocarcinoma*, arises from bile-duct epithelium within the liver which has a much lower metabolic activity. The diazo-dye, butter yellow and some other substances are capable of inducing carcinomas of the intrahepatic biliary epithelium in experimental animals. Man may possibly be exposed to such substances occasionally, but the definition of what is probably one of the major aetiological factors in cholangiocarcinoma has been achieved by observations on human material.

In most regions where liver cancer is highly prevalent, the vast majority of the tumours are of the hepatocellular form. Hong Kong, the neighbouring city of Canton in the Kwan Tung province of China (LIANG and TUNG, 1959), Bangkok in Thailand (BHAMARAPRAVATI and VIRRANUVATTI, 1966) and doubtless other unrecorded areas in southeast Asia are unusual in that the incidence of cancer of the intra-hepatic bile ducts also is increased. In Hong Kong about 17% of primary liver cancers are of bile-duct type (GIBSON, 1971); the ratio of cholangiocarcinoma to liver-cell carcinoma is about the same as in the West (STEWART, 1931) despite the vastly increased number of liver-cell carcinomas. In the region of Taipei in Taiwan (YEH, 1965, 1966) and in Indonesia (BONNE, 1937) cholangiocarcinoma is, however, relatively rare, just as it is in Africa.

Over the years, a good deal of evidence has been collected which points to the association of intrahepatic-bile-duct carcinoma with oriental distomiasis (Fig. 1); the evidence has been reviewed recently elsewhere (GIBSON, 1971). The liver fluke responsible for infections in Japan, Korea, China and Hong Kong is *Clonorchis sinensis*; a similar species, *Opisthorchis viverrini* causes distomiasis in Thailand. Liver fluke infections are common in these countries but are very uncommon in and around Taipei, Taiwan and in Indonesia where cholangiocarcinoma is also uncommon (YEH, 1965, 1966; BONNE, 1937).

In Hong Kong, flukes are found in about 23% of cases over 2 years of age coming to autopsy at present. Infection is based on dietary habit and so is hard to prevent; it often persists for life without giving rise to serious symptoms. None of the present forms of treatment is entirely satisfactory but, from various causes, new infections are becoming less frequent than formerly (GIBSON and SUN, 1970). Cholangiocarcinoma is diagnosed in Hong Kong almost exclusively in persons over 40 years of age and so it seems that the carcinogenic action of distomiasis works slowly; most persons harbouring clonorchis die of causes other than cholangiocarcinoma.

How clonorchiasis brings about its carcinogenic effect is unknown. Possibly the secretions of the flukes contain weak carcinogens. At no stage in their development are the flukes found within the tissues proper although their metabolic products or secretions elicit an immune reaction demonstrable by precipitation tests (SUN and GIBSON, 1968) and other techniques. Various enzymes have been identified in the metabolic products (SUN and GIBSON, 1969) that enter the bile ducts of the host and evidently gain access thereafter to the immunological system. No systematic attempt has been made to isolate carcinogenic substances from these secretions and the difficulties of establishing the full life cycle of the parasite in the laboratory limit this field of investigation at present.

Oriental distomiasis is associated with a proliferation of the biliary epithelium (Fig. 2), with an enhancement of the mucus secretion and with the new formation of goblet cells in segments of the ducts in the immediate vicinity of the flukes. Changes of this kind may possibly be an intermediate stage in the development of cholangiocarcinoma. In Hong Kong this type of carcinoma in the liver is often mucin-producing and sometimes to a marked degree. The mucin produced in clonorchiasis in man and in laboratory animals appears to be the same as that produced normally in the biliary tree (CHOU and GIBSON, 1970) but it is excessive in amount and abnormal in the level of its production in the biliary passages.

The view that this type of hyperplasia and metaplasia is a premalignant change in the biliary system is supported by the fact that the lesion which is termed "cholangiofibrosis" and which is characterised by abnormal production of mucin is found in the livers of rats when certain azo-dyes or some other carcinogens have been administered to them. Mucin-secreting cholangiofibrosis has been noted by several investigators during the evolution of hepatocellular tumours in the course of experiments in carcinogenesis (OPIE, 1944; FARBER, 1956; GUPTA, 1956). In experiments with ethionine, CHOU and GIBSON (in press) found that the mucin in cholangiofibrosis is identical in histochemical reactions with that produced normally in the common bile duct of the rat. Cholangiofibrosis then may be a precursor of the bile duct tumours that sometimes occur in place of the more usual hepatocellular tumours in experimental carcinogenesis, and particularly when butter yellow is employed.

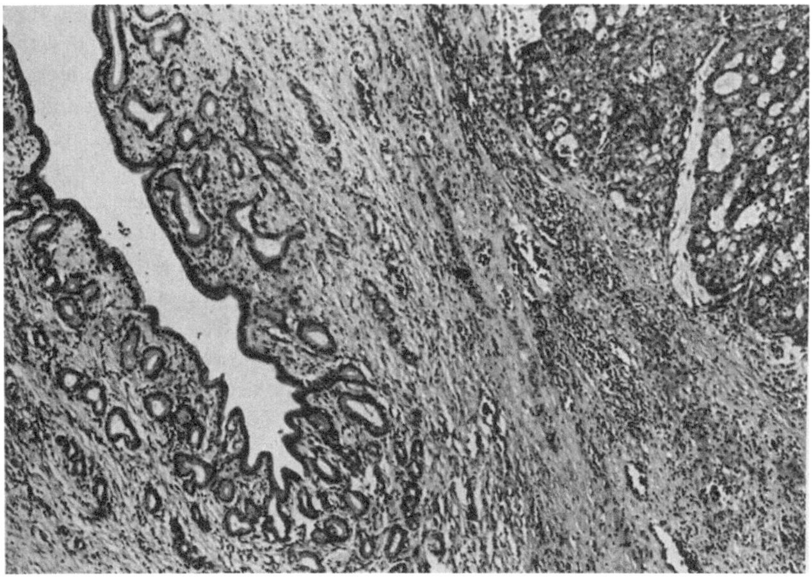

Fig. 2. Glandular proliferation and fibrous thickening in a large bile duct in long-standing clonorchiasis (left). Cholangio-carcinoma (top right) present in the neighbourhood: same case as Fig. 1. Haematoxylin and eosin; X 80

Considerably more than half of cancers of the gall bladder are associated with stones, and cholelithiasis may play a major part in the aetiology of gall bladder cancer (STEWART, 1931; HART, MODAN and SHANI, 1971). It has been suspected that gall stones contain a carcinogenic substance, but a few malignant tumours of the gall bladder have been induced in guinea pigs by procedures such as the insertion of sterile glass beads into the organ and leaving them in-situ for about 2 years (PETROV and KROTKINA, 1933). In animals which did not develop malignant tumours, polyps and other proliferations of the gall-bladder mucosa were noted. This may be compared with the epithelial proliferation and metaplasia found in the intrahepatic bile ducts harbouring *C. sinensis*, and the carcinogenic effect of that infection may have a mechanical rather than a chemical basis. The presence of stones is not apparently necessary for the induction of intrahepatic cholangiocarcinoma in man, for stones are generally absent in human clonorchiasis. Stones are encountered not uncommonly in this infection in guinea-pigs (SUN and GIBSON, 1968).

In Hong Kong, as elsewhere, *liver-cell carcinoma* is commoner than cholangiocarcinoma, and clonorchiasis, schistosomiasis and other forms of parasitism play no demonstrable part in the aetiology, either directly or indirectly through an intermediary phase of cirrhosis (GIBSON, 1971). The association of *cirrhosis* with hepatocellular carcinoma has long been established, but cirrhosis as defined by current criteria (Fifth Pan-American Congress of Gastroenterology, 1956) is not caused by parasitic diseases in Hong Kong. The sequence of cirrhosis being complicated eventually by malignancy is well documented in the West and is not in doubt. In Hong Kong, however, although cirrhosis is present in 92% of cases dying with hepatocellular carcinoma, there is very little to suggest in general, or even in individual case histories, that the cirrhosis has preceded the malignant condition. When we consider the long incubation period of malignant tumours, it seems likely that

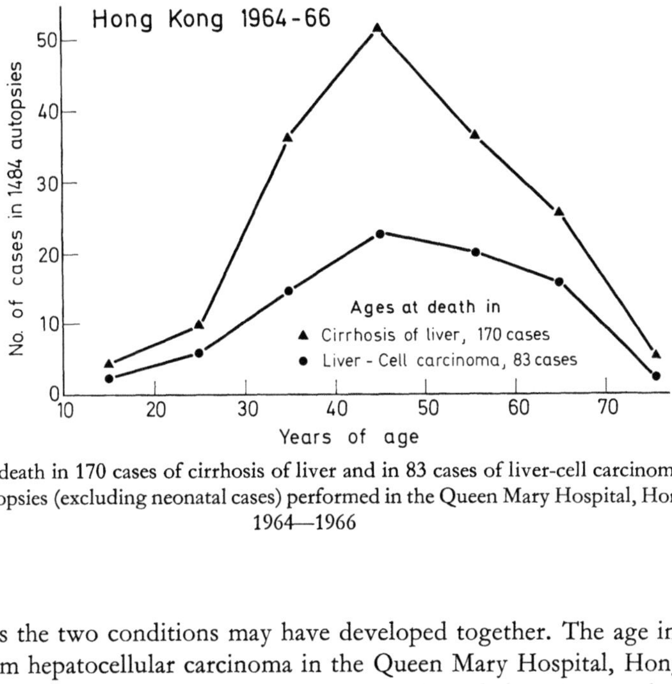


Fig. 3. Ages at death in 170 cases of cirrhosis of liver and in 83 cases of liver-cell carcinoma in 1484 consecutive autopsies (excluding neonatal cases) performed in the Queen Mary Hospital, Hong Kong, 1964—1966

in many cases the two conditions may have developed together. The age incidence of deaths from hepatocellular carcinoma in the Queen Mary Hospital, Hong Kong is very much the same as that from cirrhosis (Fig. 3) and there is a predominance of male cases in both, although this is more marked with cancer (Gibson, 1971). In the Far East generally, hepatocellular carcinoma usually runs a rapid course. For instance in Thailand death occurs in histologically proved cases on average 1.3 months after the disease is diagnosed by a physician and 4 months after the onset of symptoms; the association of cirrhosis does not affect the duration of illness (Shank *et al.*, V), and a preceding phase of illness that could be ascribed confidently to cirrhosis is, as a rule, absent.

In experiments with chemical carcinogens on rats it is common to find that effective agents can produce either cirrhosis or carcinoma or both. When diethylnitrosamine is given to young male rats, hepatocellular carcinomas are induced within a few months (Fig. 4). In some current experiments with this substance Dr. Lily Ma in our laboratory has found only a few instances in which cirrhosis was present in addition to the tumour; the cirrhosis does not appear to have preceded the carcinoma but to be an associated condition. Possibly then in searching for the cause of hepatocellular carcinoma in Hong Kong, we are searching for a cause of cirrhosis also. The association of the two conditions is too frequent to be fortuitous, but it is evidently not a simple relationship of cause and effect.

Cirrhosis in Hong Kong is not very different from that seen in other tropical locations. In most cases there is very little fat and the stigmata of alcoholism or of other nutritional factors are absent. The liver is commonly shrunken and the nodules of regeneration are rather small but the disease is progressive. There is rarely any direct evidence that infectious hepatitis has caused the cirrhosis in Hong Kong, but hepatitis is not uncommon there and acute cytolytic necrosis, usually also of unknown aetiology, is probably more frequent than in Britain.

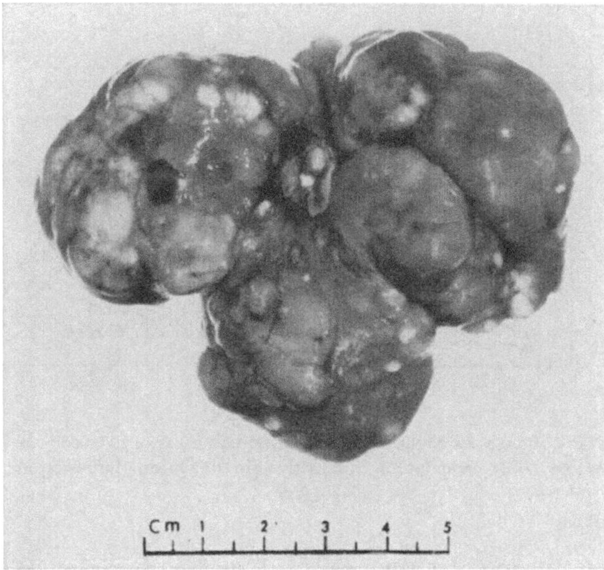


Fig. 4. Hepatocellular carcinoma in liver of 34-week-old male rat given a total of 105 mgm. of diethylnitrosamine by intraperitoneal injections from 4 to 18 weeks of age. The liver weighed 59 gm. Metastases were present in the lungs

HUTT (1971) and PRINCE (1971) have reviewed the evidence for and against the view that viral hepatitis causes cirrhosis. Discussing the "hepatitis associated" or "*Australia*" *antigen*, discovered by BLUMBERG in 1964, PRINCE (1971) concluded that "the availability of what appears to be a specific means for identification of at least a proportion of those persons who carry serum hepatitis virus chronically makes possible for the first time a controlled prospective study designed to determine the risk of chronic liver disease in such persons". Another speaker will be discussing the subject of Australia antigen but we may be permitted here to note the variability in the incidence of positive tests for Australia antigen in patients with liver carcinoma in different reports and in different parts of the world, for instance 40% in Uganda (VOGEL *et al.*, 1970) and 2.6% in Singapore Chinese (SIMONS *et al.*, 1971). The results of tests in Hong Kong (SMITH and BLUMBERG, 1969) indicate that the situation there is similar to that in Singapore Chinese. How far these differences in results reflect differences in technique or differences in the relationship of viral hepatitis to liver-cell cancer in different areas is quite uncertain. At all events, the antigen persists in the blood of some groups of patients with carcinoma as well as in some with cirrhosis, whatever its aetiological role may be. On-going research will show whether or not Australia antigen can exert an influence comparable to that of chemical substances which can produce either carcinoma or cirrhosis or both in animal experiments.

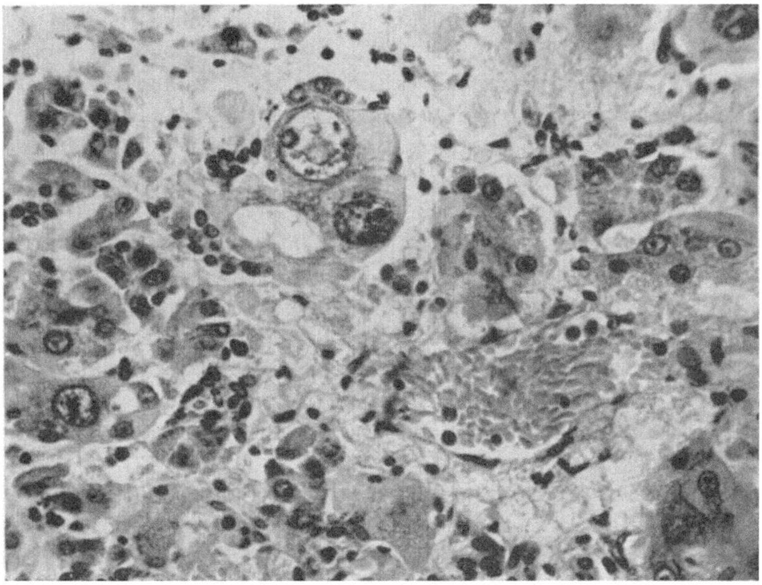

Fig. 5. Bizarre liver cells with giant nuclei, nuclear inclusions and cytoplasmic vacuolation in the centrizonal region: neighbouring liver cells have atrophied; from a male rat dying after 4 doses of 0.25 mgm. of Senecio alkaloids per kgm. Haematoxylin and eosin X 300

Many circumstances modify the effects of hepatotoxic and carcinogenic agents in animals and this may well be true of the human situation also. Carcinogens and liver toxins may have an additive effect. Environmental temperature affects the incidence of acute necrosis in dietary deficiency in rats; the incidence is greatest at higher temperatures (NAFTALIN, 1951). Young animals are more susceptible to many agents than old. PEACOCK (1957) reviewed experiments showing the influence of diet on butter-yellow carcinogenesis and similar considerations may have a bearing on human cancer. Male animals are more susceptible to many agents than females, just as male cases predominate in human cirrhosis and liver-cell cancer. In Hong Kong the predominance is 3.1:1 for cirrhosis, and 6.8:1 for carcinoma. In Thailand also there are about 6 male cases of cancer of the liver to each female one (BHAMARAPRAVATI and VIRRANUVATTI, 1966; SHANK *et al.*, V). This suggests that in the search for a causative factor in human liver cancer, we should take account of hepatotoxic elements in the environment.

Many of the present-day inhabitants of urban Hong Kong have spent long periods of their lives in a rural environment and this is true nowadays of many large cities in the tropics. SHANK and his colleagues (V) found no evidence of a difference in the incidence of primary liver cancer in the rural and the urban populations of Thailand that they surveyed. Some naturally occurring biological products such as *pyrrolizidine alkaloids* have attracted considerable attention as a source of chronic liver disease. BRAS, JELLIFFE and STUART (1954) drew attention to the association of these alkaloids present in native remedies in the West Indies with a form of acute liver disease there and SCHOENTAL, HEAD and PEACOCK (1954) and SCHOENTAL and HEAD (1957) induced liver tumours in rats with alkaloids of this type. The alkaloids may be present in milk and so can affect suckling animals (SCHOENTAL, 1959). Marked cytological abnormalities (Fig. 5) can be produced by single doses with lasiocarpine (SCHOENTAL and MAGEE, 1957) as well as subacute and chronic liver changes (SCHOENTAL and MAGEE, 1959). Pyrrolizidine alkaloids are present throughout the world in a number of plant genera as well as the genus *Senecio* in which they are most familiar in Britain, and it is possible that they are present in some of the herbal remedies so often used by persons in Hong Kong. Unfortunately, reliable information on the composition of such remedies is hard to come by. Most of the constituents are imported from unknown sources to Hong Kong and doubtless vary from time to time even in relatively standard remedies. In any case the yield and range of extractable alkaloids varies even in one species according to the time of collection and the location of growth. We are, in fact, unable to confirm or deny the importance of pyrrolizidine alkaloids in the aetiology of hepatocellular carcinoma in Hong Kong.

Another source of hepatotoxic agents is contamination of food by *toxigenic fungi* and especially of rice, the staple in the Far East. MIYAKE and colleagues (1960) investigated the effects of *Penicillium Islandicum, Sopp* present in rice imported to Japan shortly after World War II. They isolated luteoskyrin from this yellowed rice and were able to produce toxic liver injuries and cirrhosis in rats but no metastasising tumours with the substance. The discolouration imparted by the fungus is such that the contaminated material is unlikely to be eaten when better rice is available. Broken rice grains, which are particularly susceptible to contamination, are bought only by the poorer classes, but I am not aware of any data to suggest that primary liver cancer has a marked predilection for the poorer classes. This particular incident has apparently not been repeated but similar incidents involving other toxigenic fungi probably pass unrecorded in other areas of Asia from time to time and the occurrence is probably not unique.

A fungus which is commonly present in foodstuffs and which has been investigated more fully than *Penicillium* is *Aspergillus Flavus*. The potential of Aflatoxin to cause liver damage and tumours in animals is well known and several investigations have been carried out, or are still in progress, to evaluate its possible role as a cause of human liver cancer. Recently we took part in a joint project with the Massachusetts Institute of Technology to assess the degree of fungal contamination of market foodstuffs in Hong Kong in comparison with those in Thailand.

In more than 3,000 food samples from both places *A. flavus* was the commonest contaminating fungus; *A. glaucus* and species of *Penicillium*, *Fusarium* and *Rhizopus* were also encountered. Among 162 isolates, 49 proved to be toxigenic in tests on rats. A high proportion of certain foods such as rice, (51% of samples in Thailand and 40% of samples in Hong Kong) beans, peanuts and corn were contaminated by one or more species of viable fungus (SHANK *et al.*, I). Formed aflatoxins were present most frequently in peanuts and also found in some grains and other foods in Thailand. Beans of various kinds were the chief carriers of aflatoxins in Hong Kong, and aflatoxin contamination was less frequent and at lower levels than in Thailand. Rice was seldom contaminated by aflatoxins and the presence or absence of aflatoxins in the food samples did not correlate well with the fungi isolated from them at the time of collection (SHANK *et al.*, II). Evidently considerable amounts of aflatoxin can be ingested with food by the inhabitants of both countries.

SHANK and his colleagues (III) then measured the actual amounts of aflatoxin ingested with meals in 144 selected families over certain periods in three areas of Thailand and calculated the annual mean intake per kilogram of body weight per day for each individual on a family meals basis. In the Singburi area, north of Bangkok, this intake ranged from 73—81 nanograms, equivalent to 20—30% of the comparable intake values that induce a nearly 100% liver tumour incidence in rats following continuous exposure. In the Songkhla area the average annual intake was 10—14 times less than in Singburi. It is particularly noteworthy that the higher level of aflatoxin intake was found in Singburi which is reported to have a high liver-cancer incidence, while in Songkhla, where the measured intake was much lower, the incidence of liver cancer is also low (SHANK *et al.*, IV). ALPERT *et al.* (1971) found a similar situation in Uganda, where the distribution of aflatoxins in foods stored for consumption correlated with the pattern of incidence of liver cancer, in that aflatoxin contamination was greatest in areas with highest incidence of the disease.

Another speaker will be discussing aflatoxin as a possible cause of liver cancer and it would be inappropriate to refer here to any more of the extensive work that is going on in other regions of high liver-cancer incidence. At least in southeast Asia, however, it appears at present that contamination of foodstuffs with aflatoxins is likely to prove of significance in the aetiology of the disease.

Another group of carcinogenic substances that may be found in foodstuffs are the *Nitrosamines*. In a recent review of the N-nitroso compounds as a possible human health hazard, MAGEE (1970) points out that there is no published report of any animal species that is resistant to carcinogenesis by these agents and no reason to believe that man is not susceptible. Liver-cell carcinoma with a marked tendency to metastasise can be induced regularly in rats by repeated intraperitoneal injections of diethylnitrosamine (Fig. 4) or more quickly and simply by replacing their drinking water at all times with 0.0075% aqueous solution of the carcinogen. If 4-week-old males are used, liver tumours can be detected 10—20 weeks after the start of the experiment (MA; personal communication). When liver tumours are induced in monkeys with diethylnitrosamine, alpha-foetoprotein appears in the serum just as in human liver-cell cancer (HULL *et al.*, 1969).

Field studies to investigate the possibility of human exposure to nitrosamines have been few and existing analytical methods are not entirely satisfactory, but a start has been made by MCGLASHAN, WALTERS and MCLEAN (1968) who found material with the properties of nitrosamines in amounts which might well be carcinogenic in locally distilled alcoholic drinks in Zambia. This is of special interest because some of the nitrosamines are among the few carcinogens known to induce carcinoma of the oesophagus in animals and this tumour has become common in recent years in the Bantu population of Africa. In any case measurement of ingestion of nitrosamines is unlikely to reflect the effective exposure of man to these compounds. Nitrites used for food preservation can combine with secondary amines in foods to form nitrosamines at a low pH and under the conditions existing in the mammalian stomach. In reviewing this work Magee (1970) referred to studies on the formation of nitrosamines from secondary amines in the presence of nitrates by bacterial action and drew attention to the widespread occurrence of alkali nitrates in the environment. In view of the exceptionally strong carcinogenic action of some of the N-nitroso compounds in inducing carcinoma of the liver, the possibilities of their acting on the human liver should be investigated further.

## References


Alpert, M. E., Davidson, C. S.: Mycotoxins: a possible cause of primary carcinoma of the liver. Amer. J. Med. **46**, 325—329 (1969).

Alpert, M. E., Hutt, M. S. R., Wogan, G. N., Davidson, C. S.: Association between aflatoxin content of food and hepatoma frequency in Uganda. Cancer **28**, 253—260 (1971).

Belamaric, J.: Malignant tumours in Chinese. Int. J. Cancer **4**, 560—573 (1969).

Bhamarapravati, N., Virranuvatti, V.: Liver diseases in Thailand: an analysis of liver biopsies. Amer. J. Gastroent. **45**, 267—275 (1966).

Blumberg, B. S.: Polymorphisms of serum proteins and the development of isoprecipitins in transfused patients. Bull. Acad. Med. (N.Y.) **40**, 377 (1964).

Bonne, C.: Cancer and human races. Amer. J. Cancer **30**, 435—454 (1937).

Bras, G., Jelliffe, D. B., Stuart, K. L.: Veno-occlusive disease of the liver with nonportal type of cirrhosis, occurring in Jamaica. Arch. Path. (Chicago) **57**, 285—300 (1954).

Chinese Medical Association: Society of Pathology and Departments of Pathology of 38 Medical Colleges and Hospitals: statistical analysis of 1,979 autopsies of malignant diesase. Chin. J. Path. **4**, 174—181 (1958), (in Chinese).

Chou, S. T., Gibson, J. B.: The histochemistry of biliary mucins and the changes caused by infestation with *Clonorchis sinensis*. J. Path. **101**, 185—197 (1970).

Chou, S. T., Gibson, J. B.: A comparative histochemical study of rat livers in alpha-naphthyl-isothiocyanate (ANIT) and DL-Ethionine intoxication. In press.

Doll, R., Payne, P., Waterhouse, J.: Cancer Incidence in Five Continents. U.I.C.C. publication. Berlin-Heidelberg-New York: Springer 1966.

Fifth Pan-American Congress of Gastroenterology: La Habana, Cuba, January 20—27, 1956. Report of the Board for classification and nomenclature of cirrhosis of the liver. Gastroenterology **31**, 213—216 (1956).

Farber, E.: Carcinoma of the liver in rats fed ethionine. Arch. Path. **62**, 445—454 (1956).

Gibson, J. B., Sun, T.: Clonorchiasis. In: Pathology of Protozoal and Helminthic Diseases. Ed. R. A. Marcial-Rojas. Baltimore: Williams and Wilkins 1970, pp. 546—566.

Gibson, J. B.: Parasites, liver disease and liver cancer. In: Liver Cancer. I.A.R.C. Scientific Publications, No. 1. Lyon: International Agency for Research on Cancer 1971, pp. 42—50.

Gupta, D. N.: Nodular cirrhosis and metastasising tumours produced in the liver of rats by prolonged feeding with thioacetamide. J. Path. Bact. **72**, 415—426 (1956).

Hart, J., Modan, B., Shani, M.: Cholelithiasis in the aetiology of gall bladder neoplasms. Lancet **1971 I**, 1151—1153.

Hull, E. W., Carbone, P. P., Gitlin, D., O'Gara, R. W., Kelly, M. G.: Alpha-foetoprotein in monkeys with hepatoma. J. nat. Cancer Inst. **42**, 1035 (1969).

Hutt, M. S. R.: Epidemiology of human primary liver cancer. In: Liver Cancer. I.A.R.C. Scientific Publications, No. 1. Lyon: International Agency for Research on Cancer 1971, pp. 21—29.

KENNAWAY, E. L.: Cancer of the liver in the negro in Africa and in America. Cancer Res. **4**, 571—577 (1944).

LIANG, P. C., TUNG, C.: Morphologic study and etiology of primary liver carcinoma and its incidence in China. Chin. med. J. **79**, 336—347 (1959).

MA, LILY: Personal communication, 1971.

MCGLASHAN, N. D., WALTERS, C. L., MCLEAN, A.E.M.: Nitrosamines in African spirits and oesophageal cancer. Lancet **1968 II**, 1017.

MAGEE, P. N.: Toxicity of nitrosamines: their possible human health hazard. Fd. Cosmet. Toxicol. **9**, 207—218 (1970).

MIYAKE, M., SAITO, M., ENOMOTO, M., SHIKATA, T., ISHIKO, T., URAGUCHI, K., SAKAI, F., TATSUNO, T., TSUKIOKA, M., SAKAI, Y.: Toxic liver injuries and liver cirrhosis induced in mice and rats through long-term feeding with Penicillium Islandicum, Sopp growing rice. Acta path. jap. **10**, 75—123 (1960).

NAFTALIN, J. M.: Interactions between environment and diet in the production of acute liver necrosis in the rat. J. Path. Bact. **63**, 649—666 (1951).

OPIE, E. L.: The pathogenesis of tumors of the liver produced by butter yellow. J. exp. Med. **80**, 231—246 (1944).

PEACOCK, P. R.: Carcinogenesis. In: Cancer; ed. R. W. RAVEN, Vol. I. London: Butterworth & Co. 1957, p. 65.

PETROV, N., KROTKINA, N.: Experimentelles Gallenblasen- und Lebercarcinom. Z. Krebsforsch. **38**, 249—263 (1933).

PRINCE, A. F.: Role of viruses in chronic liver disease in man an animals. In: Liver Cancer. I.A.R.C. Scientific Publications, No. 1. Lyon: International Agency for Research on Cancer 1971, pp. 51 to 57.

SCHOENTAL, R.: Liver lesions in young rats suckled by mothers treated with the pyrrolizidine (senecio) alkaloids, lasiocarpine and retrorsine. J. Path. Bact. **77**, 485—496 (1959).

SCHOENTAL, R., HEAD, M. A., PEACOCK, P. R.: Senecio alkaloids; primary liver tumours in rats as a result of treatment with (1) a mixture of alkaloids from S. Jacobea, lin.: (2) Retrorsine: (3) Isatidine. Brit. J. Cancer **8**, 458—465 (1954).

SCHOENTAL, R., HEAD, M. A.: Progression of liver lesions produced in rats by temporary treatment with pyrrolizidine (senecio) alkaloids and the effects of betaine and high casein diet. Brit. J. Cancer **11**, 535—544 (1957).

SCHOENTAL, R., MAGEE, P. N.: Chronic liver changes in rats after a single dose of lasiocarpine, a pyrrolizidine (senecio) alkaloid. J. Path. Bact. **74**, 305—319 (1957).

SCHOENTAL, R., MAGEE, P. N.: Further observations on the subacute and chronic liver changes in rats after a single dose of various pyrrolizidine (senecio) alkaloids. J. Path. Bact. **78**, 471—482 (1959).

SHANK, R. C., WOGAN, G. N., GIBSON, J. B.: Dietary aflatoxins and human liver cancer. I. Toxigenic molds in foods and foodstuffs of tropical Southeast Asia. Fd. Cosmet. Toxicol., (in press).

SHANK, R. C., WOGAN, G. N., GIBSON, J. B., NONDASUTA, A.: Dietary aflatoxins and human liver cancer. II. Aflatoxins in market foods and foodstuffs of Thailand and Hong Kong. Fd. Cosmet. Toxicol., (in press).

SHANK, R. C., GORDON, J. E., WOGAN, G. N., NONDASUTA, A., SUBHAMANI, B.: Dietary aflatoxins and human liver cancer. III. Field survey of rural Thai families for ingested aflatoxins. Fd. Cosmet. Toxicol., (in press).

SHANK, R. C., GORDON, J.E., WOGAN, G. N., BHAMARAPRAVATI, N.: Dietary aflatoxins and human liver cancer. IV. Incidence of primary liver cancer in two municipal populations of Thailand. Fd. Cosmet. Toxicol., (in press).

SHANK, R. C., GORDON, J. E., WOGAN, G. N., SIDDHICHAI, P., SUBHAMANI, B., BHAMARAPRAVATI, N.: Dietary aflatoxins and human liver cancer. V. Duration of primary liver cancer and prevalence of hepatomegaly in Thailand. Fd. Cosmet. Toxicol., (in press).

SIMONS, M. J., YAP, E. H., YU, M., SEAH, C. S., CHEW, B. K., FUNG, W. P., TAM, A. Y. O., SHAMUGARATNAM, K.: Australia antigen in Singapore Chinese patients with hepatocellular carcinoma. Lancet **1971 I**, 1149—1151.

Smith, J. B., Blumberg, B. S.: Viral Hepatitis, Postnecrotic Cirrhosis and Hepatocellular Carcinoma. Lancet **1969 II**, 953.

Sun, T., Gibson, J. B.: Antigens of Clonorchis sinensis in experimental and human infections: an analysis by gel-diffusion technique. Amer. J. trop. Med. Hyg. **18**, 241—252 (1968).

Sun, T., Gibson, J. B.: Metabolic products of adult Clonorchis sinensis: their composition and antigenic potential. J. Helminth. **43**, 395—402 (1969).

Stewart, M. J.: Precancerous lesions of the alimentary tract. Lancet **1931 II**, 565—572, 617—622, 669—674.

Vogel, C. L., Anthony, P. P., Mody, N., Barker, L. F.: Hepatitis associated Antigen in Ugandan patients with hepatocellular carcinoma. Lancet **1970 II**, 622—624.

Yeh, S.: Some geographic pathology aspects of common diseases in Taiwan. Part I and II. Int. Pathology **6**, 81—85 (1965); **7**, 24—28 (1965 and 1966).

# Recent Techniques and Hypotheses in the Epidemiology of Liver Cancer

A. J. Tuyns

International Agency for Research on Cancer, Lyon, France

## Introduction

Primary liver cancer, which can be so easily provoked in laboratory animals by a variety of chemical agents, is not a common disease in man, except in Africa. Although spontaneous primary hepatoma is rare in Western Europe and in the United States, it is commonly observed in Asia and Latin America and is exceedingly frequent in some parts of Africa.

There are various hypotheses which seem to be consistent with the observed distribution of liver cancer throughout the world; yet the possibilities of testing these hypotheses are limited. At a recent symposium held in Kampala, Uganda, these hypotheses were reviewed in the light of available experimental and clinical evidence. It was agreed that the two best hypotheses at present in the African context were:

a) food contamination—by aflatoxin or other mycotoxins, and

b) viral hepatitis.

Whether these agents directly cause cell damage leading to cancer, or whether there is an intermediate phase of cirrhosis, is still debatable; whether these two agents can, independently, provoke liver cancer in man, or whether they need to be associated, is still unknown. Fig. 1 summarizes the present position.

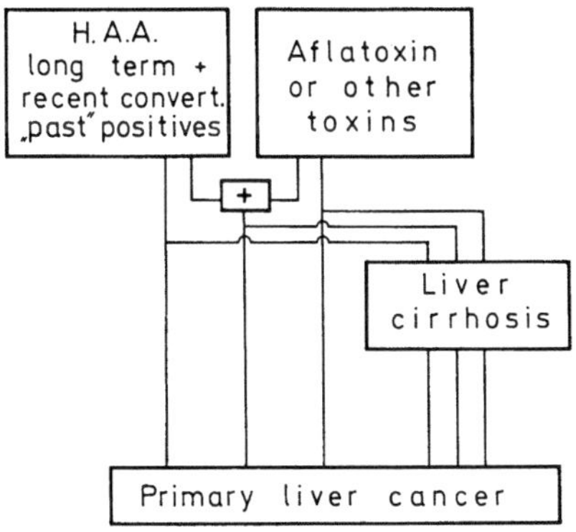


Fig. 1

A number of studies have provided arguments in favour of, or against the role of each of these agents. Most of them are experimental and clinical. So far, there is no good epidemiological evidence of a causal relationship between any of these agents and liver cancer in man.

Epidemiological studies on the subject are difficult, particularly in Africa; they are hampered by major difficulties in obtaining adequate measurement of occurrence of the disease and of exposure to any one of the suspected agents.

However, recent developments have provided new tools for such investigations. The purpose of this paper is to discuss the application of some new techniques in field studies and to describe some of the work that the International Agency for Research on Cancer has initiated in this context.

## The Use of the Alpha-foetoprotein Test as a Tool for Diagnosing Primary Hepatoma and for Measuring the Frequency of the Disease

### 1. Alpha-foetoprotein (AFP) and Primary Liver Cancer

In 1963, Abelev [1] described the presence of an alpha-foetoglobulin in the serum of mice with hepatoma. Tatarinov [2], one year later, demonstrated the presence of a similar protein in human patients with spontaneous primary hepatoma and suggested that it might be used as a diagnostic procedure. Preliminary studies in USSR and Dakar (where primary liver cancer is particularly frequent), indicated that the new serologic test was, indeed, of a great interest.

On these premises, a comprehensive study was set up by IARC for the evaluation of the test, in seven places throughout the world. Sera were collected from 231 patients with primary hepatoma and from 555 controls. Testing was performed blindly and independently by three investigators and the results reviewed by a group of those who participated in the study [3]. Alpha-foetoprotein was found in 75% of patients with histologically confirmed hepatoma. A careful analysis of 12 false positives revealed that two referred to teratocarcinoma of testicles and that, for the ten others, liver cancer could not be excluded on the basis of the information available. It was concluded that the test was highly specific for liver cancer and that its use "in epidemiologic surveys should provide information on the natural history of embryonic antigen production in liver cancer and its relevance to suspected aetiologic factors".

### 2. Use of the Alpha-foetoprotein Test as a Diagnostic Tool in Population Surveys

A survey was set up by IARC in Dakar to examine approximately 10000 male adults working in the main factories of the city. In the course of 1969 these individuals were enrolled and bled for the detection of alpha-foetoprotein. Further collections of sera took place at four-monthly intervals for a total duration of two years. Various local difficulties imposed changes in the original planning and some groups were dropped and replaced by groups of the Senegalese army. In addition, it became clear after the third bleeding that too much insistence in obtaining blood samples might result in losing substantial numbers of individuals under study. As follow-up information was considered more important than the actual testing, every effort was made to keep track of individuals. By the end of the study, the percentage of bleedings had dropped considerably, but the figure for losses at sight was minimal and did not exceed 4%.

The discovery of nine cases of primary hepatomas in the study population indicated that detection, based on a screening campaign, is feasible and that it permits a direct measurement of occurrence of the disease. The computation of an accurate incidence rate will require a precise determination of the population at risk in terms of years of observation; this work is under way. It is possible to state, even at this stage, however, that the annual crude incidence rate in this adult male study population is not inferior to 45 per 100000. For technical reasons, this rate may be regarded as the most accurate ever obtained in Africa.

## 3. Alpha-foetoprotein and Clinical Development of Liver Cancer

1. The relationship between the presence of AFP in the sera of hospitalized patients with a hepatoma and the various clinical, anatomical and histological characteristics of the tumour, have been thoroughly investigated by the Dakar group [4]. The following parameters were investigated: age, clinical form (tumoral, versus malignant cirrhotic type), volume of tumour, weight of tumour, duration of evolution, various histological criteria (differentiation, cellular necrosis, intrahepatic thrombosis, cholostasis, aspect of extra-tumoral tissue). For each parameter examined, the proportion of alpha-foetoprotein positives was roughly the same. By no existing criterion can the "positive" tumours be distinguished from the "negative". There were cases who were first negative and then became positive in the course of the disease. In a few exceptional cases, the test was occasionally negative after a long period of positivity, but this could be ascribed to a temporary drop in the titre of antigen present.

2. The analysis of our nine cases provided some additional information [5] on the relation in time between appearance of alpha-foetuin in the serum and that of clinical symptoms. Our material differs from the other series published so far, by the way in which cases were identified *either* by a positive blood test *or* by the appearance of clinical signs, while, in the other series, the cases under study were always hospitalized cases, i.e. cases which had already developed clinical signs. By definition, these cases could be studied as to simultaneous presence of AFP or as to ulterior development of such a positivity, but could not provide information on AFP positivity preceding clinical signs.

In our Dakar population study, three cases were picked up by the serological test *before* the appearance of clinical symptoms; the six other cases were detected either by traditional consultation for liver symptoms or at the clinical examination organized within the study for checking the absentees; three of the latter cases developed AFP positivity in the course of the disease, two refused hospitalization and could not be further investigated and one remained negative until he died.

In one of the three cases identified by the AFP test only, in the absence of symptoms, a laparotomy was performed; a small cancer was found in the left liver lobe which was removed. The patient, however, died one month later with generalized metastases.

The respective proportions of hepatomas with and without alpha-foetoprotein (6 cases positive versus one negative and two unknown) are in line with previous clinical studies. One new finding is that in three of the six positives, alpha-foetoprotein was present in the serum before the appearance of clinical symptoms. This adds a time dimension to the relationship between clinical symptoms and presence of AFP in the blood.

The lack of parallelism between volume of the tumour and production of AFP is already known. This is confirmed by our Dakar study since, in three cases the tumour was not clinically detectable while AFP was already present. These observations are in agreement with the experimental work of Gusev and Engelhardt [6], who showed that in human hepatomas, only certain cells are capable of producing AFP and that the proportion of these cells is independent of size and extension of the tumoral tissue.

3. A practical implication of all these findings is that some hepatomas never produce AFP; some others do produce AFP at a stage where the clinical development of the tumour excludes any therapeutic measure. There are hepatomas, however, which start producing AFP at an early stage of their development; in such cases the search for AFP may be considered as a valid detection technique [5]. Even though we obviously failed in our study to alter the course of the disease, the theoretical possibility of picking up very early cases which might be saved by surgery or other therapeutic measures is not unlikely. It is, further, not unreasonable to assume that more sensitive methods of determination may permit detection at an even earlier stage. Whether this assumption is true is now being tested using sera collected in another population survey which IARC is carrying out in Ivory Coast.

As to using AFP testing as a public health screening technique, it would be premature to recommend it for the time being. This, however, may have to be re-evaluated if we ever succeed in determing selective high risk groups.

## Food Contamination by Aflatoxin and Other Mycotoxins as an Agent of Liver Cancer in Man

This hypothesis is based on strong laboratory evidence. Human exposures were difficult to estimate until recently. Dr. C. A. Linsell and Dr. F. Peers in the IARC Regional Centre in Nairobi, Kenya, have solved this technical problem; they have carried out a field survey which is described separately by their authors [7].

## The Hepatitis Associated Antigen (H. A. A.)

In Africa, liver hepatoma is often associated with liver cirrhosis [8]. It has also been shown that acute hepatitis may be a cause of cirrhosis [9]. Hepatitis has been claimed to create liver damage which may develop into cancer with or without passing through the stage of cirrhosis, but this theory, which has been defended by the Dakar Group as early as in 1953 [8] could not be adequately documented as long as acute hepatitis was a clinical concept subject to considerable individual variation. With the discovery of the Australia antigen—now commonly referred to as Hepatitis associated antigen (H.A.A.)—which seems to be closely related with infectious hepatitis at least in Africa, the situation has changed.

This is not the place to discuss the uncertainties as to the nature of H.A.A., its relationship to the various types of infectious hepatitis, the significance of the presence of H.A.A. in the sera of healthy individuals, nor the difficulties in comparing results obtained by authors using different techniques. For the purpose of the present paper what matters is that we now have a tool permitting an objective detection in man of an antigen related to hepatitis.

There is evidence that the prevalence of H.A.A. positives is much higher in Africa where liver cancer is common, than in the Western world. There is also concurrent evidence that the H.A.A. is much more frequently present in the sera of patients with hepatoma than in control groups; this was found independently by two groups of investigators working on Ugandese [10] material and on Dakar [11] material respectively. More recently, the same finding was reported from Singapore [12].

Although this type of association may simply indicate a greater susceptibility of hepatoma patients to H.A.A., or alterations of their immunological response to the antigen, it is, nevertheless, consistent with the hypothesis that chronic carriers of H.A.A. are at greater risk for liver cancer.

To decide between the two possibilities, one has to know the sequence of events in time. If we want to test the hypothesis of H.A.A. carriers being at greater risk for liver cancer, then we have to design a prospective study, by which this increased risk can be demonstrated. The problem is to define suitable groups of chronic H.A.A. carriers and control groups, and to organize the follow-up so as to measure risks of developing cirrhosis and/or liver cancer in both groups. However, before embarking on such a study, which is likely to be a long-term one, it is necessary to know more about some basic epidemiologic features of the "H.A.A. disease".

Surprisingly enough, very little is known about the basic epidemiology of "H.A.A. disease" in Africans. Available prevalence data refer to highly selected groups (blood donors, hospital patients, the army etc.) and there are no data on H.A.A. prevalence in a normal African population, and a forciori, no data on incidence and conversion, which imply repeating bleedings at regular intervals of time. We are not even sure that there are such people as "chronic carriers" and, if they do, in fact, exist, how they can be defined in terms of time (duration). Such basic information is, of course, a prerequisite to defining a potential high risk group of H.A.A. carriers, as opposed to normal or negative groups, which would serve for a further prospective study.

IARC is now engaged in such preliminary work, using sera collected in two representative groups of population in the Ivory Coast. This was primarily designed as a liver cancer detection study based on the AFP test; it differs from the Dakar study in that it refers to a rural population with little medical facilities, apart from the visiting teams who collect the blood. Another major difference refers to the unselective nature of the study population, which is made of representative samples of people living in the two main components of the country, i.e. the Savanna in the North and the tropical forest in the South. In addition food samples are collected in the study areas for the measurement of aflatoxin. Aliquots from the sera are stored and constitute adequate material for the determination of prevalence and incidence of H.A.A.

Once this basic work is done, and provided we find it possible to define chronic H.A.A. carriers, then it will become possible to plan the prospective study mentioned previously. This study would enable us to clarify the respective relationships of liver cirrhosis and of liver cancer to viral hepatitis and to aflatoxin exposure.

## Conclusion

New techniques have recently become available for detecting liver cancer, for measuring aflatoxin in food, and for detecting H.A.A. in the serum. These techniques lend themselves to use in field studies. It has now become possible to measure liver cancer occurrence, exposure to aflatoxin and to H.A.A. in population studies; thus, adequate epidemiological investigation can now be designed for testing the two major hypotheses on the aetiology of liver cancer in Africa. Several such studies have already been initiated by IARC in Africa and more are under preparation.

Considering the time and effort that so many investigators have already spent in studying unsuccessfully liver cancer in Africa over the last 25 years, it would be a sound investment to start as soon as possible the prospective studies that are needed. Even though it may take a long time—perhaps 10 to 12 years—to get answers, at least by that time we, or our successors, would have valid answers.

## References

1. ABELEV, G. I., PEROVA, S., KHRAMKOVA, N., POSTNIKOVA, Z., IRLIN, I.: Production of embryonal α-globulin by transplantable mouse hepatomas. Transplant. Bull. **1**, 174—180 (1963).
2. TATARINOV, Y.: Detection of embryospecific α-globulin in the blood sera of patients with primary liver tumors. Vopr. Med. Chimii **10**, 90—91 (1964).
3. O'CONOR, G. T., TATARINOV, Y., ABELEV, G. I., URIEL, J.: A collaborative study for the evaluation of a serologic test for primary liver cancer. Cancer **25**, 1091—1098 (1970).
4. MASSEYEFF, R., SANKALE, M., ONDE, M., MENYE, A., CAMAIN, R., QUENUM, C., MAYDAT, L., MATTERN, P., ANCELLE, J. P., LEBLANC, L.: Valeur de la recherche de l'Alpha-1-foetoprotéine sérique pour le diagnostic du cancer primitif du foie. Bull. Soc. méd. Afr. noire Langue franç. **13**, 537—548 (1968).
5. TUYNS, A., LEBLANC, L.: Primary liver cancer: time relationship between appearance of alpha-foetoprotein in the serum and clinical symptoms. (In press.)
6. GOUSSEV, A. I., ENGELHARDT, N. V., MASSEYEFF, R., CAMAIN, R., BASTERIS, B.: Immunofluorescent study of alpha-foetoprotein in liver and liver tumours. II localisation of AFP in the tissues of patients with primary liver cancer. Int. J. Cancer **7**, 207—217 (1971).
7. LINSELL, C. A.: The Aflatoxins and Human Liver Cancer. (This Volume).
8. Symposium on primary cancer of the liver in Africa, Kampala, 1956. Acta UICC **13**, 515—975 (1957).
9. CHARMOT, G., CAMAIN, R., GIUDICELLI, P.: Place de l'hépatite épidémique ictérigène dans l'étiologie des cirrhoses tropicales. Bull. Soc. Path. exot. **46**, 847—860 (1953).
10. VOGEL, CH. L., ANTHONY, P. P., MODY, N., BARKER, L. F.: Hepatitis-associated antigen in Ugandan patients with hepatocellular carcinoma. Lancet **1970**, II, 621—624.
11. PRINCE, A. M., LEBLANC, L., KROHN, K., MASSEYEFF, R., ALPERT, M. E.: S.H. antigen and chronic liver disease. Lancet **1970**, II, 7675, 717—718.
12. SIMONS, M. J.: Personal communication.

# The Aflatoxins and Human Liver Cancer

C. A. LINSELL and F. G. PEERS

Nairobi Regional Centre International Agency for Research on Cancer, Nairobi, Kenya

The possible role of natural and synthetic chemical carcinogens in the aetiology of human liver cancer has been reviewed recently by MAGEE (1971). The synthetic chemical carcinogens generally have little relation to the situation in man and remain laboratory shelf carcinogens with the interesting exception of the nitrosamines. The possibilities among the natural carcinogens, however, appears more promising and the pyrrolizidine alkaloids from Senecio and Crotalaria plants, the glycosides from the cycads, the toxic agents from rice contaminated by Penicillium islandicum, and the aflatoxins from the Aspergillus moulds have been the subject of much endeavour during the last decade.

The aflatoxins are metabolites of certain strains of Aspergillus flavus and their isolation following fatalities in 1960 among domestic birds and fish is now a familiar story. The possible association with human liver disease was first made by LE BRETON (1962) soon after the isolation of the toxin and was later expanded by OETTLE (1965) who, reviewing the aetiology of hepatocellular cancer particularly in relation to the African situation, considered that the mycotoxin hypothesis fitted the data better than any other. The known areas of high incidence are those where bad storage of dietary staples can provide the critical microclimate for propagation of the mould and elaboration of the toxin. The first isolations were from groundnuts and whilst these remain a natural substrate of choice, the aflatoxins are readily found on corn, wheat, soya beans, rice and other crops. Contamination of market samples and home-stored dietary staples in Africa, potential sources of human consumption, has been reported (ALPERT, 1968; COADY, 1965). In late 1968, the Nairobi Regional Centre of the International Agency for Research on Cancer decided to design field studies to test the possible association of the aflatoxin and human liver cancer. After preliminary dietary surveys and field feasibility trials, a study area in Kenya—the Murang'a district of the Central Province—was chosen for the initial project. It was decided that the project must be based on the examination of food ready for ingestion as preliminary studies showed that rejection of patently mouldy food during the pre-cook sorting of cereals by the housewife was considerable. To enable the exposure levels and cancer rates to be compared with other areas, the study was based on a defined population. It was decided to limit the chemical analysis to the aflatoxins as sensitive and reliable methods for other mycotoxins such as sterigmatocystin, a metabolite of Aspergillus versicolor, were not available when the study started. However, to enable the samples to be examined for other mycotoxins or chemical carcinogens at a later date, they were stored at —30 °C.

The principal questions posed by this study were:

1. Were the aflatoxins ingested by the study population or was there marked loss of available toxin following food selection or cooking?

2. Was there any evidence that this possible exposure was seasonal and were occasional high levels available?

3. Could an association be shown between exposure levels and liver cancer data within the study area?

4. Could a consistent dose response relationship be demonstrated?

5. Would it be possible to remove the potential carcinogen and show a fall in the cancer rate?

The details of the Murang'a project will be reported elsewhere but briefly, households were randomised and samples of food ready for ingestion and home-brewed beers were collected over a period of eighteen months. The specimens were frozen and examined in our Nairobi laboratory for the aflatoxins, using thin-layer chromatography. Cancer registration particularly directed towards liver cancer was intensified, using the existing medical services. The introduction of the alpha-foeto protein test as a diagnostic aid greatly assisted this part of the study. To assess possible differences of aflatoxin levels within the Murang'a district, the study area was divided geographically into three altitude areas which offered varying opportunities for mould proliferation.

The main conclusions of the Murang'a study were:

1. Aflatoxin is ingested and can be measured in mixed food samples.

2. There was no seasonal effect on levels nor were occasional high levels detected in this study area.

3. The association between aflatoxin exposure levels and liver cancer data within the Murang'a district was sufficiently significant to justify further registration of cancer cases in the study area.

4. These field studies show that it is feasible to test the proposed relationship in rural populations and that using the same methodology, studies in areas with a similar cancer incidence to test the consistency of the relationship and further studies in areas with widely different incidence to test the strength of a dose/response relationship are justified.

5. Provided that the technical difficulties of collection of a representative sample of food and those associated with laboratory methods are overcome, the limiting factor of accuracy of such studies is the collection of cancer data.

6. It is considered that the possibility of removing aflatoxin from the Murang'a environment is remote but urbanisation with changes in food habits and the sources and storage of cereals may greatly reduce risk.

Currently, work on these lines is continuing in the Ivory Coast and a number of other areas are under consideration, and some proposed studies have reached the stage of preliminary feasibility surveys and field planning.

These studies, comparing exposure levels and cancer incidence, assume that the mechanism of the role the aflatoxins will play in human cancer is similar to that demonstrated so clearly in animal experiments—a dose response relationship of chronic ingestion effective at such low levels as to enable us to label it the most potent rate hepatocarcinogen known. Our experience in Africa leads us to believe that chronic ingestion might also be possible in man and, of course, could be associated with other factors such as have been proposed over the years.

The most interesting of these at the moment is hepatitis which, having some association with the Australia antigen, gives us a better opportunity to assess its role in the aetiology of liver cancer.

The possibility that cellular regeneration associated with chronic hepatitis and cirrhosis may provide susceptible targets for the action of aflatoxin has some experimental support, notably that the effects of the aflatoxins on DNA and RNA synthesis is greater in regenerating than normal liver—DE RECONDO *et al.* (1966)—and this obviously should receive attention when designing studies on man.

However, we must not neglect the important possibility raised by the work of CARNAGHAN (1967) who showed that tumours could be produced in rats after a period as long as two years following a single dose.

There is an increased susceptibility of the new-born or young animals to some chemical hepatocarcinogens, even to the extent in some cases of the agent being incapable of producing tumours in the adult animal. Although it has been shown by WOGAN (1966) that age has an effect on the susceptibility of animals to aflatoxin, little is known of the susceptibility of man to mycotoxins and with an agent showing such a wide range of toxicity and carcinogenicity as aflatoxin between and even within species, it is perhaps unwise to speculate. However, is it practical in terms of the acceptability of contaminated food to suggest that doses near an assumed toxic range could be ingested by man? If one accepts that man's susceptibility will be similar to monkeys and the primates, then the toxicity demonstrated by SVOBODA *et al.* (1966) in monkeys and our own observations in Nairobi on baboons suggest an approximately LD 50 of 3 mg/kg. Could foodstuffs be contaminated at levels to give this exposure and still be acceptable to man? It is considered unlikely in adults but possible in young children, particularly if groundnuts form a large part of the diet. With this in mind, reports of fatal cases of acute hepatitis in children associated, for some reason, with toxic rather than infectious agents, become of interest as fatal cases may represent only a small proportion of those exposed to such toxins.

The "Labrea Hepatitis" in children reported from remote regions of the Amazon was thought by DE PAOLA (1968), who has experience in liver pathology of virus infections of South America, to have a toxic aetiology.

SERCK-HANSSEN (1970) reported from Uganda a case of fatal hepatitis where available food in the patient's home showed contamination by aflatoxin at a level of 1.7 mg/kg.

A high incidence of encephalopathy and acute fatty degeneration of the viscera in children has been reported from Thailand (OLSON *et al.*, 1970). In some of these cases food heavily contaminated by aflatoxin was found in the children's home. The clinical course and pathological findings were compatible with Reye's syndrome (BOURGEOIS *et al.*, 1969 and 1971), and had remarkable similarity to the pathology of acute aflatoxin poisoning in monkey experiments by the same authors using aflatoxin produced by fungi grown from food samples from the Thai children's homes.

Material from an epidemic of hepatitis in Lourenco Marques Mozambique, an area where the highest incidence of hepatocellular cancer in the world has been reported, was reviewed by TORRES *et al.* (1970) and 44% of the epidemic cases and

25% of routine hepatitis biopsies gave rise to discussion as to whether the lesions were of toxic rather than infective origin. Again, the authors draw, for histological comparison, on considerable material from their animal experiments using the mycotoxin, sterigmatocystin, which has a similar chemical structure to aflatoxin and which has been shown to be carcinogenic (PURCHASE, 1968).

All the above authors are rightly cautious in interpreting the liver lesions as definitely of toxic origin. The difficulties of doing this on morphological grounds alone are well-known, as the liver pathology of viral infections varies so widely and as some drugs such as ipronaizid and halothane are said to produce a hepatitis-like microscopic picture. However, the supporting evidence of available mycotoxins and the similarity of toxic lesions in animal experiments would make an examination of the environment of doubtful cases valuable in areas of the world where mycotoxin contamination is likely.

It should also be recalled that the clinical symptoms of liver failure in children can be confusing as convulsions, screaming and mania followed by coma are common and jaundice may be absent. In areas poorly served by medical services, such symptoms could well result in a diagnosis of encephalitis or malaria. The suggestion, therefore, of whether the role of aflatoxin in some cases of liver cancer could be a near-lethal dose in childhood needs further study. It may well be that the background exposure to continuous small doses or even the same dose which would cause symptoms in children is tolerated by adults and it is only those children exposed to doses sufficient to modify the template activity of DNA who are a high-risk group for liver cancer in later life. Careful follow-up of cases, fortunately few in number, where children are known to have consumed aflatoxin-contaminated food may also offer valuable information.

In summary, therefore, we are still faced with the familiar problem of relating lesions produced in the rat liver to the possible situation in man. Even if we can show an association between levels of aflatoxin exposure in communities and liver cancer rates, we shall be confronted by the problems of the individual selection of cancer victims and by the ill-understood mechanisms of tumour production. Any solution of this problem certainly calls for continued correlation of laboratory and field research.

The possibility of contamination of dietary staples by the mycotoxins may frustrate exports and prevent use of available food resources in parts of the world where both of these may be vital. Therefore, the solution of whether aflatoxin is associated with human liver cancer is not only an intriguing epidemiological problem and a study which can elucidate some of the mechanisms of liver cancer but is a far-reaching economic problem for developing countries and an important issue for supplementary food programmes for children of such countries. It requires not only the resources of the chemist and the pathologist using the epidemiological method but of domestic science, crop husbandry, food storage and sociology which are, perhaps, less commonly involved in cancer research.

## References

ALPERT, M. E., DAVIDSON, C. S., WOGAN, G. N.: Gastroenterology **54**, 49 (1968).

BOURGEOSIS, C. H., KESCHAMRAS, N., COMER, D. S., HARIKUL, S., EVANS, H., OLSON, L., SMITH, T., BEEK, M. R.: J. med. Ass. Thailand **52**, 553 (1969).

BOURGEOIS, C. H., SHANK, R. C., GROSSMANN, R. A., JOHNSON, D. O., WOODING, W. L., CHANDAVIMOL, P.: Lab. Invest. **24**, 206 (1971).
CARNAGHAN, R. B. A.: Brit. J. Cancer **21**, 811 (1967).
COADY, A.: Ethiopian M. J. **3**, 173 (1965).
DE PAOLA, D., STRANO, A. J., HOPPS, H. C.: Int. Path. **9**, 43 (1968).
DE RECONDO, A. M., FRAYSSINET, C., LAFARGE, C., LE BRETON, E.: Biochim. biophys. Acta. (Amst.) **119**, 322 (1966).
LE BRETON, E., FRAYSSINET, C., BOY, J.: C. R. Acad. Sci. (Paris) **255**, 784 (1962).
MAGEE, P. N.: I.A.R.C. Publication **1**, 110 (1971).
OETTLE, A. G.: S. Afr. med. J. **39**, 817 (1965).
OLSON, L. C., BOURGEOIS, C., COTTON, R., HARIKUL, S., GROSSMANN, R., SMITH, T.: Amer. J. Dis. Child. **120**, 1 (1970).
PURCHASE, I. F. H., VAN DER WATT, J. J.: Fd. Cosmet. Toxicol. **6**, 555 (1968).
SERCK-Hanssen, A.: Arch. Environm. Hlth. **20**, 729 (1970).
SVOBODA, D., GRADY, H., HIGGINSON, J.: Amer. J. Path. **49**, 6 (1966).
TORRES, F. O., PURCHASE, I. F. H., VAN DER WATT, J. J.: J. Path. **102**, 163 (1970).
WOGAN, G. N.: Bact. Rev. **30**, 460 (1966).

# Latent Carcinoma of the Prostate

IVAR LIAVÅG, THORSTEIN B. HARBITZ, and OLAV A. HAUGEN

Diakonissehusets Hospital, Department of Surgery and Ulleval Hospital, Department of Pathology, Oslo, Norway

Carcinoma of the prostate is defined as *latent* when it is detected at autopsy or in surgical specimens from patients in whom carcinoma was clinically not suspected. When symptoms and/or signs have aroused suspicion of prostatic malignancy, the term *clinically manifest* carcinoma of the prostate is used.

Carcinoma of the prostate is now the most frequent form of cancer among Norwegian men, accounting for 19 per cent of all new cases of malignant neoplasms in men in the period 1964—1966 (The Cancer Registry of Norway, 1969). The annual number of new cases of prostatic carcinoma has increased from 708 in 1960 to about 900 in 1970. This increasing number of registered cases is mainly due to an increase in the mean age of the male population during this period (PEDERSEN, 1971). During the last 10 to 15 years, the age-specific incidence rates of prostatic carcinoma in men under 70 years of age have remained nearly constant. After this age, however, there has been a slight increase. There are reasons to believe that this increased incidence can be ascribed to improvement in diagnosis and higher autopsy rates.

There is a great discrepancy between the occurrence of latent and clinically manifest carcinoma of the prostate. At autopsy, prostatic carcinoma is frequently found in elderly men, whereas prostatic carcinoma as a cause of death is relatively rare. However, in patients with clinically manifest carcinoma of the prostate, there is a high risk of subsequent death from the malignancy: Within a mean of two and a half years after the diagnosis is made, three fourths of the patients are dead (JOHNSON, 1962).

From the study of latent carcinoma, information can be obtained about the natural history of prostatic carcinoma and the relation between histological pattern and clinical course.

## Histological Criteria of Prostatic Carcinoma

The generally accepted criteria of malignancy should also be applied in the diagnosis of latent prostatic carcinoma. The evidence of malignancy is based on an evaluation of 1) cellular irregularities, 2) atypical glandular structures and 3) tissue invasion. Absolute criteria of malignancy are 1) invasion of perineural spaces, 2) invasion of blood vessels, 3) local or capsular invasion and 4) periprostatic invasion or distant metastases. In latent carcinoma of the prostate it may be difficult to tell whether true local or capsular invasion is present. When conclusive invasive properties can not be recognized, the structures should not be regarded as carcinomas. For these lesions we suggest the term *atypical glandular proliferations.*

## Frequency of Latent Prostatic Carcinoma

Several autopsy and biopsy studies of prostatic carcinoma have been carried out in Norway during the last decade (Table 1). In two autopsy series of patients 40 years old or more, latent carcinoma was found in 26.5 and 32.0 per cent, respectively. The age-specific prevalence of latent carcinoma in these studies is similar to that reported from Denmark (STARKLINT, 1950), Great Britain (FRANKS, 1954), U.S.A. (BUTLER, BRAUNSTEIN, FREIMAN and GALL, 1959) and Japan (KARUBE, 1961; OOTA, 1961). On the other hand, the death rates of prostatic carcinoma in Japan differ significantly from those in the aforementioned countries (WYNDER, MABUCHI and WHITMORE, 1971).

The frequency of latent carcinoma is substantially higher in autopsy than in biopsy series (Table 1). In three Norwegian series of patients treated for urinary obstruction, the percentage of latent carcinoma (stage I) varied from 1.2 to 4.8 (Table 1). The lower frequency of latent carcinoma in biopsy material is mainly due to the fact that transurethral or open prostatectomy leaves the peripheral parts of the gland behind in which carcinoma is likely to occur.

Table 1. Frequency of latent prostatic carcinoma in autopsy and biopsy series of Norwegian men

| Authors | Material | No. of cases | No. with carcinoma | % |
|---|---|---|---|---|
| LIAVÅG (1967) | Autopsy | 340 | 90 | 26.5 |
| HARBITZ and HAUGEN (1971 a) | Autopsy | 206 | 66 | 32.0 |
| JOHNSON (1962) | Biopsy | 1434 | 17 | 1.2 |
| ANDERSEN (1959, 1971) | Biopsy | 6189 | 142 | 2.3 |
| MILLER and SELJELID (1971) | Biopsy | 566 | 27 | 4.8 |

Table 2. Occurrence of prostatic carcinoma in Norwegian men operated on for urinary obstruction

| Authors | No. of cases | Prostatic carcinoma | % | Latent carcinoma [a] |
|---|---|---|---|---|
| JOHNSON (1962) | 1434 | 139 | 9.7 | 12.2 |
| ANDERSEN (1959, 1971) | 6189 | 796 | 12.9 | 17.8 |
| MILLER and SELJELID (1971) | 3636 | 427 | 11.7 | 30.0 |

[a] In % of all prostatic carcinomas.

In biopsy series, the occurrence of latent carcinomas as percentage of all prostatic carcinomas ranged from 12.2 to 30 per cent (Table 2). BOJSEN (1961) found that the percentage reported in the literature showed a similar variation, though in most series latent carcinoma accounted for about 10 per cent of all prostatic carcinomas. The variation in the reported frequency of latent carcinoma in biopsy series is probably mostly due to differences in the diagnostic ability of the surgeons and different histological criteria of cancer.

In an autopsy study (HARBITZ and HAUGEN, 1971 a), atypical glandular proliferations were found in 10 per cent of the prostates studied. MILLER and SELJELID (1971) observed marked or slight atypical glandular proliferation in 8.1 per cent of cases operated on for urinary obstruction. Of 100 cases (2.8 per cent) with marked atypia which were followed for 7 years after the operation, 4 died from prostatic carcinoma within 5 years. The significance of these atypical structures is not clear, but they might represent premalignant lesions.

## Relationship between Prostatic Carcinoma and Age

The frequency of latent carcinoma found at autopsy increases with age, approaching 50 per cent in patients 80 years old or more (Table 3). The age-specific incidence rates of all prostatic carcinomas also increase steadily with age (The Cancer Registry of Norway, 1969).

Table 3. Occurrence of latent prostatic carcinoma by age in an autopsy series (LIAVÅG, 1967)

| Age | No. of autopsies | No. with carcinoma | % |
|---|---|---|---|
| 40—49 | 25 | 2 | 8.0 |
| 50—59 | 54 | 11 | 20.0 |
| 60—69 | 122 | 28 | 23.0 |
| 70—79 | 91 | 26 | 28.6 |
| 80—89 | 45 | 21 | 46.7 |
| 90—99 | 3 | 2 | 66.7 |
| Total | 340 | 90 | 26.5 |

In an autopsy study, LIAVÅG (1967) found that the weight of prostates with latent carcinoma or benign hyperplasia increased steadily with age. After the age of 60, prostates with latent carcinoma weighed significantly more than those showing benign hyperplasia only (Fig. 1). The weight of the latent carcinoma itself also

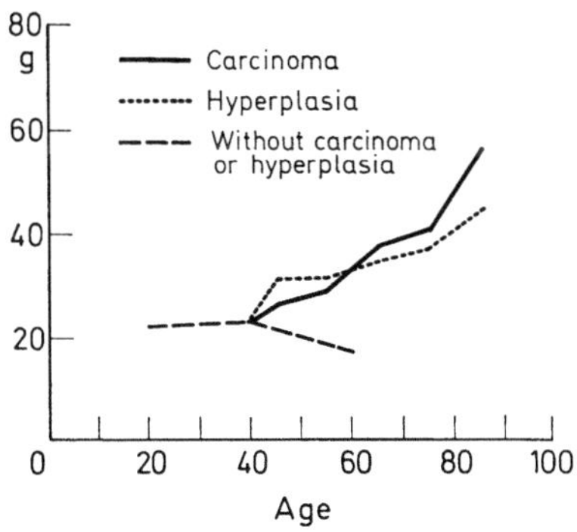


Fig. 1. Mean weight of prostates without carcinoma or hyperplasia, with benign hyperplasia, or with latent carcinoma in relation to age of the patients (LIAVÅG, 1967)

increased with age to a peak in the eighth decade (Fig. 2). Furthermore, the frequency of cellular atypia and undifferentiated growth in glands with latent carcinoma increased with age (Table 4). These findings are supported by other autopsy studies (STARKLINT, 1950; LUNDBERG and BERGE, 1970). Hence, large tumours are associated with marked cellular atypia and a high frequency of undifferentiated growth. These observations are probably of importance in the treatment of patients with carcinoma of the prostate.

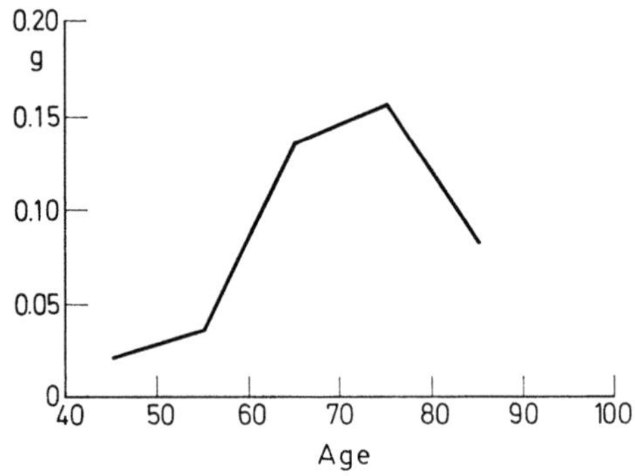


Fig. 2. Mean weights of 83 latent carcinomas in relation to age of the patients (LIAVÅG, 1967)

Table 4. Frequency of undifferentiated growth in latent prostatic carcinoma by age (LIAVÅG, 1967)

| Age | No. of prostates | | |
|---|---|---|---|
| | With carcinoma | With undiff. growth | % |
| 40—49 | 2 | 0 | 0.0 |
| 50—59 | 11 | 2 | 18.2 |
| 60—69 | 28 | 8 | 28.6 |
| 70—79 | 26 | 13 | 50.0 |
| 80+ | 23 | 10 | 43.5 |
| Total | 90 | 33 | 36.7 |

## Etiology and Pathogenesis

The etiology of carcinoma of the prostate is unknown, and several pathogenetic factors are probably involved.

There is strong evidence in support of a causal relationship between local atrophy and the development of prostatic carcinoma (for ref. see LIAVÅG, 1968). The local atrophy frequently seen with advancing age may be induced by inflammation, nutritional deficiencies and local ischemia. However, in an autopsy study, marked prostatitis was not more frequent in glands with latent carcinoma than in non-carcinomatous glands (LIAVÅG, 1967). In a study on blood flow of the prostate measured by means of the hydrogen polarography method, there was no significant difference in mean flow in glands with carcinoma and benign hyperplasia (HAFFNER and LIAVÅG, 1969).

Based on clinical observations (HUGGINS, STEVENS and HODGES, 1941), morphological studies of endocrine organs (SOMMERS, 1957) and biochemical analyses of human plasma and urine (BULBROOK, FRANKS and GREENWOOD, 1959; STERN, HOPKINS, WEINER and MARMORSTON, 1964) the concept of some form of endocrine imbalance in patients with prostatic carcinoma has gained wide acceptance. However, further studies in man are needed to evaluate the role of certain endocrine glands for the development of prostatic malignancy.

In an autopsy series of Norwegian men, studies of the pituitary gland, the adrenal glands, the testicles and the prostate are in progress (HARBITZ and HAUGEN, 1971b). The preliminary results indicate further evidence for structural differences in the endocrine glands of men with benign nodular hyperplasia or latent carcinoma of the prostate. Before the age of 70 years, men with latent prostatic carcinoma had significantly lower mean testicular weights than patients with benign nodular hyperplasia. On the other hand, the latter showed a significant decrease of mean testicular weights with age, whereas no such decrease was found in patients with latent carcinoma of the prostate. The mean pituitary weights were about the same in latent carcinoma and in benign hyperplasia. Patients with latent carcinoma showed a higher frequency of small pituitary adenomata. The mean adrenal weight in patients with latent carcinoma which was not accompanied by benign hyperplasia was significantly higher than in patients with prostates showing benign hyperplasia only.

The incidence of prostatic carcinoma is higher in Western than in Eastern Europe, in U.S. Negroes compared with African Negroes, and in Japanese immigrants to the United States compared with native Japanese (WYNDER, MABUCHI and WHITMORE, 1971). This strongly suggests that environmental factors play a role in the pathogenesis of prostatic carcinoma.

It has recently been shown in rats and men that there is a selective uptake of androgen by the prostate. Further, the demonstration of androphilic macromolecules in prostatic tissue indicates the presence of specific androgenic receptors in the prostate (TVETER, 1970; TVETER, UNHJEM, ATTRAMADAL, AAKVAAG and HANSSON, 1970). It has already been shown that certain compounds inhibit the action of testosterone by competing for androgenic receptors in the prostate (TVETER, 1970 for ref.). It is therefore possible that certain environmental factors might inhibit or enhance the action of testosterone in the prostate.

## Histological Relationship between Latent and Manifest Prostatic Carcinoma

In a previous study by STARKLINT (1950), no histological differences between latent and manifest carcinoma of the prostate could be demonstrated. In our studies, the same histological types were observed both in latent and in clinically manifest prostatic carcinomas. However, the frequency of undifferentiated tumours were higher, and cellular atypia more marked in manifest than in latent carcinomas. Dedifferentiation was found to increase with the size of the tumour. Latent carcinomas were usually small, whereas the manifest carcinomas were large, commonly involving the whole prostate. Thus, the structures of latent and manifest prostatic carcinomas were essentially the same, but differences in size, differentiation and cellular atypia were present.

## Biological Relationship between Latent and Manifest Prostatic Carcinoma

The question whether latent prostatic carcinoma may develop into clinically manifest carcinoma is of great interest.

In an autopsy study (Liavåg, 1967) of patients previously subjected to prostatic surgery for urinary obstruction, latent prostatic carcinoma had been diagnosed in 3 patients at the time of operation. Within a course of 5 to 18 years they all died with manifest carcinoma of the prostate. The clinical course or latent prostatic carcinoma was studied in two series by Bauer, McGavran and Carlin (1960) and Miller and Seljelid (1971). Within 13 and 7 years, respectively, after the diagnosis was made, about 30 per cent of the patients were dead from prostatic carcinoma. Small and well differentiated lesions had a more favourable prognosis than large and poorly differentiated tumours.

It seems justified to conclude that latent carcinomas have the histological characteristics and biological properties of manifest carcinomas. However, the majority of latent carcinomas are small, well differentiated and slowly growing tumours in old men, and no further treatment is required.

Prostatic cancer in advanced stages is only amenable to palliative treatment. Our aim should therefore be to diagnose these tumours in an early stage before they have progressed beyond the scope of radical cure. When the age of the patient and the histological pattern of the tumour indicate an unfavourable prognosis, radical treatment is only possible when the cancer remains within the confines of the prostate. On the other hand, when manifestations of the carcinoma are unlikely to appear, a wait and see attitude should be adopted.

## References

Andersen, R.: Carcinoma of the prostate. Clinical observations and treatment. Acta chir. scand. Suppl. **246**, pp. 74 (1959).

Andersen, R.: Personal communication, 1971.

Bauer, W. C., McGavran, M. H., Carlin, M. R.: Unsuspected carcinoma of the prostate in suprapubic prostatectomy specimens. A clinicopathological study of 55 consecutive cases. Cancer **13**, 370—378 (1960).

Bojsen, F. K.: Om cancer prostatae. Köbenhavn: Munksgaard 1961, pp. 193.

Bulbrook, R. D., Franks, L. M., Greenwood, F. C.: Hormone excretion in prostatic cancer: An attempt to correlate urinary hormone excretion and clinical state. Brit. J. Cancer **13**, 45—58 (1959).

Butler, J., Braunstein, H., Freiman, D. G., Gall, E. A.: Incidence, distribution, and enzymatic activity of carcinoma of the prostate gland. Arch. Path. **68**, 243—251 (1959).

Franks, L. M.: Latent carcinoma of the prostate. J. Path. Bact. **68**, 603—616 (1954).

Haffner, J. F. W., Liavåg, I.: Blood flow of the hyperplastic and neoplastic human prostate measured by hydrogen polarography. Scand. J. Urol. Nephrol. **3**, 271—275 (1969).

Harbitz, T. B., Haugen, O. A.: 1971 a; 1971 b. To be published.

Huggins, C., Stevens, R. E., Jr., Hodges, C. V.: Studies on prostatic cancer. II. The effect of castration on advanced carcinoma of the prostate gland. Arch. Surg. **43**, 209—223 (1941).

Johnson, J. A.: Histological diagnosis and prognosis in patients operated upon for prostatic obstruction. Acta chir. scand. Suppl. **286**, pp. 25 (1962).

KARUBE, K.: Study of latent carcinoma of the prostate in the Japanese based on necropsy material. Tohoku J. exp. Med. **74**, 265—285 (1961).

LIAVÅG, I.: Carcinoma of the prostate. Oslo: Universitetsforlaget 1967, pp. 151.

LIAVÅG, I.: Atrophy and regeneration in the pathogenesis of prostatic carcinoma. Acta path. microbiol. scand. **73**, 338 —350 (1968).

LUNDBERG, S., BERGE, T.: Prostatic carcinoma. An autopsy study. Scand. J. Urol. Nephrol. **4**, 93—97 (1970).

MILLER, A., SELJELID, R.: Cellular atypia in the prostate. Scand. J. Urol. Nephrol. **5**, 17—21 (1971).

OOTA, K.: Latent carcinoma of the prostate among the Japanese. Acta. Un. int. Cancer **17**, 952—957 (1961).

PEDERSEN, E.: Personal communication, 1971.

SOMMERS, S. C.: Endocrine changes with prostatic carcinoma. Cancer **10**, 345—358 (1957).

STARKLINT, H.: Undersögelser over latent og manifest prostatacancer. Köbenhavn: Munksgaard 1950, pp. 130.

STERN, E., HOPKINS, C. E., WEINER, J. M., MARMORSTON, J.: Hormone excretion patterns in breast and prostate cancer are abnormal. Science **145**, 716—719 (1964).

The Cancer Registry of Norway: Cancer registration in Norway. The incidence of cancer in Norway 1964—1966. Oslo 1969.

TVETER, K. J.: Studies on selective uptake and metabolism of testosterone-$^3$H in the prostate and the seminal vesicles of the rat. Oslo: Universitetsforlaget 1970.

TVETER, K. J., UNHJEM, O., ATTRAMADAL, A., AAKVAAG, A., HANSSON, V.: Androgenic receptors in rat and human prostate. Adv. Biosci. **7**, 193—207 (1970).

WYNDER, E. L., MABUCHI, K., WHITMORE, W. F., Jr.: Epidemiology of cancer of the prostate. Cancer **28**, 344—360 (1971).

# Mortality and Morbidity of Prostatic Carcinoma

G. DHOM and M. HOHBACH

Pathologisches Institut der Universität des Saarlandes, Homburg/Saar, Germany

Prostatic carcinoma and its importance on the aging man have been occupying pathologists around the world for a long time. We therefore would like to make some comments regarding morbidity and mortality from the point of view of the pathologist engaged in routine diagnostic pathology. We want in particular to discuss the question of morbidity as the statistician and epidemiologist are relying primarly upon the histologic finding of the pathologist.

We owe to MUIR and NECTOUX (1971) a world-wide review on figures on mortality and morbidity of prostatic carcinoma. These figures show a considerable variation (Fig. 1). The highest age-adjusted morbidity-rate is found among the black population

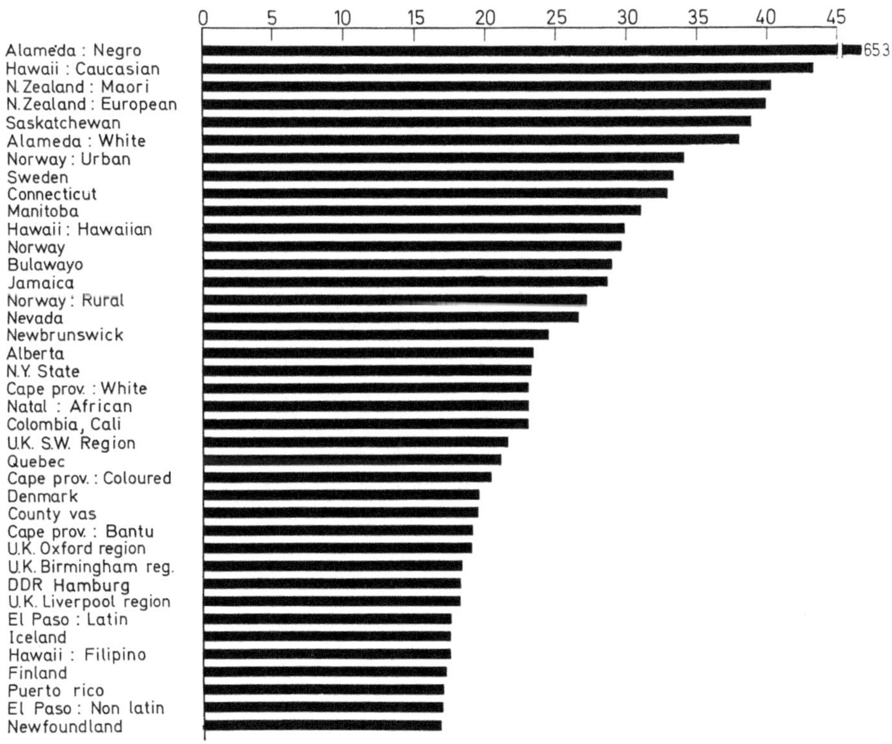


Fig. 1a

of Alameda/California, the lowest among the oriental population of Singapore. Among the European countries (Fig. 2) Norway and Sweden are way at the top with a morbidity rate of 34.1 and 33.5 respectively, it is even higher among the urban population of Norway as compared to rural population. Among the other European countries we see a gradual but significantly increasing incidence from East to West as well as a lower incidence in some rural areas compared with urban population.

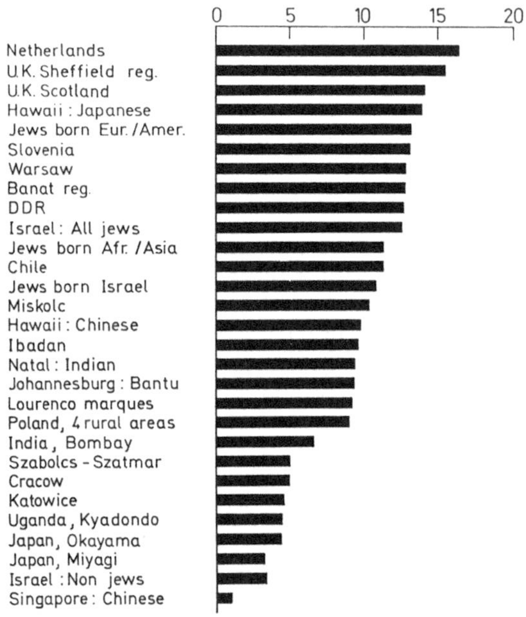


Fig. 1b

The figures on mortality of prostatic carcinoma in general follow this pattern. Again the coloured population of the USA is at the top with a rate of 21.9, followed by South Africa, Sweden and Norway. By far the lowest figures are again found in the oriental countries of Japan, the Philippines, and Taiwan.

The factors that cause these extreme differences of incidence of prostatic carcinomas are today still completely unclear. KING and others (1963) compiled a few (Table 1). Age certainly is of major significance, all other factors must up to now be considered as either quite uncertain or questionable regarding their significance for prostatic carcinoma.

May I add at this point some figures from the Saarland, the small state in which our department is located. Aside from Hamburg it is the only state in the Federal Republic that has its own cancer registry. The age distribution of the male population above 40 years of age (Fig. 3) is quite similar to that of the standard population of the USA, this age group accounts for 36% of the total male population compared to 34.8% in the USA. The annual mortality rate of men rises from 0.53% among the 40 to 50 years group to 31% in those over 90 years. 1139 men died of cancer—exclud-

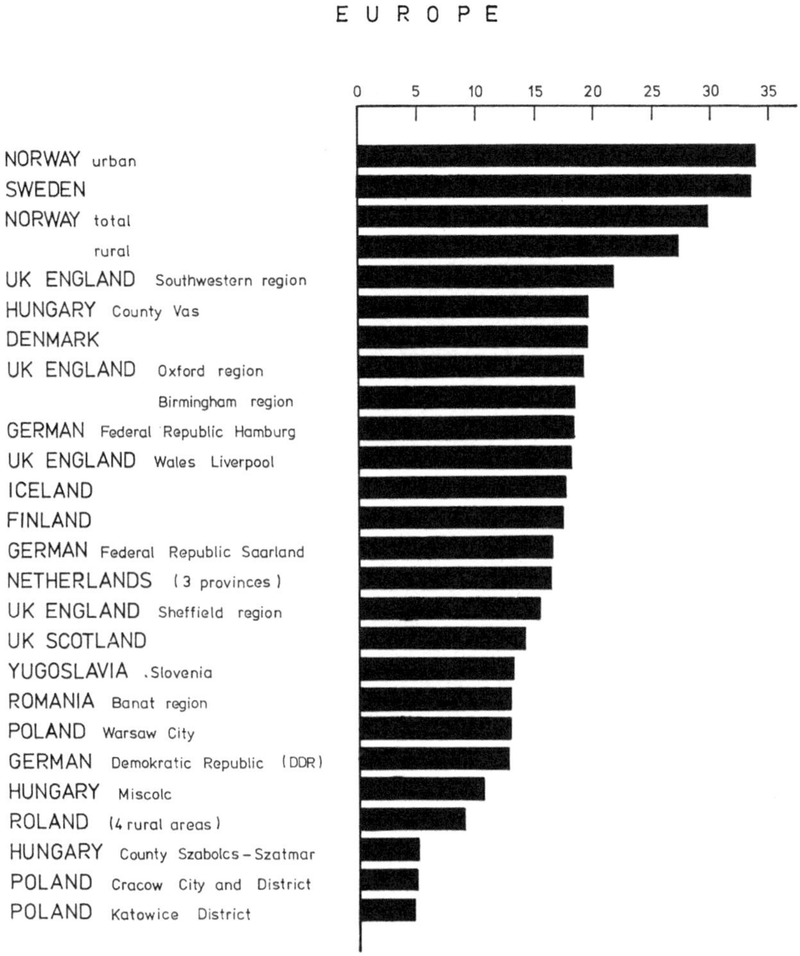


Fig. 2. Age adjusted morbidity rates for prostate cancer

ing diseases of the hemopoetic system. The mortality from carcinoma in general therefore is 18% after 40 years of age or 0.5% of all living men over 40 years of age. Prostatic carcinoma accounts for 7.4% of this cancer mortality. Up to 90 years of age this incidence of prostatic carcinoma is increasing to more than 20 %. Fig. 4 shows the relative frequency of prostatic carcinoma among the 7 most common localisations of cancer for the years 1966 to 1968. Prostatic carcinoma ranks 3rd both in men alive with cancer and those that died.

These raw figures tell nothing about the particular epidemiology of prostatic carcinoma, and I would like to show now, how very much we are still at the first stage of an epidemiologic study, that is to determine the true frequency of prostatic carcinoma in our population.

In conducting such an epidemiologic study of prostatic carcinomas there are obstacles that are certainly harder to tackle than would be the case in cancer of other localisations. For most cancers there is a correlation between the frequency

Table 1. Summary of factors associated with cancers of the prostate and male genital organes (King *et al.*, 1963)

| Factor | Type of Association |
|---|---|
| Age | Geometrical increase from the critical age (40—50) to upper limits of life |
| Race | Higher frequency among Negroes than among whites since 1940's; low frequency among Orientals and Indians; higher frequency among Japanese Americans than among Japanese in Japan |
| Geographic area | Higher northern than southern frequency among whites and nonwhites; low mortality differential between urban and rural areas and between metropolitan and non-metropolitan counties |
| Nativity | Lower frequency among foreign than native-born whites; higher frequency among migrants than among residents of the country of origin |
| Religion | Frequency highest among Protestants, lowest among Jews and intermediate among Catholics; higher frequency among Occidental than among Oriental populations in Israel |
| Marital status | Higher frequency among the ever married than among single persons, particularly the widowed and divorced, and among the married with children; higher urban than rural frequency among the married |
| Socio-economic status | Generally no regular socio-economic gradient; high frequency among professionals, low frequency among manual workers, agricultural workers, miners, and clerical and kindred workers. (The numbers in most occupational groups are small) |
| Familial aggregation | High frequency among male relatives of prostatic cancer decedents |

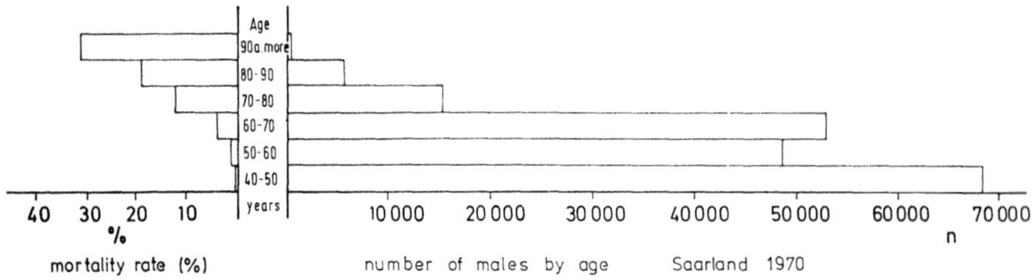


Fig. 3

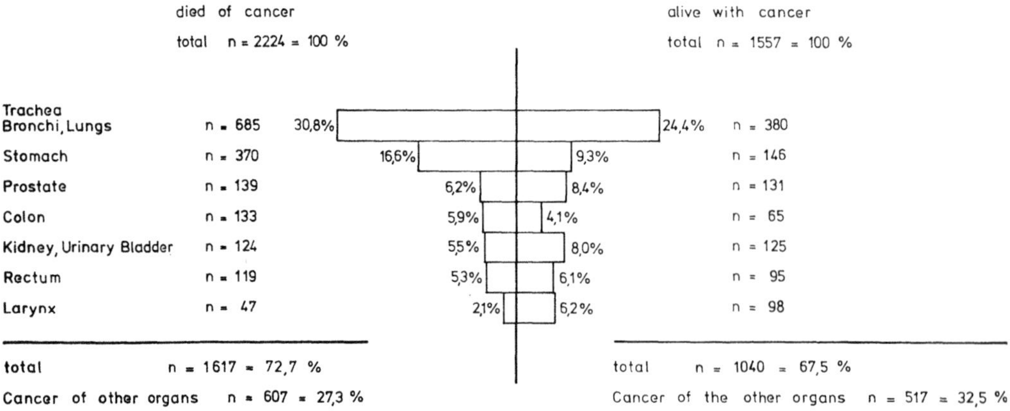


Fig. 4. Morbidity and mortality of cancer. Males 1. 6. 66 — 31. 12. 68 (Source: Statistisches Amt des Saarlandes)

of clinical, bioptic and autoptic findings. Prostatic carcinoma, however, is found in series of rountine autopsies 8 times more frequently than would be expected from the rate of mortality of prostatic carcinoma (ASHLEY, 1965). This is to be explained on the basis of the very variable degree of biologic malignancy. Latent cancerous foci grow very slowly in the prostate, their size and frequency is therefore primarly related to age (FRANKS, 1954; 1956). In most cases, death interrupts the natural history of this tumor. LIAVÅG (1967) found among 103 prostatic carcinomas only 13 that had been diagnosed during live. Assuming an incidence of 30% of latent prostatic carcinoma in males over 50, we would arrive at a figure of around 58,000 men with latent prostatic carcinoma in our small state, the Saarland. In 1970 92 cases of carcinoma were discovered clinically and histologically, and 83 deaths from prostatic carcinoma were registered. This would mean, that during this year 0.3% of the men that can be suspected as having a latent carcinoma either died of or showed clinical manifestations of prostatic carcinoma. We shall see that this figure is not the real incidence of carcinomas that can be detected clinically, but that we shall have to expect higher numbers. The epidemiologist and statistician, however, in evaluating their data, have to take into consideration the unfortunate fact, that two processes of different malignant potential appear in statistics lumped under the single designation of carcinoma:

1. Latent carcinoma with slow growth and low malignant potential.
2. Carcinomas that can be detected clinically, with locally infiltrating growth and metastases and therefore high malignant potential.

When as pathologists we discover a clinically unsuspected carcinoma in surgical material—according to MOSTOFI (1970) this happens in about 14% of BPH-prostatectomies—we generally do not know, whether we are dealing with a tumor of high or low malignant potential.

The epidemiology—and especially the figures for morbidity—of prostatic carcinoma are therefore significantly influenced by the difficulties of clinical detection and histologic verification.

The mortality rate in addition is influenced by the autopsy rate as prostatic carcinoma often will impress clinically as metastasising cancer with unknown primary and such cases of course can only be detected at autopsy.

The main factors which influence the morbidity rate are:

1. Number of older men that had a physical examination.
2. Experience of the clinician.
3. Type of bioptic procedure.
4. Uniform evaluation of histologic findings.

Now that a systematic cancer prevention program for detection of rectal and prostatic carcinoma in males has been initiated in the Federal Republic, an ever increasing number of rectally palpable prostatic carcinomas will be discovered, that otherwise would have remained among the large group of unsuspected carcinomas. The mere propagation of rectal examination will therefore increase the rate of morbidity. Until a short time ago, rectal examination was widely considered as sufficient for a diagnosis of cancer. Now we demand with good reason histologic verification of a suspected carcinoma. The rate at which prostatic carcinoma is included in a biopsy specimen, depends upon the methods employed.

TUR specimens will include only such prostatic carcinomas that already have progressed pretty far towards the center or the rare cases, that start in the center. 65% of the cancers, however, are located in the posterior parts of the gland and 20% in the peripheral parts of the lateral lobes (Fig. 5). Smaller carcinomatous foci are therefore not included in TUR specimens. It was only after the introduction of punch and aspiration biopsy techniques that it was possible to detect these tumors without radical procedures. Here I want to show with some figures from the years 1968 to 1971 how the incidence of cancer in the surgical material of a pathology department is shifted on account of introduction of these methods. The Fig. 6 shows, arranged according to age, our biopsy material of TUR's and prostatectomies. Each column represents an age group of one year. In 1971 the months January to September have been evaluated.

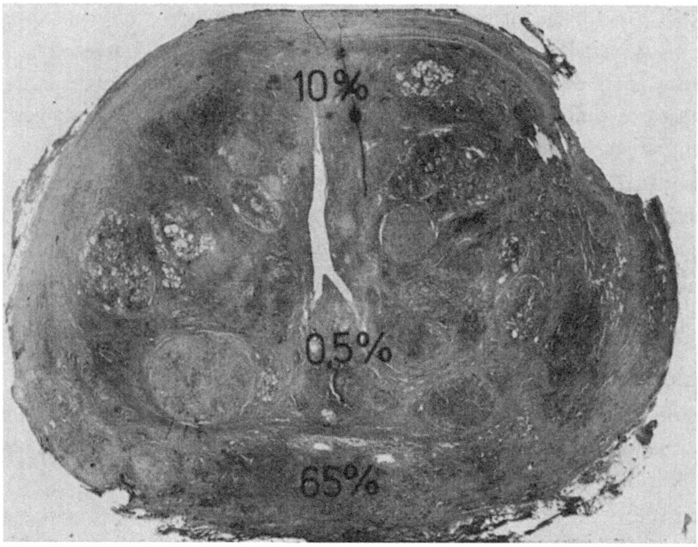


Fig. 5

Among the higher age groups too the incidence of carcinoma is low, among a total of 764 tissue samples it is 12%. The material from needle-biopsies on the other hand (Fig. 7) gives a quite different picture. There has been a marked increase in the number of biopsies especially among those patients between 50 and 70 years of age. There is no significant increase in the numbers of carcinomas detected in the two lower age groups. The highest incidence of carcinoma is found among the groups between 60 and 70 years of age. We found 104 carcinomas out of a total of 285 biopsies. These are 36% of the cases or 3 times the number of what was detected in material from TUR's (Table 2).

The well-known increasing incidence of prostatic carcinoma with age does not show up at all in the TUR specimens, whereas it is quite obvious in the needle biopsies (Fig. 8). So it is quite evident, that the morbidity rate of prostatic carcinoma

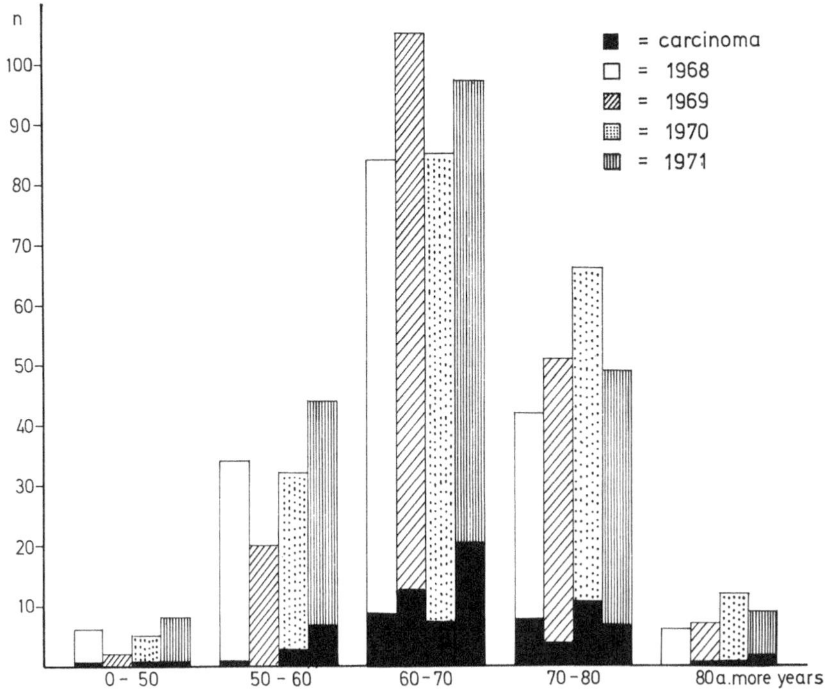


Fig. 6. Suprapubic prostatectomy and TUR 1968—1971

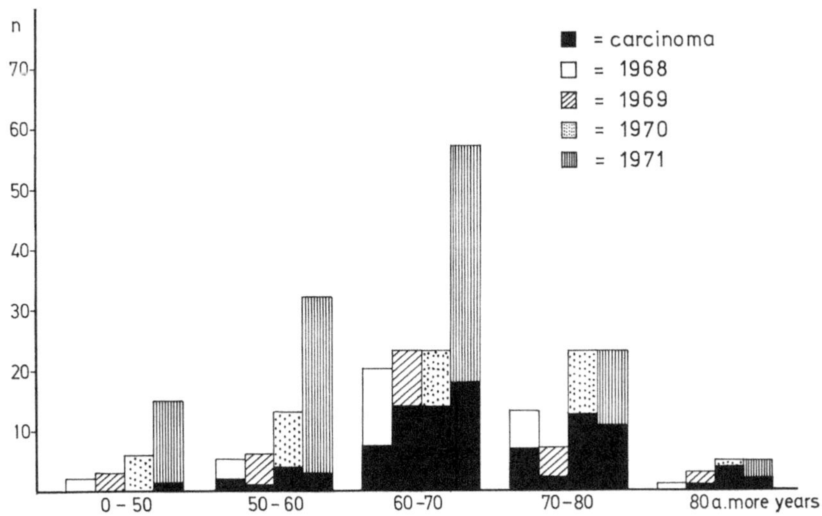


Fig. 7. Needle biopsies of prostate 1968—1971

Table 2. Percentage of carcinoma in biopsy material of the prostate obtained by different methods (Pathol. Institut, Homburg, Germany)

| 1968—1971 | 0—50 | 50—60 | 60—70 | 70—80 | 80 a. more years | total |
|---|---|---|---|---|---|---|
| Needle biopsy | | | | | | |
| Total | 26 | 56 | 123 | 66 | 14 | 285 |
| Carcinoma | 1 | 10 | 53 | 33 | 7 | 104 |
| % carcinoma | 3 | 17 | 43 | 50 | 50 | 36 |
| Transurethral a. suprapubic (TUR) | | | | | | |
| Total | 21 | 130 | 371 | 208 | 34 | 764 |
| Carcinoma | 3 | 11 | 50 | 30 | 4 | 98 |
| % carcinoma | 14 | 8 | 13 | 14 | 11 | 12 |
| Needle biopsy + TUR | | | | | | |
| Total | 47 | 186 | 494 | 274 | 48 | 1049 |
| Carcinoma | 4 | 21 | 103 | 63 | 11 | 202 |
| % carcinoma | 8 | 11 | 20 | 22 | 22 | 19 |

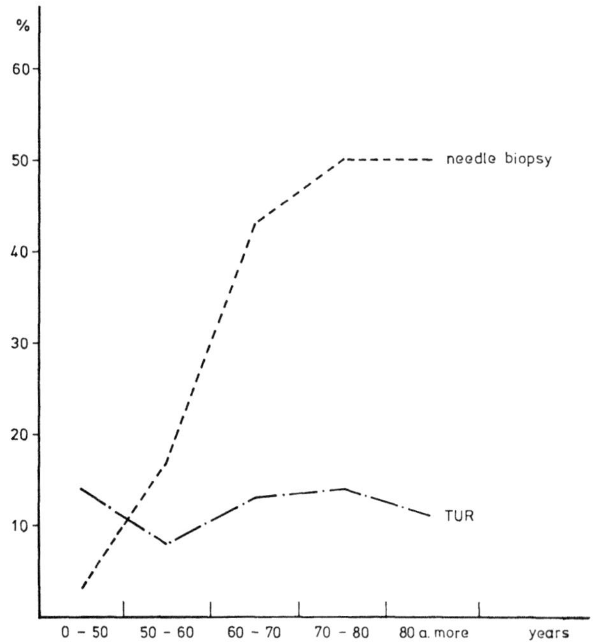


Fig. 8. Incidence of carcinoma of the prostate in biopsy material 1968—1971

is to a high degree dependent upon the diagnostic activity of our clinical colleagues. 3 times as many carcinomas are detected after introduction of needle biopsy. This also effects directly the figures of our cancer registry to which we report every case of carcinoma. In the Saarland there was in 1969 only 1 patient with carcinoma of the prostate among 1000 men over 70 years of age, 1970 this figure rose to 2.4/1000. In 1971 this figure will be higher still. This clearly shows, how the morbidity rate of prostatic carcinoma in epidemiologic studies is dependent upon the clinical activity and histopathologic diagnosis. In our country, many pathologists still receive material from TUR's and prostatectomies only, but no punch or aspiration biopsies. In such areas the morbidity rate of prostatic carcinoma will be low.

I believe, that we shall know the true frequency of clinically detectable prostatic carcinoma only after a large number of men have been examined clinically under the cancer prevention program and cases of suspected carcinoma been biopsied. In order to obtain sufficient material for this, the German urologists and pathologists are planning a separate register for prostatic carcinoma, where all cases of prostatic carcinoma in the Federal Republic, that have been verified clinically and by biopsy are to be collected and evaluated. We hope that this study which is to extend over several years, will provide us with better material for epidemiologic studies of prostatic carcinoma, then are available up to now.

## References

ASHLEY, D. J. B.: On the incidence of carcinoma of the prostate. J. Path. Bact. **90**, 217—224 (1965).

FRANKS, L. M.: Latent carcinoma of the prostate. J. Path. Bact. **68**, 603—615 (1954).

FRANKS, L. M.: The natural history of prostatic cancer. Lancet **1956 II**, 1037—1039.

KING, H., DIAMOND, E., LILIENFELD, A. M.: Some epidemiological aspects of cancer of the prostate. J. chron. Dis. **16**, 117—153 (1963).

LIAVAG, I.: Carcinoma of the prostate. Oslo: Universitetsforlaget 1967.

MOSTOFI, C.: Diagnostic aspects of the prostatic carcinoma. Report on the occasion of the Symposium Prostatic Carcinoma in Homburg (1970) (unpublished).

MUIR, C. S., NECTOUX, J.: The occurrence of prostatic cancer. A world-wide survey. Epidemiology Unit, International Agency for Research on Cancer, 16, Avenue Maréchal Foch, 69 Lyon 6e/ France (1971).

# The Incidence of Carcinoma of Prostate: An Epidemiological Survey

L. M. FRANKS

Department of Cellular Pathology, Lincoln's Inn Fields, London, Great Britain

Although I have been interested in prostatic cancer for many years I feel that I am here under false colours. I am neither a statistician nor a epidemiologist. Figures, particularly in statistical tables, induce a state in me bordering on catalepsy. You cannot, therefore, expect from me a critical analysis of mortality tables, relative incidence data and other such abstruse data. Dr. LIAVÅG has dealt with the behaviour of one type of prostatic cancer, and Professor DHOM has discussed very specific intracellular changes. I shall be concerned with the more general problem of the distribution of prostatic cancer in different populations and the factors which may influence this distribution. Several other workers have studied this problem. As a general rule each has found one or more apparent relationships which require more information before they can be accepted or disproved. Unfortunately in almost every case further investigation tends to refute the original association, with two exceptions. The exceptions are of course the low incidence of clinical cancer in Japan and the influence of age, about which I shall say more later.

## Definition of Terms

Before we can usefully discuss the problems of prostatic cancer we must define our terms, as there is still some confusion about the meaning of the descriptive qualifications we apply to the disease. As we have heard, under the microscope and to the naked eye all cases of prostatic cancer are similar, but biologically—that is in the patient—three types can be distinguished:

### 1. Clinical Cancer

Any case in which a firm clinical diagnosis of prostatic cancer is made and confirmed by histology should be decribed as a clinical cancer.

### 2. Latent Cancer

These tumours by definition exist but do not become manifest, i.e. they produce no clinical evidence of disease. They are found *incidentally*.

### 3. Occult Cancer

These tumours manifest themselves by their metastases. The primary tumour remains hidden (occult).

These definitions have no direct relationship to size, growth rate, histological structure, local invasion or distant metastases. They are concerned *only* with the method of presentation.

## Sources of Statistical and Epidemiological Data

The data on which most recent studies are based are 3 series of figures. The first is a UICC Report on Cancer Incidence in five continent (1966 and 1970). The second is a book by Clemmesen (1965) "Statistical Studies in Aetiology of Malignant Neoplasms" which is a report from the Danish Cancer Registry. The third is by Segi and his colleagues (1969) "Cancer Mortality for Selected Sites in 24 Countries". I have also made use of an exhaustive, but so far unpublished world-wide survey by Dr. C. S. Muir and Janine Nectoux of the Epidemiology Unit of the International Agency for Research on Cancer. Two other extensive reviews on epidemiological factors affecting prostatic cancer are those of King and his colleagues (1963) and Wynder *et al.* (1971). My paper will be mainly concerned with an analysis of this and other material.

## Effects of Race on Tumour Incidence

The difficulties involved in any comparative study on cancer incidence in different countries are well known. Even in a country like Denmark, which has a fairly homogeneous population, is small and has a well established system of medical care, both in general practice and in hospitals, there are wide variations in tumour incidence at different sites, as reported to a central cancer registry (Clemmesen, 1955). Differences between rural areas, small towns and large towns may be due to differences in diagnostic facilities, the availability of histological and autopsy services, and so on. Fashions in diagnosis, particularly histological, may produce an apparent but spurious increase in incidence of a given tumour. The prostate of course is a good example of this. Prostate glands from men over 50 are very commonly found to have "latent" cancers on histological examination. Thus, increasingly effective histological studies will increase the incidence of prostatic cancers diagnosed. These must find their way into the total incidence figures since histologically there is no way of distinguishing them from any other cancer. Similarly, there appears to be an increased incidence of cases of prostatic cancer in patients with bladder tumours. It is possible that this only reflects the increased likelihood of a prostatic examination in patients being routinely examined for another genito-urinary cancer (Clemmesen and Nielsen, 1956). Even assuming that all cases are diagnosed correctly and reported to a central registry they must be related to the total population so that accurate census figures are also required. Given that the conditions in Denmark are likely to be the best which can be obtained in an imperfect world there are still variations in incidence in cancers of various sites which follow a Poisson distribution (Nielsen, 1955) so that figures for a sufficiently long period must be collected.

In less well developed societies these problems are even more marked. An obvious problem in the investigation of a disease of the elderly in such a society is that only a small proportion survives to reach old age. Although this may be corrected statistically it cannot allow for an element of selection. A less obvious problem is concerned with the social acceptance of illness. This is well illustrated in a series of cases reported from Indonesia by TAN (1961). He showed that prostatic hyperplasia and cancer were present quite frequently in an Indonesian population, although clinical prostatic disease was said to be very rare. In biopsies from 337 patients over 40 years old, prostatic cancers were found in 28, and 55 of 208 patients were found to have benign nodular hyperplasia. Further questioning of these Indonesian patients showed that they did indeed have complaints but they had grown accustomed to their symptoms and had accepted them as a natural thing in their lives. Any interpretation of statistics on the incidence of prostatic disease must therefore be treated with caution and it must take into account factors of this sort in addition to the more obvious causes of under-diagnosis in less prosperous societies.

Even taking these possible sources of error into account there seem to be some remarkable racial and geographical differences in incidence. The racial incidence of prostatic cancer was discussed by STEINER (1954) who reviewed the earlier work on this subject. It has been recognised for over 40 years that the clinical disease was very rare in the yellow races. NAGOYA (quoted by STEINER, 1954) reported that in over 12,000 autopsies in Tokyo only 5 prostatic cancers were found (0.45% of all cancers in males). In China too the incidence was low: no case in 106 autopsies or in 303 surgical specimens (HEINE, 1931) and only one case in 821 histologically diagnosed carcinomas (HU and CH'IN, 1936). STEINER also reported that the disease was rare in Filipinos and Mexicans. More recent work has amplified and extended these findings. Mortality and morbidity data are similar. The only consistent finding is the low incidence in yellow races but there is a remarkable variation in incidence in other races. The highest rate (age adjusted morbidity rate) is that for negros in one particular area of the United States—Alameda Country—of 65.3 while the whites in the same area have a rate of 38.0. This compares with a rate for 10 USA cities of 49.9 for non-white and 34.8 for whites. The regional variations are even more striking varying from 17.1 for non-Latin Texans to 37.8 for urban inhabitants of Iowa. The extremes in Canada range from 17.0 in Newfoundland to 39 in Saskatchewan. In South and Central America Chile has a rate of 11.3 and Colombia 23.3. Other continents show a similar variation. In Africa the rate varies from 4.4 in Uganda to 29.1 in Rhodesia. There are apparently inexplicable variations such as rate for Bantu in Cape Province of 19.2 as compared with 9.4 in Bantu in Johannesburg. The rate in Indians (6.5 in Bombay, 9.4 in Natal) is low, as is that in Eastern Europe (e.g. Poland, 4.6—12.8) and Israel (3.1 for non-Jews to 10.8—13.2 for Jews). New Zealand has a consistently high rate—40.0 for Europeans and 40.3 for Maoris. The Japanese in Japan have a consistently low rate (3.2—4.3). There are no comparable figures for China but the rate for Chinese in Singapore is 0.9.

## Significance Differences in Racial Distribution

It is difficult to place any reliance on minor differences but the incidence in yellow races is so greatly and consistently lower than in other groups that it can be confidently accepted, even though more critical studies may introduce minor variations in detail. It seems likely too that the high incidence in some groups of American negroes and in New Zealand can probably be accepted. The significance of lesser differences, e.g. between Eastern and Western Europe is less certain. If the differences are due to environment they should be affected by migration. Unfortunately results at present available are confusing. HAENSZEL and KURIHARA (1968) made an exhaustive comparison of the incidence of cancer and other diseases in Japanese in Japan, Japanese immigrants in the United States (Issei) and their U.S. born offspring (NISSEI and SANSEI). The pattern of change in incidence was not consistent. The stomach cancer incidence remained about the same but colon cancer incidence increased. Breast cancer in women remained low. Prostate cancer incidence rose but to nowhere near the incidence in Caucasians. The figures given by HAENSZEL and KURIHARA (1968) are:

| | (age specific mortality rates) | |
|---|---|---|
| | 65—74 years | 75 years and over |
| Japan | 11.6 | 28 |
| Issei | 40.2 | 130.0 |
| U.S. whites | 92.6 | 307.5 |

There are no figures as yet for descendants of Japanese migrants. The original paper should be consulted for details and for a discussion of the influence of an "imported environment".

Other migrants from low incidence areas, particularly from Eastern Europe, also show a rise in incidence (WYNDER *et al.*, 1971). This American experience with migrants and the high incidence in 2 dissimilar racial groups in New Zealand suggests that possible environmental factors may be concerned. Yet other figures, e.g. from Hawaii where significant environmental factors appear to vary little between the races give widely varying incidence between the races:

| | | | |
|---|---|---|---|
| Caucasians | 43.4 | Japanese | 13.9 |
| Hawaians | 30.0 | Chinese | 9.8 |
| Filipinos | 17.6 | | |

A final but important point is that the incidence of latent cancers is much higher than that of clinical cancers in all races. Even in the yellow races it is not uncommon (e.g. MISA, 1961; TAZAKI, 1962). Again, exact figures are not available but an international co-operative study organized by Dr. TULINIUS of the IARC and now in progress, should give us definite information on the relative incidence.

## The Effects of Age on Incidence

The age-associated incidence of prostatic cancer is also established beyond any reasonable doubt. It is a disease of the elderly and is rare before the age of 50 years. The incidence then increases rapidly. For clinical cases DOLL (1968) has summarised figures of rate of increase in 11 different areas and discussed figures for selected areas in Great Britain in more detail. The pattern seems to be similar in all areas for which satisfactory statistics are available. LITTLE (1964), using figures from Connecticut and New York, calculated a serial rate of increase which illustrates the pattern very well. Between 20—29 and 30—39 age groups the incidence doubled. Between the 30—39 and 40—49 year groups the rate increased 9.5 times. Between 40—49 and 50—59 years the increase was 18 fold. Between 50—59 and 60—69 the increase was 6 fold, i.e. 2052 times the rate of the 20—29 year group. Between 60—69 and 70—79 there was a further increase of 3.3 times, and over 80 an increase of 1.9 times. The slowing of the rate in patients over 80 years may be of significance even though the figures are small since there is some evidence to suggest that the disease may be "less malignant" in these patients, i.e. metastases are less frequent and death is less often due to cancer (FRANKS, 1956).

ASHLEY (1965) has shown that there is a somewhat similar rate of increase for latent cancers, using 4 series of cases; 1 from Germany (GAYNOR, 1938), 2 from the United Kingdom (ANDREWS, 1949; FRANKS, 1954) and 1 from Texas (HALPERT *et al.*, 1963). When the data were plotted on a double logarithmic scale there was a straight line relationship between frequency and age, the frequency varying with the 3rd power of the age. When a similar plot was made for clinical cancers a similar relationship was found but the slope was steeper, corresponding to the 7th power of the age. According to the "multiple hit" theory of carcinogenesis originally proposed by ARMITAGE and DOLL (1957), ASHLEY suggests that this supports the idea that latent cancer is the result of smaller number of hits than clinical cancer.

DOLL (1968) discusses the mathematical basis for the multiple hit theory and concludes that:

1. a rapid and progressive increase in incidence of cancer with age suggests that the tissue is regularly exposed to a carcinogenic agent over a long period.

2. For those cancers that increase rapidly in incidence with age, the relationship between incidence and age can be described by the equation:

$$I = b(t - w)^k$$

where $I$ is the incidence, $t$ is the age, $w$ is the sum of the pre-exposure period and the time between the beginning of the tumour and clinical recognition, $b$ is proportional to the mean daily dose of the agents, and $k$ is approximately 4. $(T - w)$ can also be defined as the duration of effective exposure and $b$ as the mean dose per mitotic cycle.

3. An unusually rapid increase in incidence with age may be due to a long pre-exposure period, a prolonged development time or a reduction in the exposure of successive cohorts to environmental carcinogens.

Frankly, I find it difficult to follow the mathematics of these arguments but I present them to you as an example of the way in which such statistical studies can provide a model which can be tested experimentally. The original papers should be consulted for further information.

## Other Factors Influencing Incidence

Many other factors have been considered. These include socioeconomic status, marital status, fertility, social and sexual habits, previous diseases, height, weight, hair distribution, religion, place of birth, family history, diet, blood group and others (summarised by KING *et al.*, 1963 and WYNDER *et al.*, 1971). No significant relationship has been found.

## The Significance of Age and Racial Incidence

The presence of latent cancers even in low incidence groups suggests that, accepting the multi-stage hypothesis of carcinogenesis, the initiation stage may occur commonly. As DOLL (1968) suggests, the increasing frequency with age may be due to the increased exposure to a hypothetical carcinogen, or it may be a direct or indirect consequence of the process of aging. The further development of the neoplastic process may then depend on promoting factors which may be environmental or genetic. The fact that other hormone-related cancers such as breast, ovary and endometrium are also low in Japan (WYNDER *et al.*, 1971 and others) does suggest that there may be a possible common endocrine basis. This again may be due to differences in the endocrine environment, i.e. hormone secretion pattern, or to differences in cellular responsiveness. Both are well known phenomena in different strains of experimental animals. Although differences in endocrine pattern have been reported in Japanese, there is little information about other low incidence groups.

In the high incidence groups WYNDER *et al.* (1971) found that inflammatory disease of the prostate was very common in American negroes but there is no evidence for this in other high incidence groups.

In summary there is still no convincing evidence which explains the differences in racial and age incidence. As in so many other fields in cancer research, all the information is not yet available but it seems likely that both genetic and environmental factors are involved.

## References

ANDREWS, G. S.: Latent carcinoma of the prostate. J. clin. Path. **2**, 197 (1949).

ARMITAGE, P., DOLL, R.: A two-stage theory of carcinogenesis in relation to the age distribution of human cancer. Brit. J. Cancer **11**, 161 (1957).

ASHLEY, D. J. B.: On the incidence of carcinoma of the prostate. J. Path. Bact. **90**, 217 (1965).

CLEMMESEN, J.: The Danish cancer registry. Under the national anti-cancer league. Dan. med. Bull. **2**, 124 (1955).

CLEMMESEN, J., NIELSEN, A.: Cancer incidence in Denmark 1943—1953. Dan. med. Bull. **3**, 33 (1956).

CLEMMESEN, J.: Statistical studies in the aetiology of malignant neoplasms. Copenhagen: Munksgaard 1965, Vols. 1 and 2.

DOLL, R., PAYNE, P., WATERHOUSE, J.: UICC Cancer Incidence in Five Continents. Vol. I. A technical report. Berlin-Heidelberg-New York: Springer 1966.

DOLL, R.: The age distribution of cancer in man. In: Thule International Symposia — Cancer and Aging, p. 15. Stockholm: Nordiska Bokhandelns Förlag 1968.

DOLL, R., MUIR, C., WATERHOUSE, J. A. H.: UICC Cancer Incidence in Five Continents. Berlin-Heidelberg-New York: Springer 1970, Vol. II.

FRANKS, L. M.: Latent carcinoma of the prostate. J. Path. Bact. **68**, 603 (1954).

FRANKS, L. M.: The spread of prostatic cancer. J. Path. Bact. **72**, 603 (1956).

GAYNOR, E. P.: Zur Frage des Prostatakrebses. Virchows Arch. Abt. A, Path. Anat. **301**, 602 (1938).

HAENSZEL, W., KURIHARA, M.: Studies of Japanese migrants. 1. Mortality from cancer and other diseases among Japanese in the United States. J. nat. Cancer Inst. **40**, 43 (1968).

HALPERT, B., SHEEHAN, E. E., SCHMALHORST, W. R., SCOTT, R.: Carcinoma of the prostate. A survey of 5000 autopsies. Cancer **16**, 737 (1963).

HEINE, J.: Über Geschwülste bei Chinesen. Z. Krebsforsch. **33**, 529 (1931).

HU, C. H., CH'IN, K. Y.: A statistical study of 2179 tumors occurring in the Chinese. Chin. med. J. (Peking) **50**, 43 (1936).

KING, H., DIAMOND, E., LILIENFELD, A. M.: Some epidemiological aspects of cancer of the prostate. J. chron. Dis. **16**, 117 (1963).

LITTLE, C. C.: The relation of age to the incidence of cancer of certain sites. Proc. nat. Acad. Sci. (Wash.) **52**, 865 (1964).
MISA, Y.: A histopathological study on latent carcinoma of the prostate among the Japanese. Jap. J. Cancer Clin. **7**, 304 (1961).
MUIR, C. S., NECTOUX, J.: The occurrence of prostatic cancer. W.H.O. Study Group 1971, (personal communication).
NIELSEN, A. cited by CLEMMESEN, J. Dan. med. Bull. **2**, 124 (1955).
SEGI, M., KURIHARA, M., MATSUYAMA, T.: Cancer mortality for selected sites in 24 countries. No. 5 (1964—1965). Department of Public Health, Tohoku University School of Medicine, Sendai, Japan, August 1969.
STEINER, P.: Cancer: race and geography. Baltimore: Williams and Wilkins 1954.
TAN, R. E.: Prostatic disease in Indonesia. J. Urol. **86**, 428 (1961).
TAZAKI, H.: Pathological studies on the prostate glands of Japanese, with special reference to latent malignancy. Keio J. Med. **11**, 253 (1962).
WYNDER, E. L., MABUCHI, K., WHITMORE, W. F.: Epidemiology of cancer of the prostate. Cancer **28**, 344 (1971).

# Correlates of Histologic Differentiation of Carcinoma of the Penis.

## Results from a Five Year Survey in Uganda, 1964—1968

R. SCHMAUZ [1]

Deutsches Krebsforschungszentrum, Heidelberg, Germany

Uganda, which is about 300 miles square and lies astride the equator, is a small country full of ecological and demographical contrasts. The altitude varies from two to nearly 17,000 feet, the climate changes from hot desert through temperate lacustrine areas to alpine pasture land, and there are more than 30 tribes in a population of only nine million people (Atlas of Uganda, 1967). It was no surprise, therefore, that cancer registration, started by the Department of Pathology of the Medical School as early as 1951, should delineate most peculiar patterns of tumour geography (DAVIES and WILSON, 1954). Mapping these patterns against amount of exposure in the environment has provided clues to the aetiology of many cancers. Examples include the association of Burkitt's lymphoma with malaria (KAFUKO and BURKITT, 1970) and of hepatocellular carcinoma with aflatoxin content of foodstuffs (ALPERT, HUTT, WOGAN and DAVIDSON, 1971).

Studies done on carcinoma of the penis have revealed the protective effect of circumcision (DODGE and LINSELL, 1963). Only very few cases are registered in regions of the country where this practice is a tribal custom. The very marked variation in the uncircumcised—in some tribes the disease is as rare as in the circumcised—seems to be determined more by the environment than by tribal affiliation. A survey covering the whole of East Africa showed that frequency of the tumour increased when there was migration from a low incidence area into an area with high incidence and vice versa (COOK and BURKITT, 1970). In Uganda the variations in incidence occurred over quite small distances. Tribes differed in incidence when living in different regions but people of different tribes inhabiting one area had a similar incidence (SCHMAUZ and JAIN, 1971).

In this communication an attempt is made to assess histologic criteria of malignancy in cases from regions of the country differing in incidence. The comparisons comprise both indigenous and migrant populations. The supposition is that environmental exposure, though as yet unidentified, is of high degree where there is a high frequency of the tumour and of low degree where the tumour is rare. Features of

1 Formerly Research Assistant, International Agency for Research on Cancer, Lyons, France

malignancy were also evaluated with regard to age of cases. The analysis shows that differentiation of the tumour does not vary with regional incidence but that there appeared to be a possible correlation with age of the cases.

## Materials and Methods

Since 1962 the Kampala Cancer Registry has filed details on cases from the whole of Uganda. The main source is the Department of Pathology, Makerere University, Kampala, which operates the only diagnostic laboratory of histopathology and provides a free service for the whole of the country (HUTT and BURKITT, 1965). 458 cases were ascertained during the five year period 1964—1968. Their age, tribal and regional distribution in Uganda has been detailed in an earlier report (SCHMAUZ and JAIN, 1971). The very variable pattern of incidence was categorized into regions of high, medium and low incidence (Fig. 1). Histologic assessment was

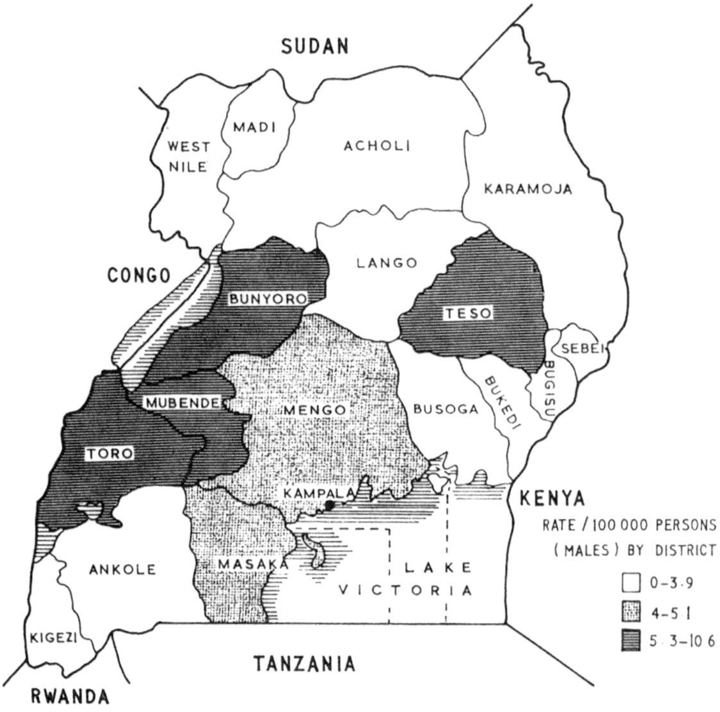


Fig. 1. Regional incidence of carcinoma of the penis in indigenous populations of Uganda

done by one person (R.S.) on several occasions. Surface areas were avoided since there tended to be more keratinisation. Verrucous and microinvasive carcinomas were not graded as only tumours with signs of frank invasion are the object of the study. Areas assessed were either deep tumour or its advancing edge. Tumour differentiation had been subdivided originally in five grades which were simplified to high, average and low differentiation for this analysis Figs. 2—4.

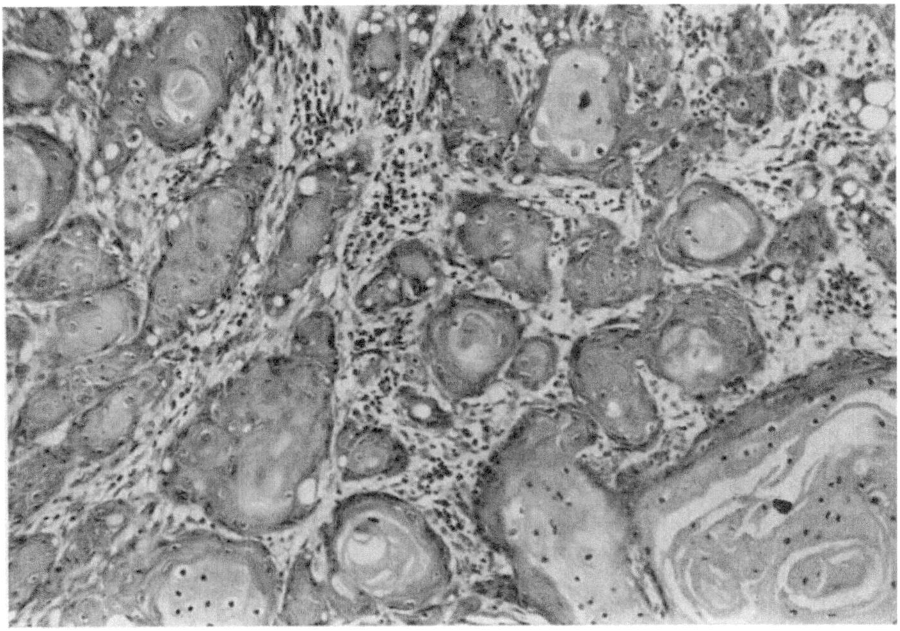

Fig. 2. Well differentiated carcinoma of the penis

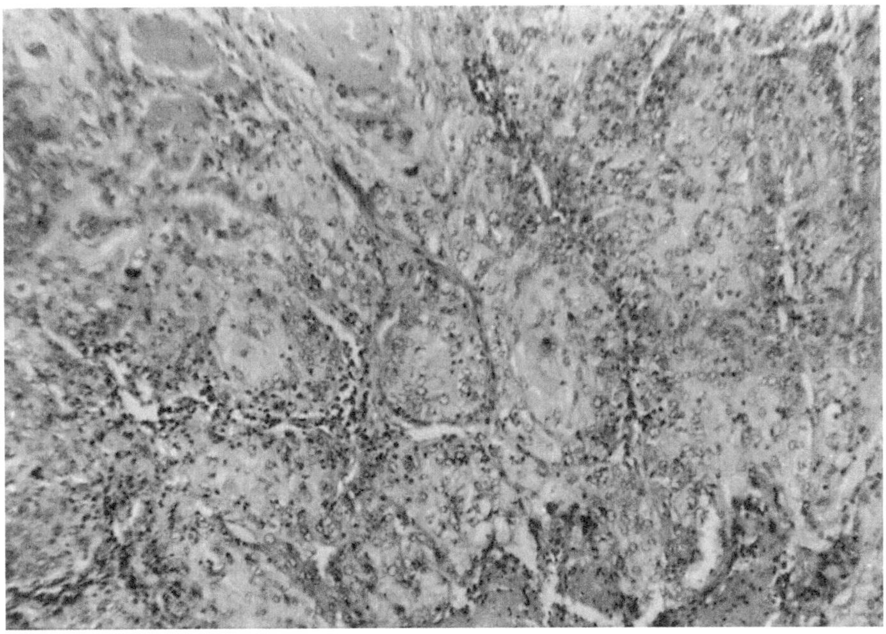

Fig. 3. Carcinoma of the penis with average differentiation

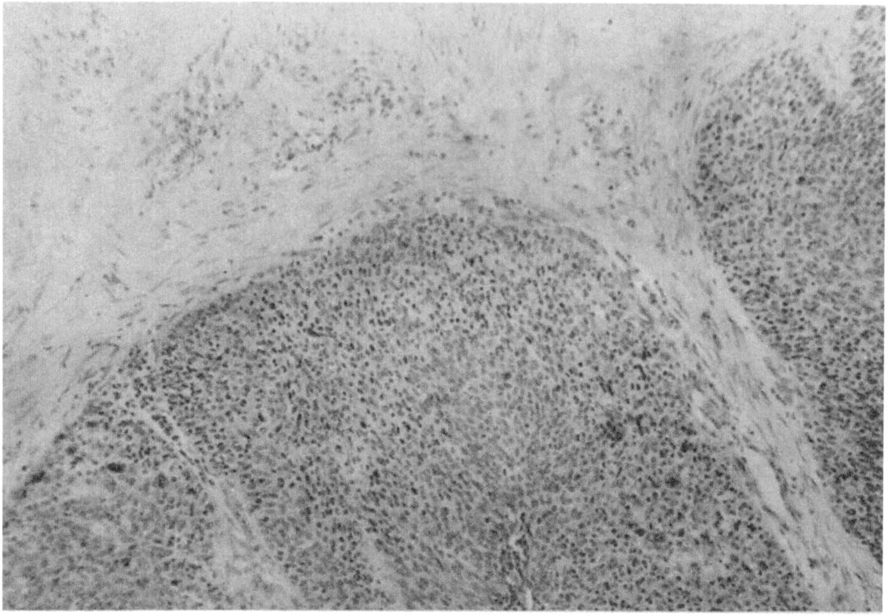

Fig. 4. Poorly differentiated (anaplastic) carcinoma of the penis. Note loss of cell differentiation and lack of keratin

## Results

Compared with other superficial carcinomas in Uganda, penile cancer is a squamous cell carcinoma with average differentiation (Table 1). Squamous cell carcinoma of the leg is better differentiated (Iversen, 1971) whereas carcinoma of the cervix is more anaplastic (James, 1971). Half of the cases of penile cancer show average differentiation. In the remainder there were slightly more high grade than low grade carcinomas. These proportions did not change over a wide range of incidence. Further, indigenous people with a presumably constant amount of exposure living in one place throughout life compare well with migrants in whom exposure must have been of varying degree.

Table 1. Percentage distribution of differentiation of carcinoma of the penis and area of incidence in indigenous and migrant populations (number of cases in brackets)

| Differentiation | | High | | Average | | Low | |
|---|---|---|---|---|---|---|---|
| Incidence rate | | | | | | | |
| indigenous populations | | | | | | | |
| High: | 5.3—10.6 | 25.6 | (31) | 52.0 | (63) | 22.2 | (27) |
| Medium: | 4.0— 5.1 | 33.9 | (37) | 45.9 | (50) | 20.3 | (22) |
| Low: | 0.0— 3.9 | 25.2 | (23) | 48.8 | (38) | 24.6 | (20) |
| migrant populations | | | | | | | |
| not computed | | 26.2 | (28) | 51.5 | (55) | 22.5 | (24) |
| Total | | 28.5 | (119) | 49.5 | (206) | 22.3 | (93) |

Age and differentiation of tumour was assessed (Table 2). In indigenous populations cases with poorly differentiated tumours were of older age when presenting than those with tumours of average and high differentiation. This trend is less obvious in migrants where the number of cases is smaller. However, there was no statistical significance between any of these mean ages. It is concluded that differentiation of carcinoma of the penis may possibly correlate with age of the case at diagnosis but that a correlation with incidence of the tumour can almost certainly be excluded.

Table 2. Mean age and differentiation of carcinoma of the penis in indigenous and migrant populations (number of cases in brackets)

| Differentiation | High | | Average | | Low | |
|---|---|---|---|---|---|---|
| Indigenous populations | 53.57 | (87) | 54.78 | (139) | 56.45 | (62) |
| Migrants | 57.14 | (28) | 54.34 | (55) | 57.42 | (24) |
| Total | 54.43 | (115) | 54.64 | (194) | 56.72 | (86) |

The difference of any two means is not statistically significant

## Discussion

The quality of data is much in question as there are shortcomings both in the collection and in the evaluation of the material. Although carcinoma of the penis is a superficial tumour and biopsy diagnosis therefore can be made readily, incidence rates most likely do underestimate its actual frequency. There is considerable shortage of doctors and hospitals throughout the country and old people—the age group at risk of the disease (SCHMAUZ and JAIN, 1971)—may be rather reluctant to seek medical attention (TEMPLETON and BIANCHI, 1972). However, under-reporting does not distort markedly the comparative incidence as these factors do not seem to act selectively in any one area of Uganda (SCHMAUZ and JAIN, 1971). Inaccuracy may be present when determining differentiation of the tumour. There could be variations both over time and in different portions of the tumour. Such changes in tumour grade, however, do not appear to be very marked. There were 39 cases during the five year period of the survey which had more than one histologic diagnosis within a month's time but only two varied in the degree of grading. By far the most inadequate data is the age recorded. No birth certificates are in use, and people give their years of life in decades or in five year periods, particularly when of older age (Fig. 5).

Whereas the distinction between high and average differentiation of a squamous cell carcinoma is made often on an arbitrary basis and may vary subject to the investigator's judgement, the presence or absence of keratin and cell differentiation is a straightforward and easily reproducible diagnostic feature. In the comparisons with other reports grade is subdivided therefore only in differentiated and anaplastic forms. As shown in Table 3 there is good agreement with the earlier study on carcinoma of the penis which found 18% of the carcinomas in Uganda to be anaplastic (DODGE and LINSELL, 1963). In the western world, where the disease is rare, anaplasia is less common, occurring only in about 10% of cases (FREW, JEFFERIES and SWINNEY, 1967; BASSET, 1952; STAUBITZ, LENT and OBERKIRCHER, 1955). This

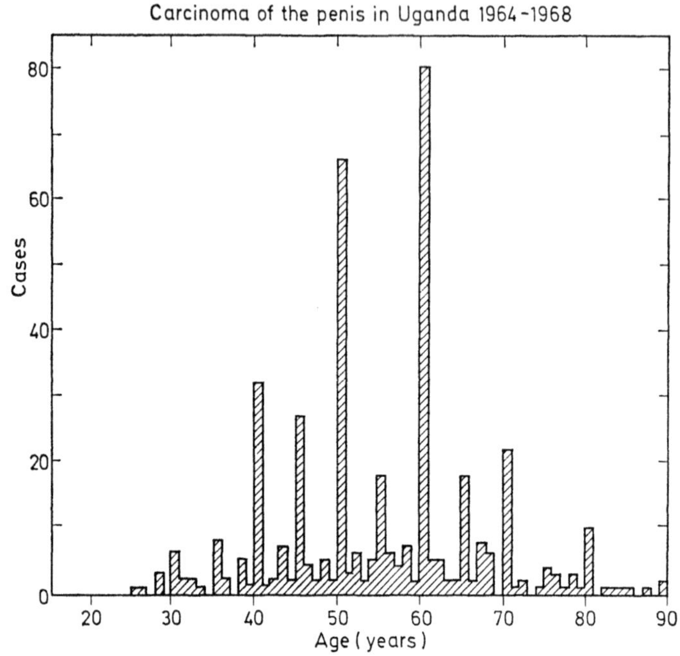


Fig. 5. Age distribution of cases of carcinoma of the penis in Uganda

Table 3. Percentage of poorly differentiated (anaplastic) carcinoma of the penis in reported series (number of cases in brackets)

| Author | Country (Registry*) | Incidence | No. of cases examined | % of anaplastic cases |
|---|---|---|---|---|
| FREW *et al.* (1967) | U. K. (Sheffield) [a] | 1.1 | 44 | 6.8 (3) |
| BASSET (1952) | U.S.A. (California) [b] | 0.6 | 62 | 11.5 (7) |
| STAUBITZ *et al.* (1955) | U.S.A. (Nevada) [c] | 0.9 | 204 | 11.6 (21) |
| DODGE and LINSELL (1963) | Uganda (Kyadondo) [d] | 3.8 | 438 | 18.3 (80) |
| Present series | Uganda (Kampala) | 2.9 | 418 | 22.3 (93) |

* Source: [a] SHONE and TROUT; [b] LINDEN *et al.*; [c] DECKER and TULARSKI; [d] DAVIES and KNOWELDEN.

could argue more than mere coincidence. However, a similar variation is not present in other carcinomas, being equally more anaplastic in Uganda than in the U.S.A. and Europe, but which differ from penile carcinoma in comparative incidence. Examples are breast cancer (DAVIES, 1970) which is less frequent in Uganda, and carcinoma of the nasopharynx (SCHMAUZ and TEMPLETON, 1972), a disease uncommon both in western countries and in tropical Africa. Thus, differentiation of penile cancer seems to be a poor correlate to incidence. This suggests that exposure in the environment does not interfere with differentiation of this tumour.

On the other hand, there are correlations reported between age and grade of tumour. Anaplastic forms of breast cancer occur more often in younger than in elderly women (TOUGH, CARTER, FRAZER and BRUCE, 1969). By contrast, transitional cell carcinoma of the bladder, the main type of bladder cancer in western countries, may show the opposite trend. Cases in the in situ stage are of younger age when presenting than cases with invasive cancer (COLE, 1971). Since there is also a correlation between stage and grade of tumour (FRIEDELL, 1971) cases with poorly differentiated carcinomas can be expected to be older than those who show high differentiation. The possibility of a correlation with age is evident in carcinoma of the penis, particularly since the ages of the cases were recorded so inaccurately (Fig. 5). It is in this direction that we must look to explain the malignancy of this tumour.

## Acknowledgements

My thanks are due to Professor DRURY and to Dr. TEMPLETON for much helpful advice during the fortnight's stay in Kampala. I am grateful to Dr. DE THÉ from the International Agency for Research on Cancer for financial support. Mr. W. SERUMAGA prepared Fig. 1 and Fig. 2. The Kampala Cancer Registry is supported by the Cancer Campaign for Research (London).

## Summary

A series of 418 cases of frank invasive carcinoma of the penis in Ugandan Africans is analysed. These were derived from the records of a country-wide biopsy survey over the five year period 1964—1968. Malignancy of the tumour as measured by histological grading did not correlate with its very variable pattern of incidence in the country. About 28% of the cases were well differentiated, 50% moderately well and 22% poorly differentiated (anaplastic), regardless of regional incidence. However, there appeared to be a possible correlation with age of cases at diagnosis. Cases in which the histology was of high grade tended to be younger than those with low grade carcinomas. It is suggested that rather than amount of exposure to the environment age could be a factor determining the malignancy of carcinoma of the penis.

## References

Atlas of Uganda. Published by the Department of Lands and Surveys: Kampala: Second Edition 1967.

ALPERT, M. E., HUTT, M. S. R., WOGAN, G. N., DAVIDSON, C. S.: Association between aflatoxin content of food and hepatoma frequency in Uganda. Cancer **28**, 253—260 (1971).

BASSET, J. W.: Carcinoma of the penis. Cancer **5**, 530—538 (1952).

COLE, P.: Personal communication (1971).

COOK, P. J., BURKITT, D. P.: An epidemiological study of seven malignant tumours in East Africa. Memor. Med. Res. Coun. (Lond.) (unpublished report, 1970).

DAVIES, J. N. P.: Epidemiology of breast cancer. Letter to the Editor. Int. J. Cancer **5**, 157 (1970).

DAVIES, J. N. P., KNOWELDEN, J.: Cancer Incidence in Uganda, Kyadondo, 1954—1960. In U.I.C.C. Cancer Incidence in Five Continents, Vol. I, Eds.: DOLL, R., PAYNE, P., and WATERHOUSE, J.A.H., Geneva: U.I.C.C. 1966.

DAVIES, J. N. P., WILSON, B. A.: Cancer in Kampala, 1952—1953. E. Afr. med. J. **31**, 395—416 (1954).

DECKER, J. W., TULARSKI, L. B.: Cancer Incidence in Nevada, 1959—1966. In: U.I.C.C. Cancer Incidence in Five Continents, Vol. II, Eds. DOLL, R., MUIR, C. S., and WATERHOUSE, J. A. H., Geneva: U.I.C.C. 1970.

DODGE, O. G., LINSELL, C. A.: Carcinoma of the penis in Uganda and Kenya Africans. Cancer **16**, 1255—1263 (1963).

FREW, I. D. O., JEFFERIES, J. D., SWINNEY, J.: Carcinoma of the penis. Brit. J. Urol. **39**, 398—404 (1967).

FRIEDELL, G. H.: Personal communication 1971.

HUTT, M. S. R., BURKITT, D. P.: Geographical Distribution of Cancer in East Africa: A new clinico-pathological approach. Brit. med. J. **2**, 719—722 (1965).

IVERSEN, O. H.: Personal communication (1971).

JAMES, P.: Personal communication (1971).

KAFUKO, G. W., BURKITT, D. P.: Burkitt's lymphoma and malaria. Int. J. Cancer **6**, 1—9 (1970).

LINDEN, G., DUNN, J. E., ARELLANO, M. G.: Cancer Incidence in California, Alameda County, 1960—1964. In: U.I.C.C. Cancer Incidence in Five Continents, Vol. II. Eds. DOLL, R., MUIR, C. S. and WATERHOUSE, J. A. H., Geneva: U.I.C.C. 1970.

SCHMAUZ, R., TEMPLETON, A. C.: Carcinoma of the nasopharynx in Uganda. Cancer **29** (1972) (in press).

SCHMAUZ, R., JAIN, D. K.: Geographical variation of carcinoma of the penis in Uganda. Brit. J. Cancer **25**, 25—32 (1971).

SHONE, S., TROUT, K.: Cancer Incidence in England, Sheffield Region, 1963—1966. In: U.I.C.C. Cancer Incidence in Five Continents, Vol. II. Eds. DOLL, R., MUIR, C. S. and WATERHOUSE, J. A. H., Geneva: U.I.C.C. 1970.

STAUBITZ, J. W., LENT, M. H., OBERKIRCHER, O. J.: Carcinoma of the penis. Cancer **8**, 371—378 (1955).

TEMPLETON, A. C., BIANCHI, A.: Bias in an African Cancer Registry. Brit. J. Cancer (in press).

TOUGH, J. C. K., CARTER, D. C., FRASER, J., BRUCE, J.: Histological grading in breast cancer. Brit. J. Cancer **23**, 294—301 (1969).

# Cervical Carcinogenesis: An Epidemiologic Model Adaptable to Control Programs

I. D. Rotkin

University of Illinois at the Medical Center, Chicago, Illinois, and School of Medicine, University of California, San Diego, California, USA

It still is held that the multistage continuum of carcinogenesis, as proposed by Berenblum [1] and developed by others, has not yet been demonstrated in application to a solid human malignancy. That such a sequence of progressive stages, from initiation through promotion, is a biologic invariance hardly is secure. Yet, the model is much more than a claim; it has been demonstrated repeatedly and by many workers with animals that adherence to 4 ordered conditions will dependably induce malignant lesions. They are 1) an adequately young animal, 2) a specific carcinogenic initiator, 3) a sufficiently long latent period, and 4) a suitably contrived cocarcinogenic event. Fitted to human solid cancers, such a theory could provide a timetable of predictable events upon which planning of primary and secondary prevention might be designed, decisions related to therapy might be strengthened, and programs of rehabilitation for survivors and their dependents might be anticipated.

*Background.* Collected epidemiologic evidence pertaining to sociocultural and biologic variables and attributes can be conformed rather convincingly to the multistage model for the most prevalent of all human female-limited carcinomas, cancer of the uterine cervix [3]. The host-agent-donor hypothesis of cervical carcinogenesis [2, 3] provides for transmission of an initiating influence from male to female during coitus. The necessary condition is that heterosexual intromission is accomplished.

Risk is substantially increased when onset of sexuality occurs during adolescence [2, 3], and also in the presence of multiple sexual consorts [3, 4]. That majorities of cervical cancer patients originate from depressed sociocultural populations is related to the excessive frequencies of these women who are described by these associated sexual variables [5]. Upon the assumption that adolescent coitus and exposure to multiple sexual partners are the pivotal factors linked with increased risk, it is possible to structure a multistage rationale for the development of cancer in cervical epithelium.

*The imperative of action subserving control.* In the sense that Cassel [6] rejects the search for validated causes in favor of interference with pathways of sociologic variables bearing demonstrated relationship to onset of disease, the rationale presented here is derived not only out of need for control, but also out of the conviction that the body of information already available regarding this one solid cancer is adequately evidential to attempt such a model.

Estimates of cancer incidence rates still hardly are reliable for most populations. Yet, if we were to project worldwide incidences of cervical cancer from known risk information, current annual world death rates from this carcinoma may approach and even exceed a quarter million. Where screening programs are carried out in crowded populations at minimal advantage, prevalences often are high enough to be considered disastrous. WAHI *et al.* [7] reported 643 cases of cervical cancer in 34,665 Hindu women, or about 1 in 55; and 46 such cancers in 4,776 Muslim women, or about 1 in 104. Frequencies even of Muslim cervical carcinomas in Wahi's study are surprisingly severe at about half of those for the contiguous Hindu population. Lifetime risk for all women in the United States is about 1 in 50 [8], and if we accept a greater than twofold risk for blacks, cervical cancer frequencies in these and other ethnic groups are extremely high. Rates also are extreme in much of the Orient, in Malaysia, in all of Latin America, in the East Indies, and in Africa.

I would agree with MACMAHON [9] that there comes a time when programs no longer may be postponed on the argument that absolute causal insight has not been achieved; and I would add that a lingering espousal of demonstrated cause-and-effect dogmas represents continuing application of single-cause dicta with germ theory origins to current problems in chronic and cultural diseases and disorders more than concern with control. It is true that epidemiologic discovery in most of the prevalent chronic diseases has been much less than eventful. Of solid cancers, only one has been researched with continuity and daring sufficient to provide a biologic floor for what I would call the *imperative of action*, the pressing need for the utilization of developed knowledge in providing an adequate, if not absolute, model for control.

*Assumptions.* In following my rationale, certain associative linkages of antecedent events with risk must be entertained for the purpose of exploring the model. These are derived from my own work and from the general literature, which is substantial for this carcinoma.

The assumptions are that:

1. Biologic activity in the cervical cellular matrix is at a maximal level during the period of adolescence, and events associated with cellular replication and the uptake of substances from the cervical milieu subside after adolescence. The rise in mitotic activity during this life period increases the probability that transformation of the cellular divisional mechanism can take place following the initiating stimulus of a carcinogenic influence, such a probability decreasing as fewer divisional events take place. I am not postulating a mutagenic effect nor alteration in the number, identity or sequential arrangement of chromosomal nucleotides since these still are hypotheses requiring demonstration. Phagocytosis of contiguous debris by cervical epithelium is demonstrated in the work of REID and his group [10] where postcoital spermatazoa were taken up in this manner. That this property can be expanded to introduced carcinogens or agentsseems likely.

2. A carcinogenic principle of some kind is required for the initiation of neoplasia in the cervix. The nature of this agent(s) still is underterminedE[1], as also is its

---

1 It is difficult so far to reconcile the discovery of serum antibodies to *Herpesvirus hominis* type 2 in association with diagnosis of cervical cancer with the claim that the virus preceded the cancer and that the cancer was initiated by the virus. These are the properties of sequence and consequence,

source, whether another previously encountered female, ambient contamination or otherwise.

3. Certain variables and attributes, some sociocultural and others biologic, appear more directly related to risk of cervical cancer than others which have been espoused in the past. These several direct events bearing relationship to risk include early coital beginnings and multiple sexual consorts. Early sexual experience, with risk rising as more males are encountered, constitutes a domain of biologic definers covering such indirect events as early pregnancy, early marriage and others in a cluster of dimensions all modified by the act of coitus. It is important to separate out such specific biologic components from the masking blanket of whole socio-cultural sets. As central a relationship as is existence in low socioeconomic strata, where risk of cervical cancer rises, such a history simply provides a network of interwoven associations the operational one of which is that onset of sexuality is accelerated in disadvantaged classes. Such further events as multiple marriages, infidelity of the female at risk, and marital separations are supportive only insofar as they provide impetus for the acceptance of additional sexual companions. The major indirect defining variables are: 1) early marriage, 2) multiple marriages, 3) low socioeconomic status, 4) ethnic classification [2].

Although the model calls for clear recognition of biologic variables, the approach to intervention would be upon social and population bases for which the biologic area of sexuality and the sociologic components of marriage, income, and education are available, together with cytologic surveillance, in planning control programs.

## The Multistage Rationale

The following section describes levels of events diagrammed in Fig. 1. It is derived from the assumptions stated above, and also from the conceptualizations of many laboratory workers, as well as the formalized construct explored by Armitage and Doll [12] and others, this time specifically in application to the human female at risk of cervical cancer.

*Candidate at increased risk.* Her identity has been developed not only during decades of demographic research, but also from what we have assumed about risk factor. In the United States she was born in the inner city of some large metropolitan center, New York or Los Angeles or Chicago or New Orleans; or perhaps in some disadvantaged setting such as a migrant population in Florida or the Imperial Valley of California; or elsewhere in the world in rural Columbia, India, Thailand or Puerto Rico. There is a better chance that she is black, Mexican, East Indian or Puerto Rican, but there is a fair possibility that she is white, poor and not well educated. From the moment that she enters the world she is sexually identified, and it is a matter of time before the males in her milieu become an environmental hazard, waiting until she barely is grown. At some time during adolescence she will yield to pressure. From the

---

both of which are required in demonstrating direct relatedness, or dependency of an effect upon a specified variable.

2 Ethnic classification is regarded as a demographic convenience in identifying populations at risk, and race is not included in the model since we are concerned with the initiation and progression of carcinogenesis. For blacks also, early onset of coitus is operational in setting up risk [11].

moment that intromission takes place she is at risk that one day she will be diagnosed with a carcinoma of the cervix, and risk rises as she engages sexually with more males, which probably she will do. The pivotal variable is onset of coitus during this time of life, at which time the male can with maximal effect contribute some kind of a carcinogen, abetted by increasing number of sexual partners, each of whom carries a discrete probability of conveying such a carcinogen to her. As more males are encountered, the probability rises that one will be a carrier.

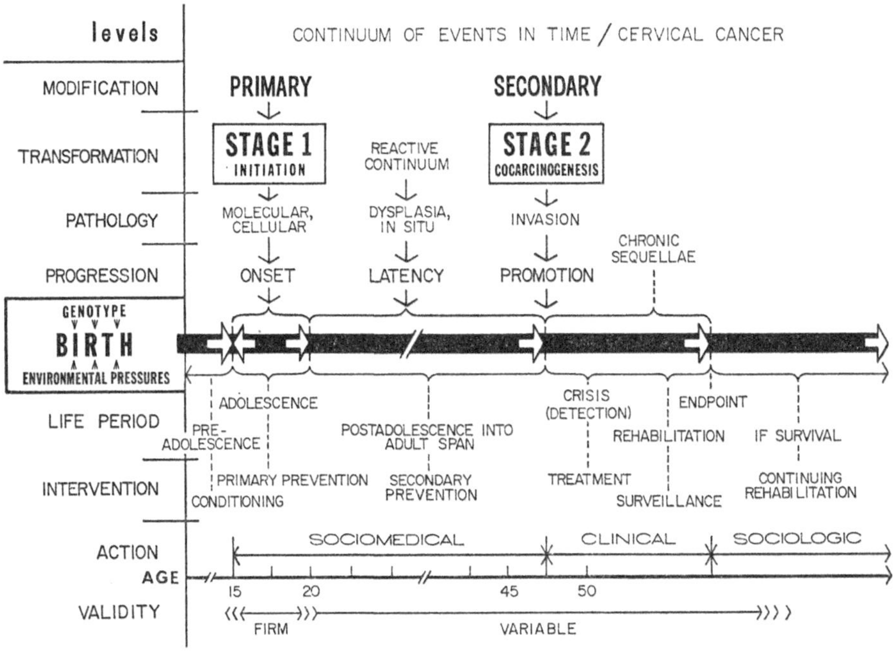


Fig. 1. The heavy horizontal bar (with arrows) represents the lifeline as it originates with conception and birth. Above the lifeline are levels describing the continuum of developing cervical carcinoma as it fitted to the multistage model of carcinogenesis, latency and cocarcinogenesis. Below the lifeline are levels associated with control of cervical cancer as conformed to the multistage continuum. Events in time are scaled by age of the candidate at risk at the bottom

Following our candidate at increased risk on Fig. 1, we can survey her in retrospect. The degree of genetic contribution to risk variance, and of environmental pressures upon the foetus, *in utero* or associated with birth, are unknown. Probably both influences can operate upon the chance that a carcinoma will arise, particularly the genetic component. Plans for intervention at this stage would be futile. The horizontal lifeline develops from birth, with arrows to delineate important markers in time. Operational levels are listed at the left, those above birth denoting development of carcinogenesis on the multistage model; those below concerned with related patterns of control. The age scale at the bottom provides sequentiality in time for the progression of carcinogenesis, and also in resolving responsibility for steps in control.

*Modification and transformation.* Our assumption is that an event of primary modification occurs during adolescence, leading to transformation of susceptible cells in the cervical matrix, with emergence of metaplastic or neoplastic epithelium from precursor cells which possess potential or capacity for malignant transformation, perhaps by genetic forecast. In theory, these cells are available to modification, in contrast to the other cells of the cervical epithelium; and it is during adolescence that they are most plentiful and active, therefore at greatest degree of exposure to an introduced carcinogen. *Initiation* follows, analogous to application of the first carcino gen to the young animal. To summarize, a transformable class of epithelium exists or arises in the cervix, an initial event endows one or more of these cells during Stage 1 with carcinogenic potential, and these cells are maximally active and numerous during adolescence. It is possible that whole areas of squamous epithelium are equally at risk, a kind of mosaic.

A period of latency follows during which dysplasias and occasional *in situ* lesions may develop. This interval may be considered a maturation period, with a duration span which also may be parallel to that of laboratory animals. Induction of carcinomas in mice requires from 20 to 40 weeks after exposure to a strong carcinogen, with a mean of about 30 weeks. The period of latency in Fig. 1 for cervical cancer, as estimated from 2 studies [3, 13], covers an average of about 30 years. Comparing a provisional lifespan of 100 weeks for a captive laboratory mouse with a 100 year lifespan for the woman under similar projected conditions of care, 1 mouse week may be conformed to 1 human year.

Latency in the initiated female is postadolescent, continues into adulthood, and ranges from about 7 to 60 years [3]. The general belief is that nothing continuous transpires during this period, but this probably is a conceptual convenience made necessary by lack of data. Much more likely latency is a *reactive continuum* during which signs of the developing lesion may be found. Since FERGUSON's [14] report of dysplasias and *in situ* carcinomas in adolescent nonvirgin girls, clinicians and pathologists have realized that precursor lesions can exist in very young women. Epidemiologic elucidation of adolescent coitus as a central risk variable [2, 3, 5] has thus been supported in emphasizing surveillance of the young nonvirgin.

*Cocarcinogenesis.* At a point during adulthood along the lifeline (Fig. 1), Stage 2 of the multistage model, a cocarcinogenic event is presumed to take place, after which the lesion is clinically detected if it is symptomologic and if care is available. The modal age for this is around 45 to 50. How the contained *in situ* lesion is promoted into malignancy, the secondary modification, is difficult to say. There is considerable security in postulating initiation by carcinogenesis, and also in demonstrating latency, but cocarcinogenesis is presumed for our purposes from the multistage model, and also from intuition derived from the distinguishing discreteness of the *in situ* and invasive pathologies. Certainly something dramatic must occur to propel the quiescent and stationary *in situ* lesion into invasion in those cases where this happens.

For a long time menopause was considered such a conditioning event, on reports that a falloff of incidence takes place after the sixth decade of life, but Fig. 1 demonstrates that this may be an artificial effect resulting from the end of the latency period. Since initiation takes place at about ages 15 to 17, and latency covers about 30 years, a large proportion of cervical cancers should arise at about the age of 45 or so, which they do. Still, altered hormonal secretion may somehow be cocarcinogenic, as also may other substances and events such as the superapplication of an inorganic ion, an organism, a carcinogenic chemical such as may be transmitted from tobacco through the vascular system to a susceptible cellular matrix, natural radiation, a breakdown of immunologic defenses, relaxation of repressors or inhibitors; or even the expansion of replicating initiated cells into voids of aging tissue. It might also be difficult to rule out some kind of emotional impact if such an event could be shown to have physiologic implications which could operate upon initiated cells.

In summary, we have here a direct conformance to the multistage sequence as it occurs in the laboratory, beginning with influences present at conception through delivery, followed by a period of maximal adolescent susceptibility, at which time we theorize a high level of metabolic uptake on the part of susceptible cells, and when a contributed contaminant carcinogen can transform or initiate susceptible cells in such a manner that a second event much later will trigger explosive and continuous proliferation. After initiation, latency follows, and then cocarcinogenesis according to the multistage theory.

The evidential quality of the assumed variables will be presented in a later paper. For now, it can be repeated that of all the events and attributes which have been proposed in the many epidemiologic and etiologic studies and surveys to date, those with any consistency on a biologic level are factors associated with sexuality, and particularly those of coital beginnings. Noncircumcision of the sexual mate as a related attribute has been abandoned by those who have weighed the evidence [3].

Marriage, early or otherwise, as a social procedure hardly delivers a curse to cervical epithelium. That early marriage shows strength in association with etiology and risk is important insofar that a large proportion of women begin coitus at about the time of marriage. Multiple marriages guarantee that there will be multiple sexual consorts, as do also to some extent broken marriages and other separations, infidelity, venereal disease, extramarital and premarital relationships, and even abortions. Gravidity and parity occurring in excess are related to earlier onset of coitus; and

3 Circumcision of all boy babies was endorsed some years ago as the universal protection against cervical cancer, yet this was a logic based upon the hope that a single cause had been found, the carcinogenicity of smegma. The few remaining supporters of intervention by programs of circumcision have transferred the assumption to an infective agent such as HVH2 which is said to be captured in the smegma matrix. Of the many studies in relating noncircumcision to risk of cervical cancer, few have convincingly demonstrated a strong role in carcinogenesis, many have resulted in negative findings, and at least one [5] has found that circumcision as a cultural practice is a defining component of subpopulations where low rates of cervical carcinoma also may exist. It is clear that the two events are found together in some populations and not in others, accounting for the differential results. The issue further has been complicated by lack of recognition that circumcision is an attribute that lends itself to comparisons between populations, providing the degree of error in classification is consistent; but not to classification itself with any degree of security. Even physicians seem to experience difficulty in classifying prepuces. At best, circumcision may be regarded as a peripheral factor with greater likelihood that a carcinogenic agent can be trapped under an adequately long prepuce, but this kind of reasoning does not apply to a viral antigen since such a virus would find harbor in a cellular matrix with or without a need for additional skin. This should not be taken as an argument against the practice of circumcision. In some males the prepuce can become associated with other pathologies, particularly carcinoma of the penis, and circumcision well may constitute generalized precautionary prophylaxis.

a woman's sociocultural station in life covers but does not particularize these variables, both sociologic and biologic.

The one pivotal variable that arises in all studies investigating it in any segment of any population, by race or by religion or by geography, is onset of coitus during adolescence, and this is the component that may be plucked out of the sociologic background. It has appeared so uniformly that should a study be reported where it does not so result, the study would be more suspect than the dominating position of early coitus in direct relation to risk variance. There is no population so far known to be afflicted with high incidence rates of cervical cancer where early coitus is not concomitant, in India, Malaysia, Africa, South America, Mexico, among rural segments, in poverty classes, among promiscuous women and those diagnosed with venereal diseases; and also among those having had earlier and more children.

The other variable that seems to persist, although not as strongly, is a plurality of sexual partners, and this conforms to another cluster of sociologic definers, including some of those associated also with early coitus, and also those with multiple marriages, infidelity and separation.

Sexual frequency seems to have no bearing upon risk. This memory-based type of information is highly insecure, and a severe level of statistical significance would be required to entertain any degree of confidence. Of about half a dozen major studies where such information was collected, only one [15] resulted in such an extreme difference, and a later study by the same first author resulted in equivalent frequencies for patients and controls. Two other studies showed similar equivalences, and one showed excesses for controls. It is highly doubtful that the quality or quantity of sexual relationships increase risk [4] except insofar as repeated sexual acts with a contaminated male may serve more effectively to initiate susceptible cells during adolescence. For males who do not carry such a carcinogenic principle, and for all males who engage in coitus with females after their adolescence, there would be little or no effect upon risk.

## The Control Levels

There is some academic interest in adapting human carcinoma data to a multistage model derived from experimental animals, not only in establishing such a parallel, but also in that human epidemiologic research has led directly back into the laboratory. This is a reversal of the usual trend, and it has resulted in the search for sexually transmissible agents, one of the possibilities being Herpesvirus type 2. Should such a viral agent be securely identified, control by immunization may eventuate and perhaps incidence will be reduced on a primary population level. Additionally, discovery of direct influences upon the transformation of cells at risk will have been expedited, and the very mechanisms whereby such cells are able to set up a pathologic autonomy will be closer to recognition, although it would be excessively optimistic to hope that a single cause might be found which, without reference to other interacting variables, could condition onset of cancer in all cases.

There is admittedly a fair amount of speculation plus some filling in of events in order to make a portion of the model work out, but the real utility of such a rationale arises when it can become applicable to desperate social situations, in this case widespread morbidity and mortality from this carcinoma. Important objectives in the control of cervical cancer are to identify candidates at increased risk, those who are most likely to reveal dysplasias and *in situ* lesions; and also, when to look for incipient disease in the cervix. Sensitivity to the notion of progressive carcinogenesis through time is crucial, *what happens and how long it takes*, even if some of the steps are fitted to demonstrated laboratory data, and to available human studies. Possible annual mortalities of a quarter million women in the world from a cancer that is almost totally controllable deserves some social appraisal, including extension of a developed model to an *action* level.

*Life periods.* The age distribution of coital beginnings around adolescence for cervical cancer patients is very tight [3], but detection of the carcinoma ranges from the early 20's into old age. Both of these events are important. The age scale at the bottom of Fig. 1 shows adolescence as a short period, reflected by a double arrow in the lifeline. Postadolescence follows and continues into adulthood. Following detection, there are the sequellae of treatment, recovery and perhaps recurrences, all leading to the endpoint where the patient survives or dies. If she survives, there are continuing social problems with which any compassionate culture must deal.

*The intervention level.* We now may return to the profile of our candidate at risk. Having been born with an endowed probability that a cervical cancer one day will be diagnosed, and with such a prospect greatly increased by early sexuality, there is opportunity for conditioning before she reaches adolescence. Preadolescence is the period when behavioral patterns are reinforced. What she does during adolescence is conditioned by what she has learned and what has been organized for her prior to adolescence. This is when matters such as early insights into sexuality, problems of parental communication with young daughters, relatedness to peer groups, and other issues bearing upon later adolescent activities are subject to resolution.

True intervention is by primary prevention insofar as it presents a secure barrier to the onset of disease by interference with the disease process. This is not feasible unless we know where, when and how to intercept pathology. In achieving this, it is indispensable to understand the contributions of every determinable event upon the onset of disease. For cervical cancer, studies consistently have upheld adolescence as the core period of initial susceptibility, and sexuality as the launching event. However, although adolescence clearly is recognizable as a period of exuberant growth, development, secretion, metabolic activity and emotional crisis, biologic entrance into and exit from adolescence varies from individual to individual, by geography, by population, and perhaps also by the complexion of societal pressures, including those of poverty, neglect, lack of education, and culturally determined timetables. For this reason, the age scale at the bottom of Fig. 1 is shown with fluid limits for adolescence around ages 15 to 20.

Studies in white populations [3, 15, 17, 18] show that excesses of cervical cancer patients experienced first coitus before age 17 compared with controls, with dilution thereafter, and the trend reversing after about age 20. The effect seems accelerated by about 2 years for blacks is some populations [11]. The level of significance for this trend in whites and blacks in exceptionally powerful, and separate subsamples from a large population are congruent [3]. Primary prevention of cervical cancer by short-term postponement of adolescent coitus would involve extremely difficult cultural strategies, including not only the transference of sublevel populations into more favorable circumstances, but also the reestablishment of the nuclear family, the maintenance of family structure and cohesiveness, solidification of the mother-daughter relationship, community wide sexual education programs on adolescent peer levels, resolution of problems associated with continuing and differently paced erotic loads of young males; and also, education directed at that segment of social scientists in which advocacy of very early sexual relationships currently is fashionable. In some cultures prevention at this level would be more formidable than in others, especially those where ritual and sexuality are combined in demonstrations of maturity.

Secondary prevention is definable as detection of early disease in relation to developing morbidity. For cervical cancer, it can take place at any time during latency with Papanicoloau smear test programs. From Fig. 1, the question of when to inaugurate smear test surveillance can be resolved has an inverse association: as a woman grows older and is found with a first negative smear, the probability of a positive second smear becomes reduced. After the modal age of cancer detection, perhaps 50, there is a decreasing likelihood that repeat smears will reveal pathology. The reasons for this are suggested by the diagram: primary modification may have taken place early in life, but if secondary modification has not already occurred, there is little chance that it will. However, a negative smear early in life does not indicate that primary modification and transformation before Stage 2 cannot yet occur. Therefore, it is advisable to continue with smears, at least until after the probability subsides that cocarcinogenesis has taken place. The precautionary position is that pathology develops at different rates, and even if most precancerous lesions are initiated during adolescence, detectable pathology may require few or many years for development. Every nonvirgin woman at any age should have a smear test; younger women should be continuously programmed for cytology. Having had negative tests over a period of years, continuing cytology stands little chance of revealing suspicion. These observations are directly in conflict with old notions in practice that smear tests need not be given to women who are young. Adolescence and youth are the best periods for secondary intervention in searching for pathology.

During adulthood the developing lesion is clinically detected if intervention has not already taken place. Cocarcinogenesis has occurred and intervention now may be construed as the act of finding pathology that precipitates the crisis reaction. For populations, especially in high risk groups, this event is *casefinding*. The technology of intervention includes modalities of treatment as the concern of the clinician for both *in situ* and invasive cancers. An awareness of cocarcinogenesis, Fig. 1, as a point in the lifeline necessary for promotion of the lesion into invasion brings the realization that many early lesions will never reach Stage 2, regressing or remaining stationary, and requiring decisions in choosing surveillance over further treatment.

A short chronic period follows and thereafter there is need for rehabilitation as another life period, and also continued supervision in watching for recurring disease. Should an *in situ* carcinoma be kept under appraisal without treatment, rehabilitation is indicated since apprehension may become phobic unless the physician elects to maintain silence regarding diagnosis.

Following the optimal five year post-treatment period, an endpoint may be positioned on the lifeline defining termination or survival. If survival, and this usually is the case where care is adequate, there is a continuing need for rehabilitation and reassurance for the patient and all who transact with her. Cancerphobia is well known to those who counsel or provide psychotherapy, and the afflicted include those in anticipation of disease as well as those in rehabilitation.

*The action level.* In planning programs for reduction of risk, morbidity and mortality of cervical cancer, it is necessary to resolve responsibility. The imperative of action is reached at the point where epidemiologic investigation has produced data and a model in the light of which further delays are neither warranted nor responsible. Responsibility for preadolescent conditioning lies with mothers, health professionals, educators and perhaps the public media. The involvement of the young girl with her peer set is so strong that coordinated educational efforts, especially in sexuality, are essential. There is a subtlety in preparing very young girls for their later sexual lives and certainly this does not include a threatening awareness of disease processes since such messages not only would be rejected and neglected, they might not even be apprehended. Maintenance of family structure can lead to open discussion and resolution of curiosity for better effect in anticipation of adolescence.

Responsibility toward the adolescent girl is shown as a sociomedical action level in Fig. 1 because it involves the setting of priorities in community health by all indicated classes of professionals. Group education in sexuality with more detail on a mature level, special concern with young girls in unfortunate settings, evaluation of mother-daughter dependencies, and high involvement activities all are indicated. It is at this time that the advantages of short-term postponement of sexual onset can be explored, but this is a delicate undertaking requiring professional skills in order that fears may not be engendered which can result in frigidity and destruction of sexual fulfillment somewhat later in life. The physician can do much to influence short postponements of sexuality, with reinforcement by community and diversionary activities. The physician also must acknowledge his share of responsibility in learning to deal comfortably with the subject of sexuality, in finding rapport with adolescent girls, in providing smear tests for those who have entered sexual lives, and in conveying information.

Following adolescence, sociomedical action extends into the span of latency. On a private level the physician can be served by the model in reaching surveillance decisions. On the community level, and also on the political level, the responsibility is for programs of casefinding and prevention by cytology and examination. The community also must appraise the preparedness of individual physicians and other professionals in collecting sexual and other types of sensitive information, and also in counseling. Classification of cytologic smears and decisions regarding diagnosis and therapeutics are specialist functions for pathologist and clinician. The superior aspect of action lies in provision of access to, and motivation toward, adequate care for all women who are at risk and who are found with disease, particularly those in identified risk groups.

With detection of the invasive carcinoma, the lifeline enters a level of strong clinical participation. Adequate medical followup is an action requirement for all so found. With survival, the sociologic action level focuses upon rehabilitation and continuing care during convalescence and anxiety periods.

*Validity*. The dependability with which such a model can be useful for control is reflected by the security with which data supports the continuum of developing disease. However, the central position of adolescent coitus as the time when the carcinoma is initiated, whether taken as a sociologic or a biologic variable, is well demonstrated in demographic and risk studies. Association of adolescent age limits with events increasing risk of initiation is shown as *firm* at the validity level in Fig. 1 to indicate that onset of disease is established at around this point in life and in this manner, but all succeeding points in the lifeline are shown as *variable* to explain the fluidity of events at any time after adolescence. Invasion of the lesion into the surrounding stroma can occur early in the third decade of life or as late as age 90. *In situ* lesions have been found in women past 80 years of age, which might indicate that some such lesions are stationary, and would further suggest a genetic component.

## Summary and Conclusions

The temporal pivot is the attribute of adolescence, supported by the probability that a carcinogenic agent will be conveyed to the milieu of the cervix by a male sexual consort. The chance of encountering such a carrier increases with more sexual mates. The direct variables increasing risk are *early coitus* and *multiple sexual partners*. Both taken together cover most other events so far associated in epidemiologic reports, including marriage, gravidity, abortions and other traumas, separations, contraception, venereal disease, and social status. In assessing the relevance of variables and attributes upon risk of disease it is necessary to distinguish between sociocultural and biologic contributions, and it hardly is useful to associate the ceremony of marriage and the misery of social disadvantage with pathology in the cervix unless the biologic definers in these domains are identified. Early marriage inaugurates early coitus; disadvantage contains early coitus as a related practice. In planning control however, intervention in social processes can reduce risk and disease frequencies provided that such planning is depended upon a biologic base, as shown in the model. Postponement of sexuality for a short period is a cultural adaptation that reduces morbidity because it has a direct influence upon initiation of carcinoma of the cervix; and cytologic programs also are directly related to the continuum of developing disease.

The one other alternative is social: to elevate depressed population segments into higher classifications of economic and educational exposure and opportunity, on the assumption that altered life patterns will result in altered life's chances and reduced incidence rates. In such a solution, the concomitant effect of reorganized sexual schedules also is directly upon the cervix.

## References


1. BERENBLUM, I.: The mechanism of carcinogenesis. A study of the significance of cocarcinogenic action and related phenomena. Cancer Res. **1**, 807—814 (1941).
2. ROTKIN, I. D.: Relation of adolescent coitus to cervical cancer risk. J.A.M.A. **179**, 486—491 (1962).
3. ROTKIN, I. D.: Adolescent coitus and cervical cancer: associations of related events with increased risk. Cancer Res. **27**, 603—617 (1967).
4. ROTKIN, I. D.: Sexual characteristics of a cervical cancer population. Amer. J. Publ. Hlth **57**, 815—829 (1967).

5. Rotkin, I. D., Cameron, J. R.: Clusters of variables influencing risk of cervical cancer. Cancer **21**, 663—671 (1968).
6. Cassel, J.: Social science theory as a source of hypotheses in epidemiologic methods. Amer. J. publ. Hlth. **54**, 1482—1488 (1964).
7. Wahi, P. N., Saraswati, M., Luthra, V. K.: Factors influencing cancer of the uterine cervix in North India. Cancer **23**, 1221—1226 (1969).
8. Stamler, J., Fields, C., Andelman, S. L.: Epidemiology of cancer of the cervix. Amer. J. Publ. Hlth **57**, 791—803 (1967).
9. MacMahon, B., Pugh, T. F.: Epidemiology principles and methods, Chapter 2. Boston: Little, Brown and Co., 1970.
10. Reid, B. L.: Cancer of the cervix uteri. Review of causal factors with an hypothesis as to its origin. Med. J. Austr. **1**, 375—383 (1965).
11. Rotkin, I. D., Taylor, W. E.: Ethnic comparability of the relation between early coital trends and cervical cancer. Cancer **23**, 458—460 (1969).
12. Armitage, P., Doll, R.: Stochastic models for carcinogenesis. In: J. Neyman (ed.) Proceedings of the Fourth Berkeley Symposium on Mathematical Statistics and Probability, Vol. IV: 4, Contributions to Biology and Problems of Medicine, pp. 19—38. Berkeley: University of California Press, 1960.
13. Aitken-Swan, J., Baird, D.: Cancer of the uterine cervix in Aberdeenshire. Aetiological aspects. Brit. J. Cancer **20**, 642—659 (1966).
14. Ferguson, J. H.: Positive cancer smears in teenage girls. J.A.M.A. **178**, 91—94 (1961).
15. Terris, M., Oalmann, M. C.: Carcinoma of the cervix. An epidemiologic study. J.A.M.A. **174**, 155—159 (1960).
16. Martin, C. E.: Marital and coital factors in cervical cancer. Amer. J. Publ. Hlth **57**, 803—814 (1967).
17. Terris, M., Wilson, F., Smith, H., Sprung, E., Nelson, J. H.: The relationship of coitus to carcinoma of the cervix. Amer. J. Publ. Hlth **57**, 841—847 (1967).
18. Wynder, E. L., Cornfield, G., Schroff, P. D., Doraiswami, K. R.: Study of environmental factors in carcinoma of the cervix. Amer. J. Obstet. Gynec. **68**, 1016—1052 (1954).

# Hormones in the Aetiology and Clinical Course of Breast Cancer

D. Y. WANG, MARGARET C. SWAIN, J. L. HAYWARD [1], and R. D. BULBROOK

Imperial Cancer Research Fund, Lincoln's Inn Fields, London, Great Britain

## Hormones in the Pre-Clinical Phase of Breast Cancer

In 1961 a prospective study was set up to test the hypothesis that the excretion of subnormal amounts of urinary androgen metabolites was related to a high risk of developing breast cancer. Urine was collected from 5,000 normal women and the excretion of androgen metabolites by women who subsequently had breast cancer was compared with that of ostensibly normal controls.

A preliminary report (BULBROOK and HAYWARD, 1967) indicated that women in whom a diagnosis of breast cancer was made tended to excrete smaller amounts of aetiocholanolone than controls matched for age, height, weight, menstrual status and parity. It was also suggested, that if 17-hydroxycorticosteroid (17-OHCS) excretion was also taken into account, the steroid abnormalities in pre-cancer cases might be multi-directional and that there might be several patterns of abnormal steroid excretion associated with a high risk of breast cancer.

Further results (BULBROOK, HAYWARD and SPICER, 1971) from this prospective study, based on 27 cases and 1506 controls, show that the characteristic abnormality in pre-cancer cases is a sub-normal excretion of androsterone and aetiocholanolone. This abnormality is present at all ages between 35 and 55 years. It is independent of the time before diagnosis of the tumour; the abnormality was found up to 9 years before diagnosis and is not a late event in the pre-clinical history of the disease. Finally, there is a direct relationship between the amount of urinary aetiocholanolone and risk of breast cancer. Women excreting less than 800 μg per 24 hrs. have approx. 5 times the risk of those excreting between 1—2 mg. per 24 hrs. The incidence curve appears to rise again for women excreting more than 2 mg of aetiocholanolone per 24 hrs., but there are not enough data to establish this point with certainty, although the finding is in keeping with the concept of multi-directional abnormalities proposed previously.

Plasma oestradiol-17$\beta$ levels have been determined in 5 women who subsequently developed breast cancer and in 31 matched controls. The oestradiol-17$\beta$ levels in the pre-cancer cases were indistinguishable from those in the control women.

---

1 Breast Unit, Guy's Hospital, London, Great Britain.

## Plasma Androgen Levels in Benign Breast Disease

If a sub-normal excretion of androgen metabolites is associated with a high risk of breast cancer, then it might be expected that women already known to have an increased risk would show similar abnormalities. Such women would include patients with benign breast disease (see Warren, 1940).

It has been shown that there is a close and significant relationship between the amount of 11-deoxy-17-oxosteroids in urine and the concentration of dehydroepiandrosterone sulphate (DS) in plasma (Wang, 1969). Accordingly, plasma levels

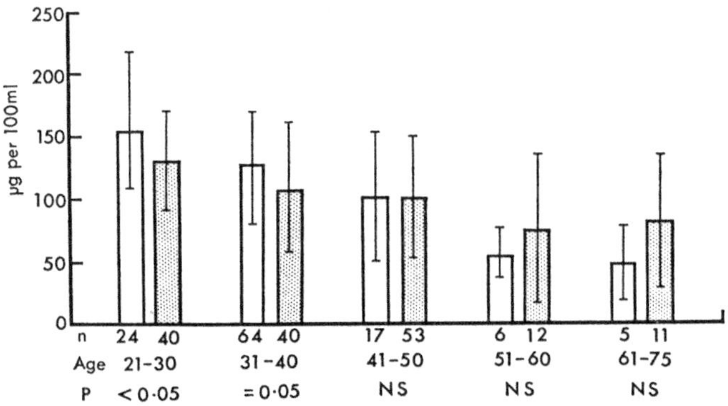


**Fig. 1. Plasma dehydroepiandrosterone sulphate and benign breast disease.** Mean levels of plasma dehydroepiandrosterone sulphate (DS) are shown for control (□) and for subjects with benign breast lesion (⁝⁝⁝) in various age groups. The number of subjects in group are indicated (n). The statistical difference between the control and benign groups in any one age group is shown (P)

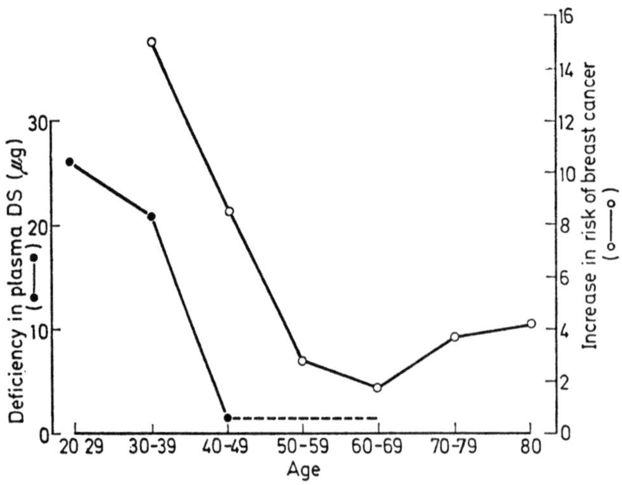


**Fig. 2. Benign breast disease and risk of breast cancer.** The increase in risk of breast cancer as calculated by Warren (1940) is shown for various age groups (o—o). Also shown is the differences, where statistically significant, in mean plasma dehydroepiandrosterone sulphate concentrations between normal subjects and patients with benign breast disease (●—●)

of DS were measured in 156 women with a variety of benign breast lesions and in 116 controls. The mean concentration of DS was significantly lower in women with benign breast disease, aged between 20—40 years compared with that of normal controls (Fig. 1). In subsequent decades the differences were not significant. The increase in risk of breast disease calculated by WARREN (1940), is shown in the Fig. 2. The results are consistent with the thesis that low plasma DS concentrations in these patients are associated with a high risk of breast cancer.

Further support for this concept has been obtained from other studies in which it has been shown that women with benign breast disease aged between 20—40 years excreted significantly less urinary aetiocholanolone than controls and also have significantly lower concentrations of total plasma 17-oxosteroids (BRENNAN, HAYWARD, DESHPANDE and BULBROOK, unpublished observations).

In a preliminary study the levels of oestradiol-17$\beta$ in plasma have been measured in 24 pre-menopausal women with benign breast lesions and in 23 controls. No significant differences were found: The plasma oestradiol-17$\beta$ concentrations appear to be normal in these patients.

At present, the relationship between steroid levels and the histological findings in the breast lesions has not been determined but this investigation is now in progress.

## Endogenous Steroids and the Clinical Course of Breast Cancer

### Early Disease

From the moment that a diagnosis of breast cancer is made a number of uncontrolled variables affect the results of any study made on the endocrine status of such patients. These include psychological stresses (KATZ, ACKMAN, ROTHWAX, SACHAR, WEINER, HELLMAN and GALLAGHER, 1970) associated with the diagnosis and entry to hospital, effects of surgery and drugs, and the general influence of illness (CHOU and WANG, 1939; ZUMOFF, BRADLOW, GALLAGHER and HELLMAN, 1971).

There is some controversy concerning androgen metabolite excretion by patients with early breast cancer (at the time of mastectomy). BULBROOK, HAYWARD, THOMAS and SPICER (1962) found that such patients excreted sub-normal amounts of urinary androsterone and aetiocholanolone ten days after mastectomy. This findings has been confirmed by various workers (MARMORSTON, 1966; BACIGALUPO and LINGK, 1968; GUTIERREZ and WILLIAMS, 1968) although not by CAMERON and his associates (CAMERON, GRIFFITHS, GLEAVE, STEWART, FORREST and CAMPBELL, 1970). Part of this confusion may have arisen because of differences in the time at which the urine was collected (i.e., pre- or post-mastectomy). Certainly BULBROOK, HAYWARD, THOMAS and SPICER (1962) studied women 10 days after mastectomy unlike CAMERON *et al.* (1970) who studied pre-mastectomy patients.

A study made on the effect of mastectomy on the concentration of plasma DS on 146 patients with early breast cancer, showed that mastectomy is generally associated with a significant decrease in the level of plasma DS (Fig. 3). The mean percentage decrease in DS is approximately 20% and highly significant ($P < 0.001$). When these values are compared with normal women (Fig. 3) the pre-mastectomy plasma DS concentrations are somewhat lower than controls, whereas, the post-operative levels are markedly sub-normal and appear to remain so in patients who have been followed for periods up to 10 months after mastectomy.

These results emphasise the importance of the timing of the collection of plasma and urine samples. At present, it is impossible to interpret these findings. The pre-operative measurements undoubtedly involve some stress factors (which include diagnosis and entry to hospital). The post-mastectomy measurements are complicated by the effects of surgery. Nevertheless, the finding of sub-normal androgen excretion before diagnosis (BULBROOK *et al.*, 1971) implies that the post-operative period may provide a better estimate of basal, non-stressed levels of androgen secretion rather than during the pre-operative period.

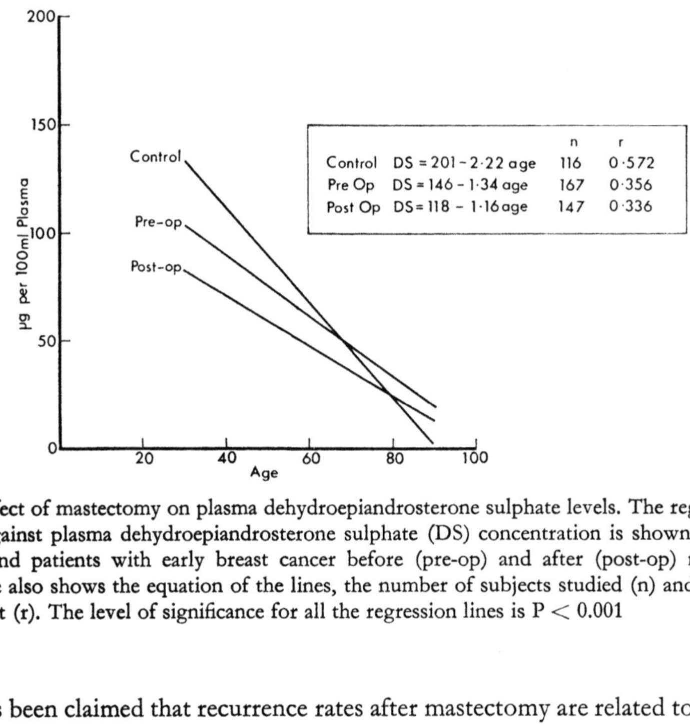


Fig. 3. Effect of mastectomy on plasma dehydroepiandrosterone sulphate levels. The regression line for age against plasma dehydroepiandrosterone sulphate (DS) concentration is shown for control subjects and patients with early breast cancer before (pre-op) and after (post-op) mastectomy. The figure also shows the equation of the lines, the number of subjects studied (n) and correlation co-efficient (r). The level of significance for all the regression lines is $P < 0.001$

It has been claimed that recurrence rates after mastectomy are related to androgen and 17-OHCS excretion. Women who excrete smaller amounts of aetiocholanolone relative to those of the 17-OHCS have tumours that recur at a faster rate than women excreting larger amounts of aetiocholanolone (HAYWARD and BULBROOK, 1968). Preliminary results obtained after mastectomy indicate that women with plasma levels of DS who are at the lower end of the range for their age have a faster rate of recurrence.

The oestrogenic status of women with early breast cancer is not clear. Some workers (BACIGALUPO and SCHUBERT, 1966; LEMON, WOTIZ, PARSON and MOZDEN, 1966; SCHWEPPE, JUNGMAN and LEWIN, 1967) have found a sub-normal excretion (mainly in the oestriol fraction). Others have found normal excretion (JULL, SHUCK-SMITH and BONSER, 1963), whilst a third group have found marginally raised amounts of urinary oestrogens (NISSEN-MEYER and SANNER, 1963; PROCOPÉ, 1968; HELLMAN, ZUMOFF, FISHMAN and GALLAGHER, 1971).

## Advanced Breast Cancer

Patients with advanced breast cancer who excrete sub-normal amounts of urinary androgen metabolites tend to respond badly to endocrine ablation (BULBROOK, GREENWOOD and HAYWARD, 1960; JURET, 1968; KUMAOKA, SAKAUCHI, ABE, KUSAMA and TAKATANI, 1968). The findings of CAMERON *et al.* (1970) are not entirely in accordance with these results in that they found that only patients with locally advanced disease showed a sub-normal excretion of androgen metabolites.

Plasma concentrations of DS have been found to be low in patients with metastatic disease (WANG, 1969) but there is no information whether the plasma steroid levels correlate with response.

In general, there appears to be little correlation between oestrogen excretion and response to endocrine ablation (see BULBROOK, 1963).

## Interpretation of Results

Urinary androgen metabolite excretion is low in the pre-clinical phase of the disease, in patients with early breast cancer and in those with the advanced metastatic disease. There is a variety of explanations for these findings. The first is that since androgen metabolite excretion decreases in many chronic diseases (CHOU and WANG, 1939), the low androgen encountered in the studies described above are non-specific to breast cancer and are due to illness, as suggested by ZUMOFF *et al.* (1971). This simplistic suggestion is improbable since by no stretch of the imagination could the pre-cancer cases be described as ill women, nor do the patients with benign breast disease fit in to any of the crude categories of "sickness" which ZUMOFF *et al.* (1971) have attempted to define. Nevertheless, their results are not without interest and certainly, as the disease advances the androgen excretion declines, and this is obviously related in part to illness (CHOU and WANG, 1939).

The second explanation for the close relation between androgenic status and breast cancer is that the androgens may be involved in the control of tumour growth. Such a control has been described for the Shinogi mouse tumour (MINESITA and YAMAGUCHI, 1965). Further, WAGNER and JUNGBLUT (personal communication) have found a receptor protein for 5$\alpha$ dihydrotestosterone in human breast tumours.

A third explanation is that the abnormalities in the androgens are simply indicative of other more fundamental changes in the endocrine environment.

In normal women, the amount of androsterone and aetiocholanolone found in the urine are highly correlated with the amounts of oestrone, oestradiol-17$\beta$ and oestriol (ADLERCREUTZ, LUUKAINEN and SVANBERG, 1967). From this, it might be argued that the sub-normal androgen excretion generally found in pre-cancer cases, reflects a sub-normal oestrogen excretion. This correlation might explain the epidemiological observation that anovulatory menstrual cycles and a degree of infertility are characteristic of patients with breast cancer (GRATTAROLA, 1964). Such a concept is entirely unexpected in view of the commonly held belief that oestrogens may be "carcinogenic" in man, as they are in the rat and mouse (HERTZ, 1957). The term "carcinogenic" is used here in a very loose sense and embraces a promoting action for the oestrogens or merely a role in controlling the rate of tumour growth.

Recent evidence shows that prolactin plays an important part in increasing the incidence of breast tumours in mice (BOOT, 1970). Tumours induced by dimethylbenzanthracene in the rat are prolactin, rather than oestrogen dependent (PEARSON, LLERENA, MOLINA and BUTLER, 1969). Since PEARSON *et al.* (1969) have shown that plasma oestrogen and prolactin levels run in parallel in the rat, under defined experimental conditions, this might imply that in the human, the presumptive low oestrogen levels may be accompanied by a low secretion rate of prolactin. The conclusion would be that in the majority of women with breast cancer, the tumours would occur in those who are subjected, not to a gross hypersecretion of factors leading to breast growth, but to a deficiency in the hormones.

The hook in the curve describing the relationship between aetiocholanolone and the incidence of breast cancer may mean that in a minority of cases hypersecretion of oestrogens and prolactin occurs. The availability of assays for plasma oestradiol-17$\beta$ (KORENMAN, PERRIN and MCCALLUM, 1969) and for human prolactin (HWANG, GUYDA and FRIESEN, 1971) means that these speculations can now be tested.

Once the disease is established, it might be expected from the above argument that tumours arising in an endocrine environment characterized by a deficiency in oestrogens, androgens and prolactin would not be susceptible to alterations in this environment brought about by endocrine ablation. This is precisely what has been found for the androgens. The reason why such tumours recur rapidly after mastectomy is not clear.

In conclusion, there is now a considerable amount of evidence that in the majority of cases a subnormal excretion of androgen metabolites is related to a high risk of breast cancer and an unfavourable clinical course of the disease. It is suggested that oestrogen levels may also be subnormal in these women and preliminary investigations have certainly not shown raised plasma oestradiol-17$\beta$ levels in pre-cancer cases or in young women with benign breast disease. The recent introduction of methods for the measurement of plasma oestradiol-17$\beta$ and prolactin in conjunction with a current prospective study in normal women means that it should eventually be possible to determine with some precision the endocrine environment associated with a high risk of subsequent breast cancer and to replace speculation with experimental data.

## Acknowledgements

The authors would like to thank Miss M. HERIAN for her highly-skilled technical assistance.

## References

ADLERCREUTZ, H., LUUKAINEN, T., SVANBERG, A.: Ann. Med. exp. Fenn. **45**, 277 (1967).
BACIGALUPO, G., LINGK, H.: Arch. Geschwulstforsch. **32**, 95 (1968).
BACIGALUPO, G., SCHUBERT, K.: Europ. J. Cancer **2**, 75 (1966).
BOOT, L. M.: Int. J. Cancer **5**, 167 (1970).
BULBROOK, R. D.: Proc. Ass. clin. Biochem. **2**, 165 (1963).
BULBROOK, R. D., GREENWOOD, F. C., HAYWARD, J. L.: Lancet **1960 I**, 1154.
BULBROOK, R. D., HAYWARD, J. L.: Lancet **1967 I**, 519.
BULBROOK, R. D., HAYWARD, J. L., SPICER, C. C.: Lancet **1971 II**, 395.
BULBROOK, R. D., HAYWARD, J. L., THOMAS, B. S., SPICER, C. C.: Lancet **1962 II**, 1238.
CAMERON, E. H. D., GRIFFITHS, K., GLEAVE, N., STEWART, H. J., FORREST, A. P. M., CAMPBELL, H.: Brit. med. J. **4**, 768 (1970).
CHOU, C. Y., WANG, C. W.: Chinese J. Physiol. **14**, 151 (1939).

GRATTAROLA, R.: Cancer **17**, 1119 (1964).
GUTIERREZ, R. M., WILLIAMS, R. J.: Proc. nat. Acad. Sci. (Wash.) **59**, 938 (1968).
HAYWARD, J. L., BULBROOK, R. D.: In: Prognostic Factors in Breast Cancer. Eds. A. P. M. FORREST and P. B. KUNKLER. Edinburgh: Livingstone 1968, p. 383.
HELLMAN, L., ZUMOFF, B., FISHMAN, J., GALLAGHER, T. F.: J. clin. Endocr. **33**, 138 (1971).
HERTZ, R.: Cancer Res. **17**, 423 (1957).
HWANG, P., GUYDA, H., FRIESEN, H.: Proc. nat. Acad. Sci. (Wash.) **68**, 1902 (1971).
JULL, J. W., SHUCKSMITH, H. S., BONSER, G. M.: J. clin. Endocr. **23**, 433 (1963).
JURET, P.: In: Prognostic Factors in Breast Cancer. Eds. A. P. M. FORREST and P. B. KUNKLER. Edinburgh: Livingstone 1968, p. 393.
KATZ, J. L., ACKMAN, P., ROTHWAX, Y., SACHER, E., WEINER, H., HELLMAN, L., GALLAGHER, T. F.: Psychosomatics **22**, 1 (1970).
KORENMAN, S. G., PERRIN, L. E., MCCALLUM, T. P.: J. clin. Endocr. **29**, 879 (1969).
KUMAOKA, S., SAKAUCHI, N., ABE, O., KUSAMA, M., TAKATANI, O.: J. clin. Endocr. **28**, 667 (1968).
LEMON, H. M., WOTIZ, H. H., PARSON, L., MOZDEN, P. J.: J. Amer. med. Ass. **196**, 1128 (1966).
MARMORSTON, J.: Ann. Acad. Sci. (N. Y.) **125**, 959 (1966).
MINESITA, T., YAMAGUCHI, K.: Cancer Res. **25**, 1168 (1965).
NISSEN-MEYER, R., SANNER, T.: Acta endocr. (Kbh.) **44**, 334 (1963).
PEARSON, O. H., LLERENA, O., MOLINA, A., BUTLER, T.: Trans. Ass. Amer. Phys. **82**, 225 (1969).
PROCOPÉ, B. J.: Acta endocr. (Kbh.) **60**, Supp. 135 (1968).
SCHWEPPE, J. S., JUNGMAN, R. A., LEVIN, I.: Cancer **20**, 155 (1967).
WANG, D. Y.: In: The Human Adrenal Gland and its Relation to Breast Cancer. First Tenovus Workshop. Eds.: K. GRIFFITHS and E. H. D. CAMERON, p. 71. Alpha Omega Alpha Press, 1969.
WARREN, S.: Surg. Gynec. Obstet. **71**, 257 (1940).
ZUMOFF, B., BRADLOW, L. H., GALLAGHER, T. F., HELLMAN, L.: J. clin. Endocr. **32**, 824 (1971)

# The Ovarian Etiology of Human Breast Cancer

Brian MacMahon and Philip Cole

Department of Epidemiology, Harvard School of Public Health, Boston, Massachusetts, USA

Knowledge of the epidemiology of breast cancer would seem to have reached the point where it should be possible to formulate and test rather specific etiologic hypotheses. To emphasize this point, we may consider one of the findings from a recently completed international collaborative study, in which histories of reproduction, lactation and illness among breast cancer cases were compared with those of women hospitalized for other diseases. The study was undertaken in seven centers representing populations with very different breast cancer incidence rates [1]. A strong association was noted between age at first birth and breast cancer risk (Fig. 1). Women who had a first child prior to age 18 had only about one third the breast cancer risk of those whose first birth was delayed until the age of 35 or later [2]. Births after the first appeared to have little or no effect on breast cancer risk, the association between total parity and breast cancer risk noted in earlier studies being a consequence of the negative correlation between age at first birth and total parity.

It has been known for many years that women in North America and Europe have about five times the breast cancer rate of those in Japan. The association between breast cancer risk and age at first birth did not explain any of the difference in incidence rates between North America and Japan, and indeed, in terms of relative risk, the association was as strong in Tokyo as in Boston.

Knowing that the risks associated with these two variables (geography and age at first birth) are independent, it follows that an American woman whose first child is born when she is over 35 years of age has about 15 times the breast cancer risk of a Japanese woman who has her first child when less than 18 years of age. This risk differential is as great as that seen in the association of cancer of the lung with cigarette smoking. Explanatory etiologic mechanisms are still lacking for both associations. While there is an important distinction between the two situations, in that the potential for prevention of lung cancer exists even in the absence of knowledge of explanatory mechanisms while the risk factors identified for breast cancer do not lend themselves to preventive measures, the observed variations in breast cancer risk appear nevertheless to offer considerable potential for preventive action if their mechanisms could be identified and are found to have alterable components.

Endocrine patterns provide one of the most obvious possibilities for investigations directed towards understanding the variation in breast cancer risk between and within populations. Nearly all investigators—clinicians, experimentalists and epidemiologists—believe that the ovary specifically plays some role in the etiology of human breast cancer. There is, however, little agreement as to the nature, mechanism or magnitude of that role. During recent years, we and our colleagues have made observations relevant to some of the issues involved. In this paper we will summarize observations that seem most pertinent to the following questions:

1. In what proportion of breast cancer cases is the etiologic role of the ovary significant?
2. Is this role important in post-menopausal as well as premenopausal breast cancer cases?
3. At what age is ovarian function most effective in producing changes in breast cancer risk?
4. Is the role of estrogenic activity that of inducing breast tumors or merely one of providing a favorable environment for the growth of tumors induced through other mechanisms?
5. What is the specific characteristic of ovarian function that relates to variation in breast cancer risk?

## Quantitative Significance of Ovarian Etiology

Several investigators have shown that women whose menopause is surgically induced have a reduced risk of breast cancer—particularly when the menopause is induced at a relatively early age [3—7]. In a recent comparison of a large series of breast cancer patients with a national probability sample of United States women [8] it was estimated that women who had surgical menopause prior to age 35 experience a breast cancer risk only one third that of women having a natural menopause—a figure quite consistent with previous estimates. From this it follows that the ovary plays an important role in at least two thirds of cases of human breast cancer.

The effect of early curtailment of ovarian activity has not been examined in humans, since castration is quite uncommon under 30 years of age, by which time women have experienced about half of the usual period of ovarian activity. In dogs, however, is has been shown that neutered bitches—usually neutered early in adult life—have only 12% of the breast cancer risk of intact animals. Furthermore, the reduction in risk is correlated with the number of estrous cycles that have occurred prior to the neutering. It has been estimated that bitches neutered prior to any estrous cycle experience less than one percent of the risk of intact females [9].

In short, the proportion of human cancer cases that depend on an intact ovary for their development is at least two thirds and may be considerably higher.

## The Ovary in Post-menopausal Breast Cancer

In the study referred to above [8], it was possible to examine breast cancer risk following surgical menopause according to age at diagnosis of cancer as well as age at menopause. Little reduction in breast cancer risk occurred in the decade following the surgical menopause, but subsequent to that decade the reduction in risk prevailed for the remainder of life (Fig. 2). Among women whose menopause was induced prior to age 35, breast cancer risk was only one third of expected even thirty and more years later—that is, when the women were in the seventh and eight decades of life. Similarly, among women with menopause induced between

35 and 44 years of age, breast cancer risk thirty years later was still only one half of that expected.

In the same study, age at natural menopause was examined. It was observed that the breast cancer risk of women whose menopause occurred at age 55 or older was approximately twice as high as that of women whose menopause occurred prior to age 45. This increased risk was as strong among women whose cancer was first diagnosed after 70 years of age as among younger groups.

The long latent period between induction and clinical appearance of human cancer is well known, and it is no surprise that the effects of etiologic events in the fourth and fifth decades of life become manifest many years later. These observations do, however, provide direct evidence that the etiologic role of the ovary is not restricted to breast tumors that become clinically apparent during the years of cyclic ovarian activity.

## Age When Ovarian Activity is Significant

There is a potentially important inconsistency between certain sets of observations in their implications to the ages during which ovarian activity appears to affect the breast cancer risk.

A number of investigators, most recently STASZEWSKI [10], have noted an inverse relationship between age at menarche and breast cancer risk. Information from the international study already referred to is summarized in Table 1. The downward trend in risk with increasing age at menarche was not seen in all centers, but the heterogeneity between centers was not statistically significant. Of course, recall of age at menarche by women in the breast cancer age range is quite unreliable; on the reasonable assumption that it is equally unreliable for cases and controls, we would conclude that the true strength of the association is underestimated in a study based on anamnestic data. In addition, even when accurately timed, menarche

Table 1. Observed and expected distribution of breast cancer cases and estimates of relative risk by age at menarche. Data from a recent international study [a]

| Age at menarche | Number of cases | | Relative risk [c] |
|---|---|---|---|
| | Obs. | Exp. [b] | |
| < 13 | 912 | 878.0 | 1.00 |
| 13– | 880 | 816.9 | 1.01 |
| 14– | 1029 | 1009.3 | 0.97 |
| 15– | 666 | 641.8 | 0.95 |
| 16– | 439 | 480.0 | 0.86 |
| 17+ | 335 | 435.3 | 0.74 |
| Total | 4261 | 4261.3 | — |

[a] Data are from the studies reported in references [11] through [17].

[b] Based on the distribution of the control series in the same center, controlled for age in ten-year age groups.

[c] Controlled for center and age at diagnosis in ten-year groups; relative to a risk of 1.0 for women reporting menarche prior to age 13.

is only a crude indicator of the beginning of cyclic ovarian activity—a fact that would tend further to weaken any true relationship between age at onset of such activity and breast cancer risk. Further evidence of the significance of the early years of reproductive life is the fact that estrogen profile differences between Asian and American women, described below, appear to be most marked among young women. There are reasons to believe that the association between age at first birth and breast cancer risk operates through an ovarian mechanism [18]. The fact that pregnancy has no protective effect when it occurs after 30 years of age (Fig. 1) suggests that the factors responsible for the protection are most important during the first half of reproductive life. All these relationships suggest the importance of the early reproductive years.

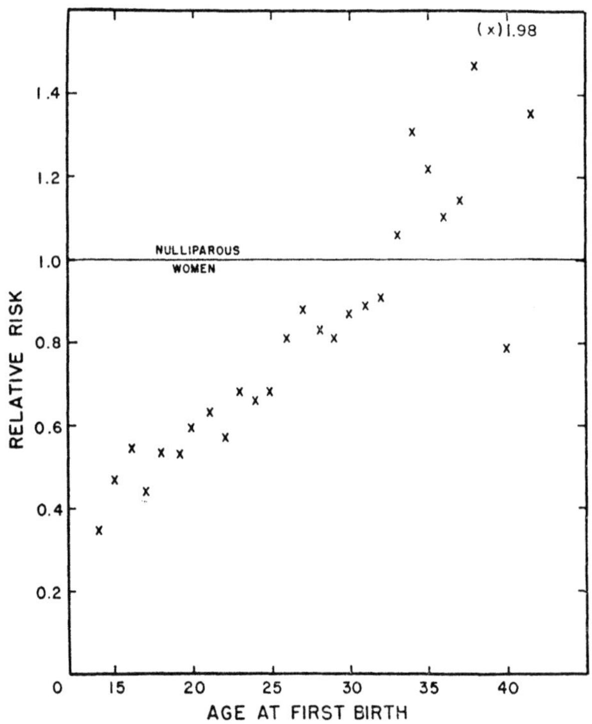


Fig. 1. Relative risk (expressed relative to a risk of 1.0 for nulliparous women) of breast cancer according to age at first birth. (Reprinted from MacMahon *et al.* [2])

On the other hand, the reduction in breast cancer risk following oophorectomy and the association of risk with age at natural menopause indicate that ovarian activity during the second half of reproductive life is also relevant.

At the present time we cannot resolve this inconsistency, but merely note that, while each set of observations tends to focus attention on one or other segment of reproductive life, the observations as a whole imply that the time period during which ovarian activity has etiologic significance may be broad. As noted below, the data on variation in estrogen profile with age are still few and the existence of differences between high and low risk populations in the older age groups cannot be excluded. It must also be recognized that even if the ovary has an etiologic role during a broad period of life the mechanism of that role may not be the same throughout the period.

## Induction or Growth Stimulation

Although the administration of estrogens to experimental animals increases tumor yield under many experimental conditions, not all experimentalists agree that estrogens are capable of actual induction of neoplasia—in contrast to providing a favorable environment for the growth of established tumors. The observations on humans suggest that some ovarian activity—whether estrogen related or not—does have a role in breast tumor induction, whether or not there is also a role in tumor growth enhancement.

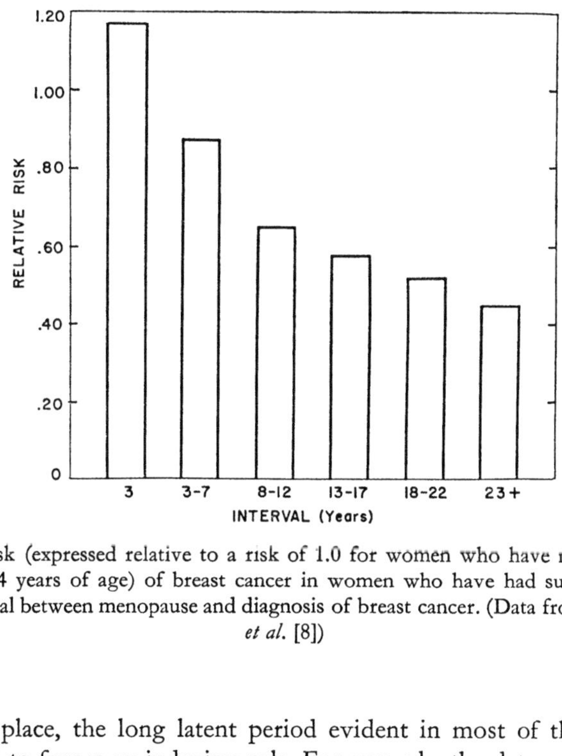


Fig. 2. Relative risk (expressed relative to a risk of 1.0 for women who have natural menopause between 45 and 54 years of age) of breast cancer in women who have had surgical menopause, according to interval between menopause and diagnosis of breast cancer. (Data from TRICHOPOULOS *et al.* [8])

In the first place, the long latent period evident in most of the relationships already referred to favors an inducing role. For example, the data on risk following surgical menopause shown in Fig. 2 suggest that the inducing role is more significant than any growth stimulating effect, since the effect of removal of a growth stimulant might be expected to decrease—rather than increase—with the passage of time. Second, the data on age at menarche in particular suggest an inducing role for some aspect of ovarian activity. It seems most unlikely that breast tumors destined to appear 40 or 50 years later already would have been induced by the time of menarche and that the higher risk for women with early menarche results solely from a few additional years of exposure to a growth enhancing agent—for example, in the case of a women aged 50, to 38 rather than 34 years of exposure. It seems more likely that the years immediately after menarche are years of high risk of tumor induction and that this period of high risk terminates with the first pregnancy. Thus, for women who bear their first child at age 22 the duration of this risk period would vary from 10 years (women with menarche at age 12) to 6 years (menarche at age 16). The relationship of these two intervals (10 years and 6 years) more closely parallels the risk of breast cancer experienced by women with menarche at age 12 relative to those with menarche at age 16.

## Nature of the Ovarian Etiologic Mechanism

For reasons that stem from some of the above observations and that have been outlined in more detail elsewhere [18, 19], we have undertaken to test the hypothesis that the nature of the estrogens produced by a women during her early reproductive years is an important determinant of her life-long breast cancer risk. In brief, the hypothesis derives from the fact that carcinogenic potential has been demonstrated for estrone (E 1) and estradiol (E 2) but not for estriol (E 3), and that E 3 has the capacity to impede certain estrogenic activities of E 1 and E 2 when administered with them. Direct tests of this hypothesis would be quite expensive and—more importantly—involve the lapse of several decades, and a number of indirect tests have therefore been initiated.

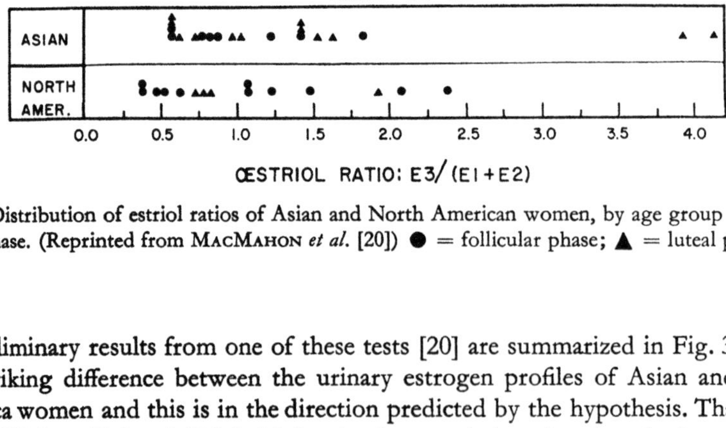


Fig. 3. Distribution of estriol ratios of Asian and North American women, by age group and cycle phase. (Reprinted from MacMahon *et al.* [20]) ● = follicular phase; ▲ = luteal phase

Preliminary results from one of these tests [20] are summarized in Fig. 3. There is a striking difference between the urinary estrogen profiles of Asian and North America women and this is in the direction predicted by the hypothesis. That is, the ratio of E 3 to E 1 and E 2 is higher in the population showing the lower breast cancer rate. Furthermore, the data suggest that the difference is particularly marked among young women, although these data are still too few to exclude the possibility that biologically significant differences also exist in older premenopausal women.

While this difference is compatible with the hypothesis postulating a carcinogenic role for certain estrogens, there are clearly many other differences between Asian and American women that could be responsible for the difference between them in breast cancer risk. BULBROOK and his colleagues have shown differences between breast cancer cases and controls in etiocholanolone excretion several years prior to the clinical appearance of breast cancer [21], and the experimental work of FURTH [22] and MÜHLBOCK [23] has suggested that trophic anterior pituitary activity may be relevant. SMITH and SMITH have suggested that even differences in estrogen profile between high and low breast cancer risk populations might merely reflect more relevant differences in pituitary activity [24]. However, laboratory work continues to accumulate on the protective role of estriol, and other anti-estrogens, against tumor induction in the rat [25]. Consideration of the epidemiologic and experimental evidence in conjunction suggests that the estrogen-fraction hypothesis is certainly worth pursuing to its resolution.

# Conclusion

Even if he makes due allowance for the brevity of this review, the reader must be impressed with the gaps in our information on the significance and nature of the role of the ovary in the etiology of human breast cancer. If these gaps were the result of research having reached a dead end, with no place to go, or of uncertainty as to whether the ovary played any role at all, they might not be surprising. But the evidence for ovarian involvement in this disease is incontrovertible, and there are many avenues still to be explored in the mapping of that involvement. Perhaps the most important aspect on which we have touched concerns the elucidation of the estrogenic or other mechanism whereby the ovarian role is mediated. From the point of view of prevention, however, an even more important issue may be the identification of the factors that are responsible for the variation in such a mechanism —for example, the variation in estrogen profile, if that proves to be the most relevant ovarian characteristic—between populations and between individual women within populations. However, until clearer evidence is obtained as to the nature of the characteristic or characteristics responsible, this further issue seems hardly susceptible to investigation.

## Acknowledgements

We wish to acknowledge our debt to the many colleagues who participated in the various studies from which data have been quoted. Their names appear in the publications referenced. Preparation of this review was aided by a grant from the National Cancer Institute, U.S. Public Health Service (5 PO 1 CA 06373).

# References

1. MACMAHON, B., LIN, T. M., LOWE, C. R. ,MIRRA, A. P., RAVNIHAR, B., SALBER, E. J., TRICHOPOULOS, D., VALAORAS, V. G., YUASA, S.: Lactation and cancer of the breast. Bull. WHO **42**, 185—194 (1970).
2. MACMAHON, B., COLE, P., LIN, T. M., LOWE, C. R., MIRRA, A. P., RAVNIHAR, B., SALBER, E. J., VALAORAS, V. G., YUASA, S.: Age at first birth and breast cancer risk. Bull. WHO **43**, 209—221 (1970).

3. Lilienfeld, A. M.: The relationship of cancer of the female breast to artificial menopause and marital status. Cancer **9**, 927—934 (1956).
4. MacMahon, B., Feinleib, M.: Breast cancer in relation to nursing and menopausal history. J. nat. Cancer Inst. **24**, 733—753 (1960).
5. Hirayama, T., Wynder, E. L.: A study of the epidemiology of cancer of the breast. II. The influence of hysterectomy. Cancer **15**, 28—38 (1962).
6. Feinleib, M.: Breast cancer and artificial menopause: a cohort study. J. nat. Cancer Inst. **41**, 315—329 (1968).
7. Dörken, H.: Häufigkeit und Bedeutung der artifiziellen Menopause bei Herzinfarkt und bei einigen Blastomen. In: Verhandlungen der Deutschen Gesellschaft für innere Medizin, 69 Congress, 1963. München: Bergmann 1963.
8. Trichopoulos, D., MacMahon, B., Cole, P.: The menopause and breast cancer risk. J. nat. Cancer Inst. **48**, 605—613 (1972).
9. Schneider, R., Dorn, C. R., Taylor, D. O. N.: Factors influencing canine mammary cancer development and postsurgical survival. J. nat. Cancer Inst. **43**, 1249—1261 (1969).
10. Staszewski, J.: Age at menarche and breast cancer. J. nat. Cancer Inst. **47**, 935—940 (1971).
11. Lin, T. M., Chen, K. P., MacMahon, B.: Epidemiologic characteristics of cancer of the breast in Taiwan. Cancer **27**, 1497—1504 (1971).
12. Lowe, C. R., MacMahon, B.: Breast cancer and reproductive history of women in South Wales. Lancet **1970 I**, 153—157.
13. Mirra, A. P., Cole, P., MacMahon, B.: Breast cancer in an area of high parity: São Paulo, Brazil. Cancer Res. **31**, 77—83 (1971).
14. Ravnihar, B., MacMahon, B., Lindtner, J.: Epidemiologic features of breast cancer in Slovenia, 1965—1967. Europ. J. Cancer **7**, 295—306 (1971).
15. Salber, E. J., Trichopoulos, D., MacMahon, B.: Lactation and reproductive histories of breast cancer patients in Boston, 1965—1966. J. nat. Cancer Inst. **43**, 1013—1024 (1969).
16. Valaoras, V. G., MacMahon, B., Trichopoulos, D., Polychronopoulou, A.: Lactation and reproductive histories of breast cancer patients in Greater Athens, 1965—1967. Int. J. Cancer **4**, 350—363 (1969).
17. Yuasa, S., MacMahon, B.: Lactation and reproductive histories of breast cancer patients in Tokyo, Japan. Bull. WHO **42**, 195—204 (1970).
18. Cole, P., MacMahon, B.: Oestrogen fractions during early reproductive life in the aetiology of breast cancer. Lancet **1969 I**, 604—606.
19. MacMahon, B., Cole, P.: Endocrinology and epidemiology of breast cancer. Cancer **24**, 1146—1150 (1969).
20. MacMahon, B., Cole, P., Brown, J. B., Aoki, K., Lin, T. M., Morgan, R. W., Woo, N. C.: Oestrogen profiles of Asian and North American women. Lancet **1971 II**, 900—902.
21. Bulbrook, R. D., Hayward, J. L., Spicer, C. C.: Relation between urinary androgen and corticoid excretion and subsequent berast cancer. Lancet **1971 II**, 395—398.
22. Furth, J.: Vistas in the etiology and pathogenesis of tumors. Fed. Proc. **20**, 865—873 (1961).
23. Mühlbock, O., Boot, L. M.: Induction of mammary cancer in mice without the mammary tumor agent by isografts of hypophyses. Cancer Res. **19**, 402—412 (1959).
24. Smith, O. W., Smith, G. V.: Urinary oestrogen profiles and aetiology of breast cancer. Lancet **1970 I**, 1152—1153.
25. Terenius, L.: Effect of anti-oestrogens on initiation of mammary cancer in the female rat. Europ. J. Cancer **7**, 65—70 (1971).

# Primary Intestinal Lymphoma: Clinical Manifestations and Possible Effect of Environmental Factors [1]

BRACHA RAMOT and AMIRA MANY

The Chaim Sheba Medical Center (Tel-Hashomer), Tel-Aviv University Medical School, Tel Aviv, Israel

Lymphoma of the small intestine can occur as a late secondary manifestation of disseminated lymphoma, or far less commonly, as a primary lesion originating in the small intestine or mesenteric lymph nodes [1—6]. The latter disease can be further subdivided into two categories: a) Solitary lymphoma that occurs most commonly in the terminal ileum and is encountered more frequently in young children, and b) Diffuse or multifocal small intestinal lymphoma, occurring most commonly in proximal small intestine encountered primarily in the older age groups. In the latter entity malabsorption has been described [3—5]. The syndrome of malabsorption in small intestine lymphoma as described by EDELMAN *et al.* (1966), occurs only rarely in the more developed countries of the Western world [7]. These authors, reviewing the medical literature of the West, were able to find only 48 cases, of which they regarded 32 as well established and 16 as probable. On the other hand, the syndrome of malabsorption in small intestinal lymphoma is not rare among certain populations whose common denominator appears to be that they are under-privileged in terms of nutrition, hygiene and medical care [7—11]. In Israel the syndrome is relatively prevalent among Arabs and among first and second generations of Jewish immigrants from mid-eastern and North Africa countries and is virtually non exsistent among Jews of European origin [7—10]. This syndrome was also described in other Mediterranean populations as, North Africa, Italy, Spain as well as in Iran, Mexico, South America and in the African-Cape-Coloured people [11—13]. The evidence thus far would seem to suggest that predisposition to primary small intestinal lymphoma is environmentally determined. One could also speculate about the unique vulnerability of certain populations due to genetic factors or a combination of environmental and genetic influences. In this work we summarized the present day knowledge on this entity and analysed the possible effects of environmental factors on its development. The possibility of abnormalities in the lymphoreticular system and its possible effect on the disease will also be discussed.

## Clinical Features of Primary Lymphoma of the Intestine in Eastern Countries

Intestinal lymphoma has been accepted as a rare cause of malabsorption by FAIRLEY and MACKIE (1937) [14]. Since that time a number of additional reports

1 Supported by the Markewitz Research Foundation.

have appeared in the literature [15—17]. It should be noted that the disease in the Western World affects usually individuals over the age of 50, with a female/male ration of 1:3. The history of malabsorption varied from several months to many years and was verified by laboratory data in many cases. In some of the patients intestinal biopsies revealed a lesion indistinguishable from celiac sprue [15, 16, 18]. On exploration, in addition to the former, malignant lymphoma of the gut or mesenteric nodes was found. Periphereal lymphadenopathy and splenomegaly were observed very rarely and abdominal masses were rarely palpated. The foregoing findings suggest rather strongly that primary small intestinal lymphoma in the Western countries is intimately related to celiac sprue. This impression is reinforced by a study performed on 202 patients with celiac sprue, followed for an average of 8.2 years [19]. 14 of these patients developed intestinal lymphoma and 13 were striken with carcinoma of the gastrointestinal tract including 6 cases with esophageal carcinoma. These findings clearly suggest that celiac sprue is related in some way to the predilection to neoplasia in general and to lymphoma in particular.

The pathological lesion in intestinal lymphoma in the Western world is not uniform. Solitary, multiple and diffuse infiltration of the small intestinal wall was observed. There was a high incidence of jejunal involvement. The abdominal nodes were usually also involved. In some patients the main pathological findings were observed in the lymph nodes and very little was seen in the intestinal wall. In two patients findings compatable with extramedullary plasmocytoma have been described [16].

## Primary Small Intestinal Lymphoma in Israel

As previously mentioned, the syndrome of primary small intestinal lymphoma in Israel is relatively common among Arabs and among Jews of Middle-Eastern and North African origin and is relatively rare in Jews of European origin. There are clear indications at present that this ethnic distribution pertains to countries outside of Israel, too. Moreover, it seems to hold true not only for primary small intestinal lymphoma with or without malabsorption but for abdominal localization of lymphoma in general [10, 20].

Primary small intestinal lymphoma as encountered in Israel differs in certain important aspects from its counter-part in the Western world. It affects primarily teen-agers and young adults with an onset at an age around 20 years. The male/female ratio is about 1.2:1. The duodenum and proximal jejunum are involved in a very striking frequency, in constrast to the primary mid-jejunal involvement in the Western world. No obvious mucosal pathology was observed in the intestinal segment uninvolved by the tumor [27], in contrast to the severe abnormalities of the mucosa in uninvolved areas of the gut in Western countries. It should, however, be stressed that no systematic study by small intestinal biopsies has been performed neither in Israel nor in any other part of the world. The most that can be said is that in Israel, concurrent celiac sprue could confidently be ruled out on histological grounds and therefore other predisposing factors should be looked for.

The macroscopic features of small intestinal lymphoma in Israel can be classified into four categories:

1. Diffuse involvement of the intestinal wall.
2. Small uniform nodular involvement.

3. Extrinsic masses or nodes with infiltration of the intestine from outside towards the lumen.
4. Interluminar multiple or single masses.

The histological pattern of intestinal lymphoma was not uniform. In about 25% of the cases a diffuse plasma cell infiltration of the intestinal wall was observed or more precisely a lymphoplasmocytic infiltration with pressure on the glands. In the other patients various types of lymphoma were observed, most of them of the histiocytic type [21]. In all the patients of the latter group a plasma cell infiltration of the mucosa was also found. However, the extent of the infiltration varied from patient to patient.

In 1968 SELIGMANN *et al.* [22] had described a syndrome of malabsorption with the histological features of plasma lymphocytic infiltration of the gut and a fragment of heavy chain of IgA (Fc fragment) in the serum. These authors studied the sera of 25 such cases, including three sent by us.

Table 1. Geographic origin of 28 patients with α-Chain disease

| | | | |
|---|---|---|---|
| *North Africa:* | | *Middle East:* | |
| Algeria | 8 | Israel | 5 |
| Tunesia | 1 | Syria | 2 |
| | | Iran | 1 |
| *South Africa:* | | | |
| Cape Coloured | 1 | | |
| *Far East:* | | *Europe:* | |
| Pakistan | 2 | South Italy | 3 |
| Cambodia | 1 | South Spain | 1 |
| | | Netherlands [a] | 1 |
| *South America:* | | | |
| Columbia | 1 | | |
| North Argentina | 1 | | |

[a] No detected intestinal involvement. Probably respiratory form.

Table 1 shows the data collected by SELIGMANN [13] and includes three additional sera studied by us during the last two months. It is clear from this table that this clinical pathological entity affects individuals not only from the Mediterranean Basin. In Israel four of the five patients listed were Arabs. The clinical features and the age and sex distribution of the cases collected by SELIGMANN are very similar to those studied by us. Furthermore, the patients with pathologic evidence of an intestinal lymphoma have an age, ethnic distribution and clinical syndrome indistinguishable from the patients with plasma cell infiltration of the gut accompanied by the IgA abnormality [9, 13]. Is this severe plasma cell infiltration and α chain abnormality a malignant process a priori, or is it an immune response of the gut to a noxious agent or agents followed by a clonal evolution of functionally abnormal plasma cells? And if so, is the stage at which the α chain disease develops, malignant, or does this still belong to a state of immunological derangement as is well known for various monoclonal gammopathies sometimes preceding the clinical picture of lymphoma. Till lately, we favoured the view that lymphoplasmocytic infiltration of the gut accompanied by a heavy chain of IgA is one type of malignant response, and histiocytic lymphoma another type of malignant response. Especially as the IgA abnormality has the properties of monoclonal gammopathy. All cases studied till now were of the type I alpha heavy chain [13]. This could be viewed similar to the variations in tissue response observed in Hodgkin's disease. On the other hand, Dr. H. RAPPAPORT considered the plasma cell infiltration in cases of heavy chain

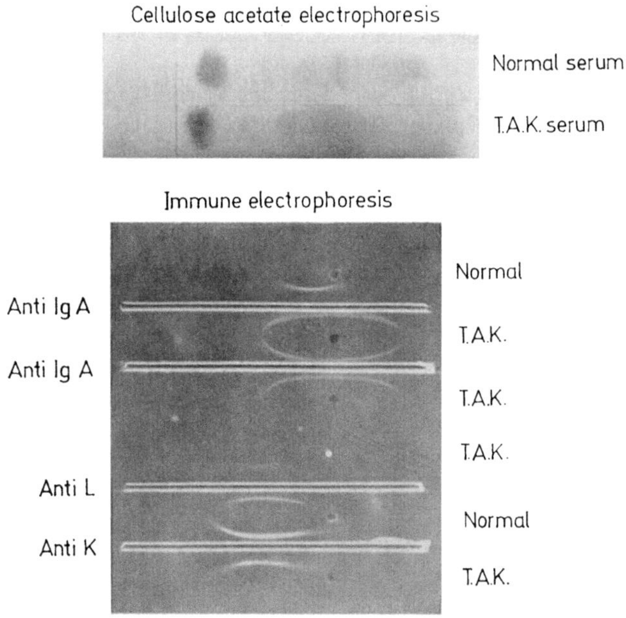


Fig. 1

of IgA, not to be malignant [21]. Lately, we have had the opportunity to study additional two young Arab patients with small intestinal lymphoma but only in one of them evident malabsorption was demonstrated. In both a heavy chain of IgA was detected (Figs. 1 and 2). The patient *without* evident malabsorption was admitted with the classical clinical picture of a diffuse reticulum cell sarcoma involving mainly the gut and abdominal lymph nodes, but the diagnosis was made from a cervical lymph node biopsy. The awareness on the one hand, and the finding of an IgA level of 400 mg-% in face of very low IgG level, 180 mg-%, was the cause for further studies which disclosed an IgA heavy chain in the serum. This case calls for awareness of the existence of a heavy chain of IgA even in diffuse lymphomas without evident malabsorption, when the abdominal lymph nodes and the gut are the main areas involved.

Furthermore, this case suggests that there might be a relationship between plasma cell infiltration of the gut with the IgA abnormality and the evolution of a malignant lymphoma later on, even outside the abdominal cavity. This problem cannot be solved at present and warrants very careful prospective studies.

In view of the very poor clinical condition of the last patient no intestinal biopsy was performed and therefore it cannot be determined whether the infiltration in the gut of this patient consists only of plasma cells.

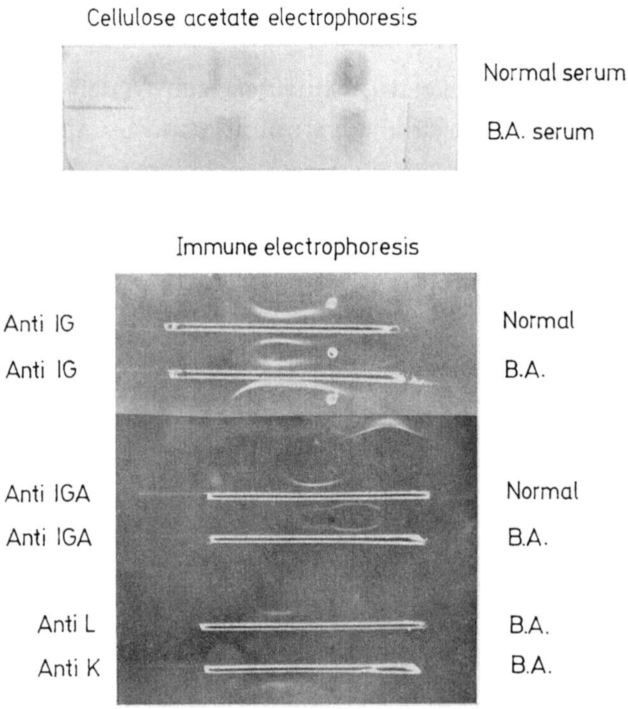


Fig. 2

## The Effect of Hereditary and Environmental Factors on the Development of Intestinal Lymphoma

In order to determine the effect of hereditary and environmental factors, a study was performed in two directions: a) Family members of ten patients with intestinal lymphoma and malabsorption were studied, b) Immunoglobulin levels were determined in a relatively large sample of the Arab population in the Gaza Strip.

No clear evidence for a protein abnormality was detected in the other family members studied, however, more studies in this direction are definitely required. As for the effect of environmental factors, the immunoglobulin levels were studied in about 600 random Arab patients. In spite of the fact that the study is still preliminary, it appears that the IgA level in the Arab population is higher than that observed in the Jewish population in Israel. If this finding will be significant the question whether chronic parasitic infections of the gastrointestinal tract, which are common in the Arab population of the Gaza Strip, is not the chronic stimulus for plasma cell proliferation in the gut and the increased level of IgA.

We may, therefore, speculate that chronic immunologic stimulation of the gut, by intestinal infestation, in under-privileged populations, leading to the develop-, ment of intestinal lymphoma may be similar to the relationship between celiac sprue and intestinal lymphoma in the Western World. This hypothesis is at present under investigation. Search for asymptomatic cases with heavy chain of IgA in individuals with chronic antigenic stimulation of the gut is needed.

## The Possible Relationship between Malabsorption, Lymphoreticular Dysfunction and Lymphoma

As already stated a malabsorption disorder seems in many instances to have preceded the development of primary small intestinal lymphoma. The former has on occasion proven to be celiac sprue, in the Western world.

There is some evidence that celiac sprue in turn may be associated with lymphoreticular dysfunction and that the latter may accompany other malabsorptive states of the small intestine.

Robb Smith (1938) described a disease entity characterized by progressive hyperplasia of the abnormal lymph nodes and termed it prohistiocytic fibrillary reticulosis [23]. The same author in 1964 pointed out the association of this entity with steatorrhea and its pathologic similarity to lymphosarcoma [24]. He suggested that the hyperplasia might be secondary to an autoimmune process in the gut which terminates in malignancy in a manner analogous to the reticulosis complicating Hashimoto's thyroiditis.

Additional information of interest from the point of view mentioned, might be gathered from the follow-up of patients with malabsorption and IgA deficiency [26], and their possible predisposition to lymphoma.

Celiac sprue has been found to be associated on occasion with splenic atrophy. A summary of 28 cases of the latter association was made by McCarthy *et al.* The diagnosis could be inferred by findings of Heinz bodies in the peripheral blood [25]. The degree of splenic atrophy was not related to the severity of malabsorption and the pathogenesis of the splenic atrophy is not known.

It will be of great interest to study the presence of Heinz bodies in the peripheral smears of patients with malabsorption in the Jewish and Arab population in general and in patients with intestinal lymphoma in particular. The present day data on patients with lymphoma suggest that splenic involvement in intestinal lymphoma with malabsorption is very rare. However, the weights of the spleens in such patients were not recorded.

Only a prospective study could be of value to determine whether any anatomic or functional abnormalities in the lymphoreticular system predispose to the development of intestinal lymphoma.

## References

1. Rosenberg, S. A., Diamond, H. D., Paslowitz, B., Craver, L. F.: Medicine (Baltimore) **40**, 31 (1961).
2. Skrimshire, J. F. P.: Quart. J. Med. **24**, 203 (1955).
3. Sleisenger, M. H., Almy, T. P., Barr, D. P.: Amer. J. Med. **15**, 666 (1953).
4. Scudamore, H. H.: Ann. intern. Med. **55**, 433 (1961).

5. KENT, T. H.: Arch. Path. **78**, 97 (1964).
6. GOUGH, K. R., READ, A. E., NAISH, J. M.: Gut. **3**, 232 (1962).
7. EDELMAN, S., PARKINS, A. R., RUBIN, C. E.: Medicine (Baltimore) **45**, 111 (1966).
8. FRAND, U. I., RAMOT, B.: Harefuah **65**, 83 (1963), (in Hebrew).
9. RAMOT, B., SHAHIN, N., BUBIS, J. J.: Is. J. Med. Sci. **1**, 221 (1965).
10. SHANI, M., MODAN, B., GOLDMAN, B., BRANDSTAETER, S., RAMOT, B.: Is. J. Med. Sci. **5**, 1173 (1969).
11. ARMIN, K.: J. med. Fac. Teheran **24**, 1 (1966).
12. BANK, S., MARKS, I. N., BOCK, O. A. A.: Proc. World Congr. Gastroenterology 3rd **2**, 344 (1967).
13. SELIGMANN, M., MIHAESCO, E., FRANGIONE, B.: (In press) 1971.
14. FAIRLEY, N. T., MACKIE, F. P.: Brit. Med. J. **1**, 375 (1937).
15. AUSTAD, W. I., CORMES, J. S., GOUGH, K. R., MCCARTHY, C. K., READ, A. E.: Amer. J. dig. Dis. **12**, 475 (1967).
16. BRUNT, P. W., SIRCUS, W., MCCLEAN, N.: Lancet **1969 I**, 180.
17. SPENCE, W. J. E., RITCHIE, S.: Canad. J. Surg. **22**, 207 (1969).
18. EAKINS, D., FULTON, T., HADDEN, D. R.: Gut. **5**, 315 (1964).
19. HARRIE, O. D., COOKE, W. T., THOMPSON, H., WATERHOUSE, J. A.: Amer. J. Med. **42**, 899 (1967).
20. HULU, N., RAMOT, B., SHEEHAN, W.: Is. J. Med. Sci. **6**, 246 (1970).
21. RAPPAPORT, H., RAMOT, B., HULU, N., PARK, J. K.: (in press).
22. SELIGMANN, M., DANON, F. HUREZ, B., MIHAESCO, E., PREUD'HOMME, J. L.: Science **162**, 1396 (1968).
23. ROBB-SMITH, A. H. T.: J. Path. Bact. **47**, 457 (1938).
24. ROBB-SMITH, A. H. T.: The classification and natural history of the lymphadenopathies. In: Lymphomas and Related Disseases, 24. Eds.: S. J. PARK and I. M. ARIEL. New York: Hoeber Medical Division 1964.
25. MCCARTHY, O. F., FRASER, I. D., EVANS, K. T., READ, A. E.: Gut. **7**, 140 (1966).
26. CRABBÉ, P. A., HEREMANS, J. F.: Amer. J. Med. **42**, 319 (1967).
27. NEUMAN, G., RUBIN, C. E.: (Personal communication).

# Detection and Assessment of Case Clustering in Burkitt's Lymphoma and Hodgkin's Disease

A. G. Baikie [1], L. J. Kinlen, and M. C. Pike

Department of the Regius Professor of Medicine, Oxford University, Oxford, Great Britain

## Introduction

Any joint consideration of Burkitt's Lymphoma (BL) and Hodgkin's Disease (HD) may, at first glance, seem unwarranted. HD was first described in 1832 and is of world-wide distribution; BL was first described only in the late 1950's and its occurrence is geographically very restricted. BL occurs in children and has distinctive clinical features; HD occurs at all ages and its diagnosis depends on histological features which themselves may be the subject of debate. BL is a neoplasm of lymphocytes, while in HD the role of lymphocytes is uncertain and complex. Despite these differences the 2 neoplasms may be considered in parallel because of the increasing circumstantial evidence for viral aetiology in both. If they are caused by viruses they may show some of the epidemiological features of infectious diseases. Recognition of these features may not only help to identify the viruses responsible but is essential to understanding the diseases themselves. Case clustering is one of the features of infectious diseases, and it is this which is the subject of this paper.

It is important to define case clustering. Three varieties of clustering have been described, all of which may be of aetiological significance.

1. Space Clustering: This is a different incidence of a disease in different areas.
2. Time Clustering: This is either a different incidence of a disease in different months or seasons of the year, or a change in the incidence of a disease in a defined area, usually for a short period. The latter may be difficult to distinguish from time-space clustering.
3. Time-Space Clustering: This is an outbreak of a disease in a limited area for a limited time, and is commonly referred to as an epidemic. Such an occurrence is usually due to an infective agent.

Two precautions must always be observed in investigating case clusters. The possibility must be considered that the observation is simply due to improvement in detection of the disease. Many factors influence the detection rate including the level of clinical awareness, the availability of diagnostic tests, hospital referral patterns, the thoroughness of the search for cases or the introduction of notification systems. An important factor which must be considered in the study of BL is the changing attitude of the African population towards seeking medical help.

---

1 On leave from the Department of Medicine, University of Tasmania, Hobart, Tasmania, Australia.

If worthwhile reports of case clustering in diseases previously unsuspected of showing this behaviour are not to be inhibited, tests of statistical significance should not be regarded as essential in the first instance. This is so because in such situations appropriate tests of statistical significance may not be available or because the mere detection of a cluster may involve bias. However, subsequent studies of the same disease must be designed to include the evaluation of the level of statistical significance. Such studies may require a great deal of work, but they are essential if the literature is not to be flooded with pseudo-clusters.

## Burkitt's Lymphoma

BL has attracted a great deal of attention since the early 1960's; a detailed review of clinical, laboratory and epidemiological features may be found in the recent book edited by BURKITT and WRIGHT (1970). We restrict our consideration to the topic of clustering of BL cases.

### Space Clustering

BL is present in significant numbers only in tropical Africa and New Guinea. This was interpreted as implicating malaria or a vector borne agent in its aetiology. The vector interpretation led to an intense and successful search for a virus in tumour tissue; in fact for a while the search was over successful, with the finding of both the Epstein-Barr virus (EBV) and Reo 3. Reo 3 appears to have been a laboratory contaminant, but EBV remains a strong candidate. Further work is required to elucidate the relationship of malaria to BL. This might take the form of case-control studies with regard to sickle cell trait and G-6-PD deficiency, both of which are known to ameliorate malarial infection. First results of such studies are encouraging (PIKE *et al.*, 1970), and the work is proceeding.

BL is known to have occurred in 2 sib pairs in Uganda (MORROW *et al.*, 1971). Rough calculations show that this is no more than would be expected by chance.

### Time Clustering

BL was not described until 1958. Consequently, a time cluster of cases must have followed its recognition just as diagnostic error preceded it.

A weak-negative association between the yearly total of BL cases and the yearly total rainfall in the West Nile District of Uganda over the last 10 years has been demonstrated (WILLIAMS, SCHNEIDERMAN and KOSIOL, pers. comm.). This is so far unexplained. It may be worthwhile to attempt to extract from the records of West Nile dispensaries the number of patients treated for malaria over this period and to associate this with the occurrence of BL cases.

There has been a marked decline in the number of cases of BL seen in the Mengo District of Uganda, from 19 cases in 1961 to 6 cases in 1968, whereas about 30 cases would have been expected on the basis of the 1961 figure taking into account the increase in population (MORROW and PIKE, unpublished). This could well be due to an increase in the use of anti-malarial drugs and could be investigated by obtaining figures for the use of anti-malarials in different parts of the country over the last decade. The results of both studies might be valuable additions to the evidence on the possible role of malaria in the aetiology of BL.

## Time-Space Clustering

This has been demonstrated in BL both in West Nile District and in Bwamba County of Uganda (WILLIAMS *et al.*, 1969; MORROW *et al.*, 1971; KAFUKO *et al.*, 1971). The Bwamba cluster consisted of the only 7 cases to have been diagnosed in that county (Fig. 1). In all 7 cases the clinical onset occurred between October 1966 and December 1968. The first case was in October 1966, the second in December 1967, and the remaining 5 in the 6 months from July to December 1968. Two of the last 5 patients were sister and brother, aged respectively 3 and 9 years, with clinical onsets in July and December. To the best of our knowledge, none of the other cases knew each other. This cluster would suggest that BL has a relatively constant and short incubation period. Such a cluster is unlikely to be due to case-to-case infection

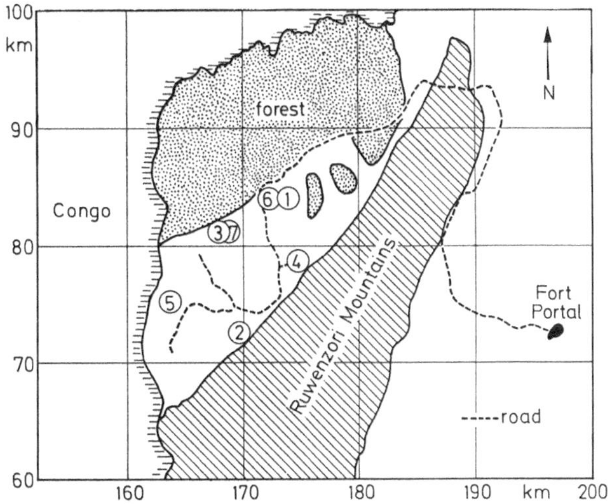


Fig. 1. Map of part of Toro District, Uganda. The area shown between the Ruwenzori Mountains and the forest is the inhabited area of Bwamba County. The place of onset of the seven known Burkitt's Lymphoma cases are marked with a numeral in time sequence of occurrence

but rather to some common aetiological factor operating for a brief period. From what we know of the epidemiology of EBV and of malaria, neither of these factors alone would explain this phenomenon. It does not follow that EBV is not an essential factor in the causation of BL. In fact, some recent evidence from the United States (LEVINE *et al.*, 1971) has made it even more likely that EBV plays a critical part in the aetiology of BL. Cases of BL are extremely rare in the United States; nevertheless they found it possible to study 11 cases satisfying the strictest clinical and microscopic diagnostic criteria. They were all found to have EBV antibodies.

When the time-space clustering in West Nile is examined, the same interpretation is possible. There were local outbreaks with a time-interval between successive clustered cases of the order of a few months.

Time-space clustering has also been sought in other areas of Uganda and in the North Mara District of Tanzania (BRUBAKER *et al.*, 1971) but without success. This absence of clusters may be a vital clue. What differences are there between West Nile, Bwamba and the rest of Uganda? The pattern of malarial infection is, we understand (MCCRAE, pers. comm.), less variable in West Nile and Bwamba than it is in those other areas of Uganda where clustering does not occur.

There is a clear need to discover some other environmental factor to account for these discrepancies. This might be achieved by examining the patterns of occurrence of other diseases in these areas. One would hope that such studies will be included in the International Agency for Cancer Research's prospective investigation now beginning in Uganda. Again, patients with BL should be questioned closely about their movements during the 2 or 3 years before the onset of their disease. This might clarify the position regarding the possibility that the disease is spread from person to person, and might in this way resolve the apparent discrepancy of time-space clustering occurring only in particular areas.

## Hodgkin's Disease

Almost any consideration of HD must take account of its several peculiarities. Firstly, age-incidence, sex-ratio, geographical pathology and histological features suggest that it may in fact be separated into 3 disease entities. Secondly, the diagnostic error may be as high as 40% in ordinary hospital practice (SYMMERS, 1968), and even experts have great difficulty in assigning cases to the histological sub-types of the disease (COPPLESON *et al.*, 1970). In addition, it must be remembered that the relationship of HD to the other malignant lymphomas—follicular lymphoma, lymphosarcoma and reticulum cell sarcoma—is uncertain. Much of the diagnostic error arises from the difficulty of distinguishing it from these disorders. There is other evidence to suggest that, especially in the elderly, HD may be separated from the other malignant lymphomas with less confidence than in the age group 15—34 years. Studies which take no account of these errors and uncertainties, or fail to describe the diagnostic criteria and the age structure of the population under consideration, are of correspondingly less value.

The suggestion of an infective origin for HD is no new hypothesis. Because of its histological and clinical features, an infective cause for the disorder was proposed as long ago as 1898 (STERNBERG, 1898). Indeed, it was slow to gain general recognition as a neoplastic disease. Consequently, with the recent increase in interest in possible viral factors in the genesis of human cancer, it is not surprising that attention should be turned to HD. Conclusive direct evidence is, of course, lacking. Some evidence suggestive of a special association between certain leucocyte antigens of the HL-A group and HD has been reported (ZERVAS *et al.*, 1970; FORBES and MORRIS, 1970). This can be interpreted equally readily as evidence of genetically determined susceptibility or as a consequence of viral alteration of the cell genome. The recent demonstration of a shared tumour antigen in two patients with HD may also be regarded as favouring viral infection (ORDER *et al.*, 1971). This result is still unconfirmed, as is the finding that so-called blastoid transformation of cultured cells from cases of HD may be associated with emergence of a herpes-like virus (EISINGER *et al.*, 1971).

A causal role has been suggested for EBV in HD, but high levels of EBV antibody have been found only in the lymphocyte depletion form of the disease (JOHANSSON *et al.*, 1970).

## Space Clustering

Major differences have been found between countries in both the incidence and mortality from HD. Thus Japan has a very low mortality rate in the younger adult age group by comparison with European countries and the United States. This is likely to be due to environmental factors rather than genetic factors since no such difference is found in Japanese and Caucasians living in Hawaii (BLAISDELL and BOXER, 1971). From Japan itself a lack of histological evidence of host response in HD has been described (ANDERSON *et al.*, 1970).

Some reported instances of space clustering of HD may be due to differences in the quality of medical care and diagnosis. Such differences usually affect the elderly more than the young and so they cannot explain the lower mortality in young adults in Japan. Nor can a lower standard of diagnosis explain certain geographic differences in mortality within the United States (COLE *et al.*, 1968).

Changes in standards of living may have determined the decline in mortality from HD in childhood in England and Wales and in the United States, while it remains relatively high in certain under-developed countries. The age incidence and histological features of HD as it occurs in several countries have recently been reviewed (CORREA and O'CONOR, 1971). Three patterns are discerned and it is suggested that these may be related to the economic status of the communities in which they occur. In Pattern I, in countries of lower economic status, there is ahigh incidence of HD in children and a predominance of histological varieties associated with a poor prognosis. In Pattern III there are higher rates in young adults and more favourable histological appearances predominate. Pattern II is intermediate.

We know of no suggestion that climatic differences are important in determining the occurrence of HD.

## Time Clustering

A seasonal peak in clinical onset of HD has been described in 2 series of hospital patients in Britain (CRIDLAND, 1961; INNES and NEWALL, 1961). These findings have been confirmed in a more broadly based study of HD in childhood in the United States (FRAUMENI and LI, 1969) and for a group of HD patients of all ages in Germany (DOERKEN, this meeting). In all 4 series there was an excess of cases presenting in December and January which, in the northern hemisphere, must suggest the possible influence of acute respiratory infection. In the earlier studies steps were taken to exclude cases in which obvious respiratory infection might have resulted in further enlargement or tenderness in already enlarged cervical lymph nodes of which the patient had been unaware. Nevertheless, this sequence of events, well recognised by JACKSON and PARKER (1947), seems the most likely explanation for the findings.

In contrast, FRAUMENI and LI (1969) have reported from the United States an excess mortality from HD in male children born in July and August. This might be due to the seasonal operation of some aetiological factor *in utero*. Evidence of previous infection might be sought in children with HD and their mothers. No such time clustering has been demonstrated as regards the months of birth of children dying of HD in Great Britain (DRAPER, pers. comm.).

Possible examples of non-seasonal clustering are few and those we know of have affected limited populations topographically demarcated and so are instances of time-space clustering.

## Time-Space Clustering

The best evidence of time-space clustering has been presented at this meeting by Davies. Much smaller apparent outbreaks have been described by Clemmesen *et al.* (1952) and by Gilmore and Zelesnick (1962), but these were only briefly reported.

When time-space clustering gives rise to familial aggregation of a disease it may be interpreted as evidence of genetic factors in aetiology. In familial cases presenting within a short time of each other, the greater the difference in ages of the patients, the more likely is an environmental influence. Unfortunately, in many of the reports of familial HD, the time interval between the cases is not stated (De Vore and Doan, 1957). However, where such details have been provided, as in the report of 13 cases by Razis and his colleagues (1959), environment is favoured more than heredity. None of the studies have suggested any simple form of inheritance of increased susceptibility to the disease. Environmental factors must certainly be invoked to explain concordance for HD in marriage partners, if this does in fact occur more often than is accountable for by chance (Mazar and Strauss, 1951).

The New York clusters show a clear-cut preponderance of adolescents and young adults amongst those involved. This may reflect social habits and opportunities for cross-infection as much as any inherent liability in that age group to pass on the infection or acquire it.

# Further Study of Time-Space Clustering in HD

The age of those involved in the New York clusters clearly suggests that in attempting to confirm these findings elsewhere it would be economical of effort to begin with cases in the 15—34 years age group. Because of the diagnostic errors and the uncertain relationship of HD to the other malignant lymphomas, cases of other malignant lymphomas should be sought amongst the contacts, even if the index cases are drawn solely from those with a histological diagnosis of HD

In attempting to assess the significance of either case-case contacts or contacts through a third party, controls are essential. There is a tendency to underestimate the number of social contacts of individuals, especially younger people, in our highly mobile society. Controls may best be provided by individuals of similar age, sex and occupation, to the index cases of HD. It may be desirable to have 2 controls for each case of HD, one living near the index case and one chosen at random.

In our preliminary work patients with a histologically acceptable diagnosis of HD are interviewed by means of a loosely structured questionnaire. Most know their diagnosis, but this is not assumed, and the disease is mentioned by name only after they have mentioned it. The primary aim of the interview is to compile a list of identifiable contacts at school or other educational institution, at work, within their own families or household, or in the course of social or other activities. Some preliminary questions are asked about the patient's well-being, his symptoms at and before diagnosis, and about previous health, including previous tonsillectomy and appendicectomy. Thereafter a systematic enquiry is pursued about schools, occupations, family including spouse and spouse's sibs, and the patient's own parental sibs. A last question invites the patient to name up to 6 close friends whose names have not already been mentioned. At each stage of the enquiry the patient is asked about the health of those named and whether he knows of the causes of death of the deceased.

A schedule of contacts is compiled from each questionnaire so that their names may be matched with the records of the Oxford Regional Cancer Registry—not for HD alone but for all the malignant lymphomas, in view of the diagnostic errors. For any contacts said to suffer from HD or a related disease, enquires will not be restricted to the Oxford Region.

Epidemiological methods alone can only suggest aetiological mechanisms. It follows that in our search for evidence of time-space clustering in HD, other evidence should be looked for. Concordance or discordance for histological type may emerge from ordinary diagnostic procedures. Maximum and minimum incubation periods will also be obvious from basic observations. Degree of contact must defy measurement. It is proposed to look for evidence of virus infection even if we do not know what viruses are likely candidates for a causal role. Despite the technical and other uncertainties of immunological phenomena, it would seem to be desirable also to study any possible clusters for the occurrence of tumour-specific antigens such as have been demonstrated in acute leukaemia, osteosarcoma, tumours of the gastro-intestinal tract, and more recently in HD itself (ORDER *et al.*, 1971).

## Statistical Tests for Time-Space Clustering

The sort of time-space clustering observed in the West Nile District BL cases can be tested for statistical significance by the method of KNOX (KNOX, 1964a, 1964b; MANTEL, 1967). This method considers each possible pair of patients and counts the number of pairs whose onsets were within some specified time of one another (say, T days), *and* whose residences at onset were within some specified distance of one another (say, D kilometers); the choice of T and D is discussed by PIKE *et al.* (1967). The test is then whether the number of cluster pairs observed is greater than would be expected on the basis of chance alone. The method is deliberately designed to be completely insensitive to either time or space clustering alone, and does not require controls for comparison.

This is clearly inappropriate for use on the New York State HD data. The dates of onset of the "clustered" cases are not particularly close together and in any case may not be the relevant dates. Similarly, the relevant address is the place of postulated contact and not the address at onset or diagnosis. An extension of the Knox method to allow for long latent periods has been developed (PIKE and SMITH, 1968), and may be applicable to HD. For this model assumptions have to be made as to the likely incubation period and the period of infectivity. This method is also insensitive to either space or time clustering and again requires no controls.

Alternatively, a test can be devised using controls, and this should be statistically more powerful. The question is whether the HD patients had more contact with each other than would be expected on the basis of chance alone. We can approach this as follows: for each HD case select 2 matched controls. (Although the method is possible with a single control for each patient, a great increase in statistical power results from having 2 controls). Thus, if there are n patients, there will be n sets of persons, each set consisting of 1 patient and 2 controls. From these 3n persons select n at random, 1 from each set. Measure the total contact C between these n persons (see below). There are $3^n$ possible random selections. If the observed C for the HD patients is statistically significantly large compared to the random distribution of C, then this is evidence for time-space interaction, and hence for the infectivity of the disease. It should be noted that the generation of C excludes all contacts between a patient and his own controls and between the controls of the same patient. This is necessary since the reason for matching is that the various matching factors influence the probability of contact between persons. The problem remains of measuring contact.

A system of scoring person-to-person contact may be developed along the following lines: direct contact within an appropriate period between 2 persons is awarded a score of 1. "An appropriate period" will be defined according to a set of rules based on assumptions about the timing of infectiousness and the length of latent period of the disease. Similarly, rules will have to be drawn up as to what constitutes significant contact. When such contact is absent, but each of the pair has had appropriate direct contact with someone in common, this indirect contact would qualify for a score of ½, say. Remoter contacts or no contact at all scores 0. More elaborate schemes are clearly possible. C is the sum of these person-to-person contacts.

Consider how this method would be applied to the problem of deciding whether 4 patients with HD have had more contact with each other than would be expected by chance. Since each case has 2 controls, there are 12 persons involved and $3^4$, i.e. 81 possible combinations of 4 persons for consideration. (As already mentioned, combinations have been excluded which involve a patient and his own controls, or the controls of the same patient.) For each combination of 4 persons, there are 6 opportunities for direct contact within pairs of this group and therefore for scoring 1 each; thus the highest possible score would be 6, and the lowest 0, while the score would be 3 if each pair had contact only through an intermediary. If the total score C for the combination of all 4 HD patients was in the top $\alpha$-% of total scores, then we could say that we had time-space clustering, with the assumed model of HD transmission, statistically significant at the $\alpha$-% level.

## References


Anderson, R. E., Ishida, K., Ii, Y., Ishimaru, T., Nishiyama, H.: Geographic aspects of malignant lymphoma and multiple myeloma. Amer. J. Path. **61**, 85 (1970).

Blaisdell, R. K., Boxer, G. J.: Ethnic comparisons of lymphomas in Hawaii: mortality rates for 1955 to 1968. Scientific Contributions, 2nd Meeting of the Asian-Pacific Division of the International Society of Haematology, Melbourne, 1971.

Brubaker, G., Geser, A., Pike, M. C.: Burkitt's Lymphoma in the North Mara District of Tanzania. (In preparation) 1971.

Burkitt, D. P., Wright, D. H.: Burkitt's Lymphoma. Edinburgh and London: Livingstone 1970.

Clemmesen, J., Busk, T., Nielsen, A.: The topographical distribution of leukemia and Hodgkin's Disease in Denmark, 1942—1946. Acta radiol. (Stockh.) **37**, 223 (1952).

Cole, P., MacMahon, B., Aisenberg, A.: Mortality from Hodgkin's Disease in the United States. Lancet **1968 II**, 1371.

Coppleson, L. W., Factor, R. M., Strum, S. B., Graff, P. W., Rappaport, H.: Observer disagreement in the classification and histology of Hodgkin's Disease. J. nat. Cancer Inst. **45**, 731 (1970).

Correa, P., O'Conor, G. T.: Epidemiologic patterns of Hodgkin's Disease. Int. J. Cancer **8**, 192 (1971).

CRIDLAND, M. D.: Seasonal incidence of clinical onset of Hodgkin's Disease. Brit. med. J. **2**, 621 (1961).

DE VORE, J. W., DOAN, C. A.: Studies in Hodgkin's Syndrome, XII: Hereditary and epidemiologic aspects. Ann. int. Med. **47**, 300 (1957).

EISINGER, M., FOX, S. M., DE HARVEN, E., BIEDLER, J. L., SANDERS, F. K.: Virus-like agents from patients with Hodgkin's Disease. Nature **233**, 104 (1971).

FORBES, J. F., MORRIS, P. J.: Leucocyte antigens in Hodgkin's Disease. Lancet **1970 II**, 849.

FRAUMENI, J. F., LI, F. P.: Hodgkin's Disease in childhood: an epidemiologic study. J. nat. Cancer Inst. **42**, 681 (1969).

GILMORE, H. R., ZELENSICK, G.: Environmental Hodgkin's Disease and leukemia. Penn. med. J. 1047 (1962).

INNES, J., NEWALL, J.: Seasonal incidence in clinical onset of Hodgkin's Disease. Brit. med. J. **2**, 765 (1961).

JACKSON, H. J., PARKER, F. J.: Hodgkin's Disease and allied disorders. New York: Oxford University Press 1947.

JOHANSSON, B., KLEIN, G., HENLE, W., HENLE, G.: Epstein-Barr Virus (EBV)-associated antibody patterns in malignant lymphoma and leukemia, I. Hodgkin's Disease. Int. J. Cancer **6**, 450 (1970).

KAFUKO, G. W., MUNUBE, G. M. R., WILLIAMS, E. H., SMITH, P. G.: Burkitt's Lymphoma in the West Nile District of Uganda, 1968—1970: Continued occurrence of time-space clustering. (In preparation) (1971).

KNOX, E. G.: The detection of space-time interactions. Appl. Statistics **13**, 25 (1964a).

KNOX, E. G.: Epidemiology of childhood leukaemia in Northumberland and Durham. Brit. J. prev. soc. Med. **18**, 17 (1964b).

LEVINE, P. H., O'CONOR, G. T., BERARD, C. W.: Antibodies to Epstein-Barr Virus (EBV) in American patients with Burkitt's Lymphoma. (In preparation, 1971).

MANTEL, N.: The detection of disease clustering and a generalised regression approach. Cancer Res. **27**, 209 (1967).

MAZAR, S. A., STRAUSS, B.: Marital Hodgkin's Disease: a review of familial incidence and of etiological factors. Arch. int. Med. **88**, 819 (1951).

MORROW, R. H., PIKE, M. C., SMITH, P. G., ZIEGLER, J. L., KISUULE, A.: Burkitt's Lymphoma: a time-space cluster of cases in Bwamba County of Uganda. Brit. med. J. **2**, 491 (1971).

ORDER, S. E., PORTER, M., HELLMAN, S.: Hodgkin's Disease: evidence for a tumor-associated antigen. New Engl. J. Med. **285**, 471 (1971).

PIKE, M. C., WILLIAMS, E. H., WRIGHT, B.: Burkitt's tumour in the West Nile District of Uganda, 1961—1965. Brit. med. J. **2**, 395 (1967).

PIKE, M. C., MORROW, R. H., KISUULE, A., MAFIGIRI, J.: Burkitt's Lymphoma and sickle cell trait. Brit. J. prev. soc. Med. **24**, 39 (1970).

PIKE, M. C., SMITH, P. G.: Disease clustering: a generalisation of Knox's approach to the detection of space-time interactions. Biometrics **24**, 541 (1968).

RAZIS, D. V., DIAMOND, H. D., CRAVER, L. F.: Familial Hodgkin's Disease: its significance and implications. Ann. int. Med. **51**, 933 (1959).

STERNBERG, C.: (Cited by JACKSON and PARKER, 1947). Z. —heilk. **19**, 12 (1897).

SYMMERS, W. ST. C.: Survey of the eventual diagnoses in 600 cases referred for a second histological opinion after an initial biopsy diagnosis of Hodgkin's Disease. J. clin. Path. **21**, 650 (1968).

WILLIAMS, E. H., SPIT, P., PIKE, M. C.: Further evidence of space-time clustering of Burkitt's Lymphoma patients in the West Nile District of Uganda. Brit. J. Cancer **23**, 235 (1969).

ZERVAS, J. D., DELAMORE, I. W., ISRAELS, M. C. G.: Leucocyte phenotypes in Hodgkin's Disease. Lancet **1970 II**, 634.

# Epidemiologic and Immunologic Considerations on the Pathogenesis of Burkitt's Tumor

GERHARD KRÜGER and GREGORY T. O'CONOR

Laboratory of Pathology, National Cancer Institute, National Institutes of Health, Bethesda, Maryland, USA

Burkitt's Tumor (BT) is identified as a malignant lymphoma composed predominantly of lymphoid cells similar to those found in the germinal centers of lymphoreticular tissues under normal conditions of antigenic stimulation [1, 2, 3]. The normal cell that morphologically most closely resembles the Burkitt tumor cell is the germinoblast of LENNERT [3, 4], and there may be only slight quantitative differences to a cell called immunoblast by DAMASHEK [5] (Figs. 1—3).

Burkitt's tumor was first described as a clinical syndrome and pathological entity in African children [6, 7] and a peculiar geographic distribution of its reported

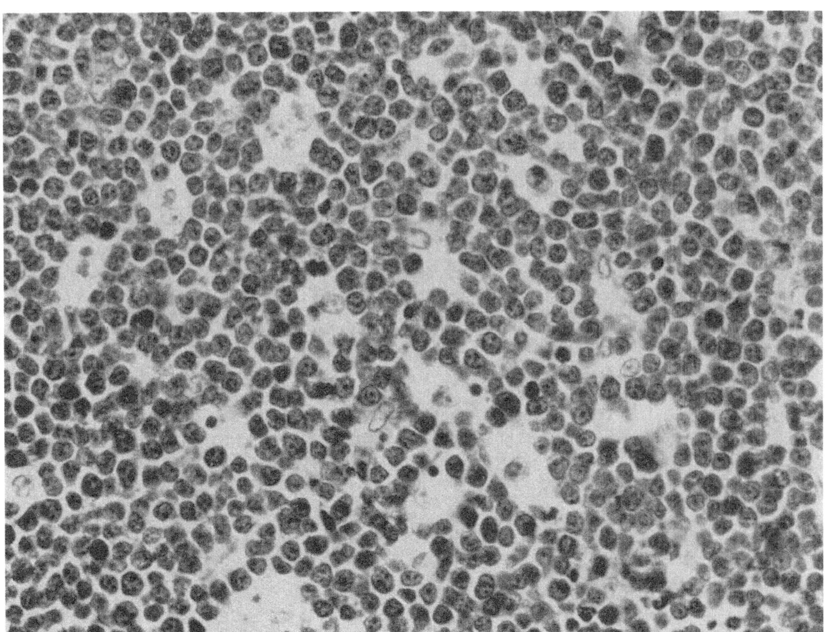

Fig. 1. Section from an abdominal Burkitt's tumor mass of a 13 year old American boy. H & E, ×400

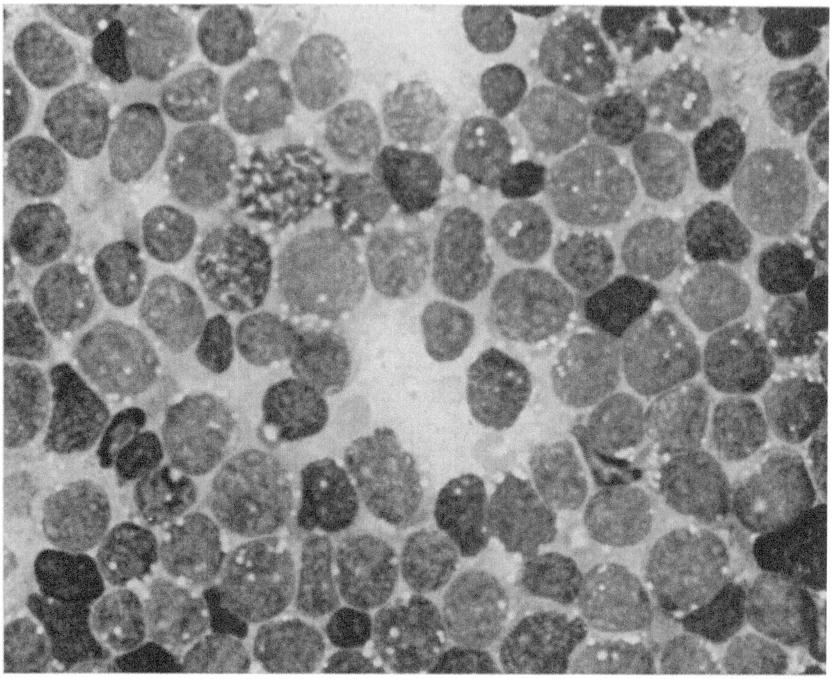

**Fig. 2.** Imprint from the same tumor shown in Fig. 1. Wright-Giemsa, ×675

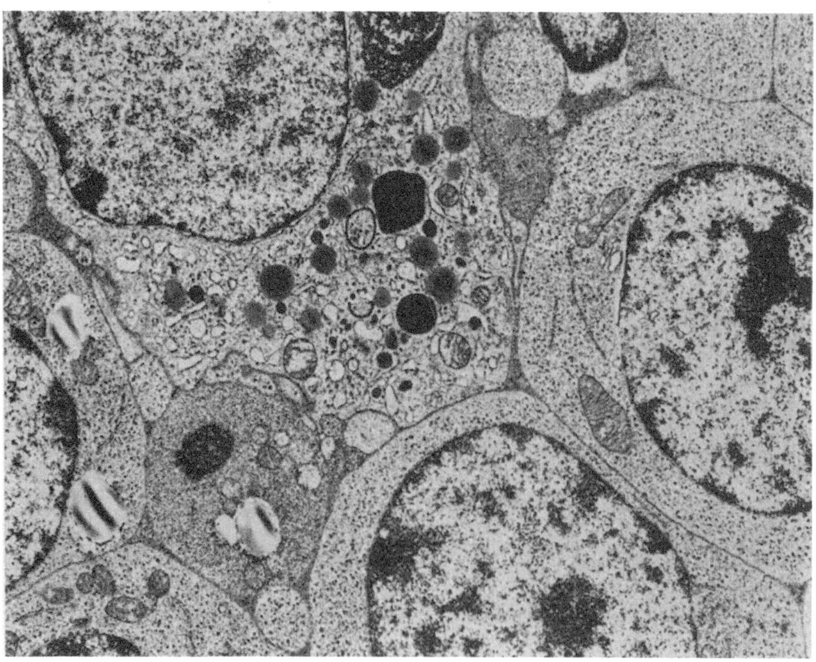

**Fig. 3.** Electron microgram of the tumor shown in Fig. 1. Uranyl acetate, ×11000

incidence soon became evident. The countries of tropical Africa, and the territories of Papua and New Guinea report significant numbers of Burkitt's tumor cases, while outside these areas only sporadic cases are diagnosed [8, 9]. In Africa high tumor frequency is limited to a belt between the tropic of Cancer and the tropic of Capricorn. Geographically the northern border is bounded by the Sahara desert, and the southern border connects Angola with Durban, South Africa. Within this region, however, the incidence of Burkitt's tumor is quite variable [10] as shown in Fig. 4.

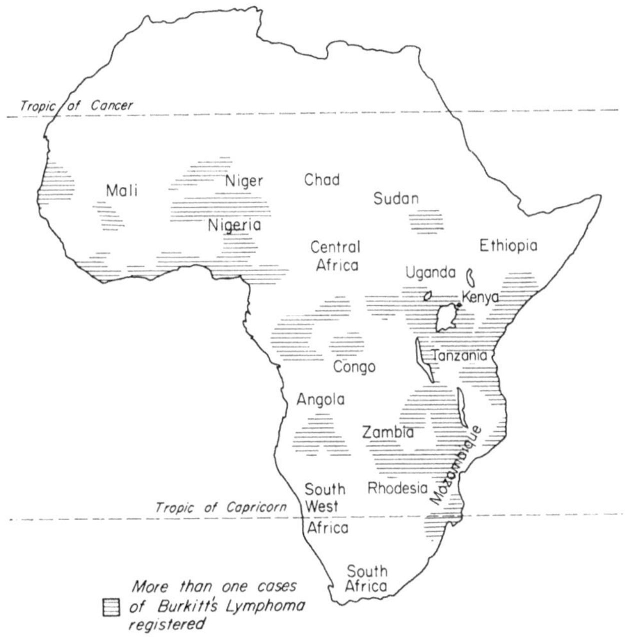


Fig. 4. Map showing clusters of Burkitt's tumor within the region of the Burkitt's tumor belt in Africa

If one concentrates on a high incidence area such as the three East African countries of Uganda, Kenya, and Tanzania (Fig. 5), several features become immediately evident. Burkitt's tumor generally does not occur in mountainous country above 1,000 and 1,500 m (i.e. about 5,000 feet). There is a predominance of Burkitt's tumor around lakes. In addition, it was observed that the tumor occurred preferentially in areas with a mean minimum temperature of 15—18 °C (i.e. about 60—65 °F). The obvious limitation of Burkitt's tumor by environmental factors led to speculations about a possible link of tumor pathogenesis with parasitic or viral infections transmitted by arthropod vectors [11]. Isolates from Burkitt's tumor revealed viruses of the arbovirus, poxvirus, picornavirus, reovirus, and herpes virus groups, but most of these were not consistently present. Mycoplasma organisms were isolated occasionally as well [12].

The herpes type Epstein-Barr virus [13] (EBV) continues to be the prime canditate for an etiological role because of its consistent association with Burkitt's tumor. This association is manifested by the repeated identification of EBV in continuous cell lines derived from the tumor and by high antibody titers to the virus or to virus related antigens recorded in virtually all African patients with the disease [14, 15, 16]. Specific antibodies to these antigens are also demonstrated in non African Burkitt's tumor patients [17, 18, 19]. In addition to Burkitt's tumor, however, variable but increased levels of antibody titer are found in patients with a number of other diseases such as infectious mononucleosis, nasopharyngeal cancer, Hodgkin's disease, and chronic lymphocytic leukemia [20, 21, 22, 23].

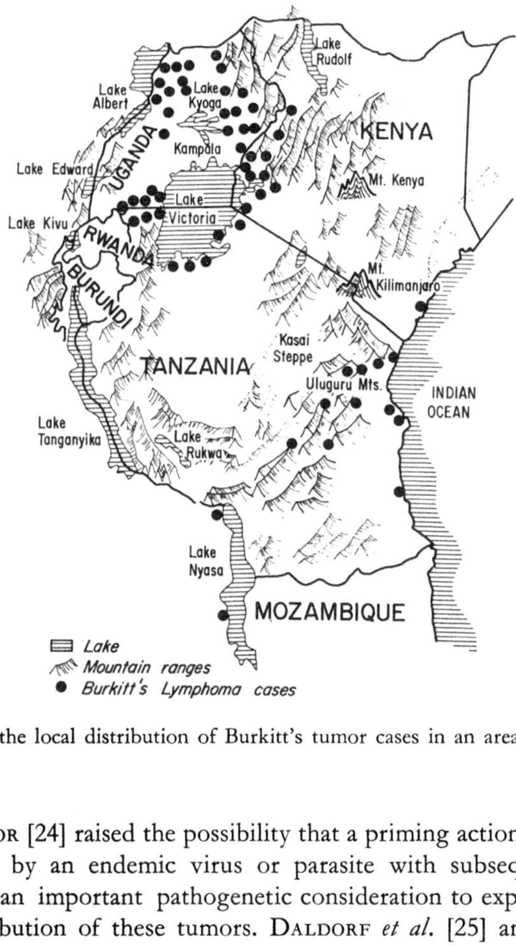


Fig. 5. Map showing the local distribution of Burkitt's tumor cases in an area of high incidence

In 1960 O'Conor [24] raised the possibility that a priming action of the reticuloendothelial system by an endemic virus or parasite with subsequent malignant change might be an important pathogenetic consideration to explain the unusual geographical distribution of these tumors. Daldorf *et al.* [25] and Linsell [26] first suggested that malaria might be an important pathogenetic factor in Burkitt's tumor. This theory was subsequently supported with data reviewed by Burkitt [27] and O'Conor [28]. Additional substantiating evidence has been supplied by Kafuko and Burkitt [29].

As shown in Fig. 6 there is a fairly close overlap of the classic malaria belt with the Burkitt tumor belt. Burkitt's tumor in significant frequency is, in fact, limited to areas with a holoendemic malaria [28].

This coincidence in geographic distribution of malaria and Burkitt's tumor, as well as the association of Epstein-Barr virus with the lymphoma, has generated a multitude of immunological and immunopathological studies and theories. Since EBV has properties of an oncogenic virus it is postulated that the antigenic stimulation of malaria produces an increase in the number of immunocompetent stem cells that are in turn sensitive to malignant transformation by the virus [28]. It has also been suggested that a simultaneous reovirus type 3 infection may serve as a cocarcinogen [30, 31]. Others stress the immunosuppressive effect of malaria infestation [32], or the persistent and unrelenting antigenic stimulation by malaria parasites [28, 33], both of which may increase the risk of lymphoreticular tissues for neoplastic transformation. Partial immunosuppression by malaria infection in man and in mice has

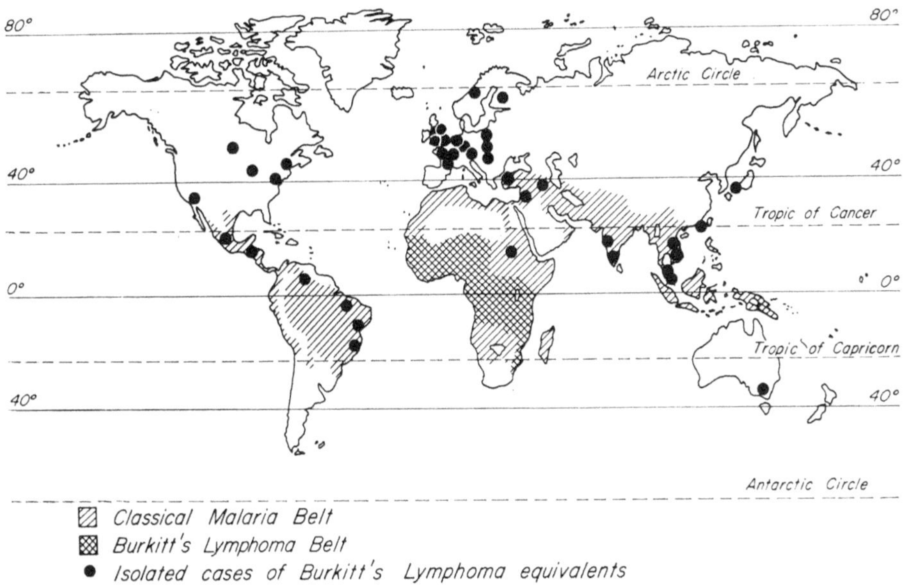


Fig. 6. Map showing the coincidence of the malaria belt with the Burkitt's tumor belt

indeed been demonstrated by several investigators [34, 35, 36, 37]. Hypergammaglobulinemia in populations where malaria is holoendemic or hyperendemic has been interpreted as an indicator of persistent antigenic stimulation [28, 38]. Another idea based on observations of the increased frequency of malignant lymphomas in immunodeficient man and animals demands a coincidence of persistent antigenic stimulation with immunosuppression as imperative for the pathogenesis of these tumors [33, 39].

A series of experiments have been carried out during the recent years which were designed to test some of these hypotheses. SIZARET *et al.* [40] studied the effect of chronic infection with plasmodium berghei in Swiss mice over an 18 month period. This form of persistent antigenic stimulation resulted in a marked and sustained elevation of gammaglobulin (Fig. 7), but no significant incidence of tumors was observed in either test or control animals. JERUSALEM [41] has claimed to have induced lymphomas resembling Burkitt's tumor in mice within six months following

Table 1

| Mouse strain | Number of animals | Antigenic stimulation | Dose | Immuno-Suppression | Dose | Malignant lymphomas Incidence [%] | Type | Latent period [months] | Lymphomas in control groups [%][a] |
|---|---|---|---|---|---|---|---|---|---|
| BALB/c | 32 | LDV[h] | $1 \times 10^{8.5}$ $ID_{50}$ | Azathioprine | 15 mg/kg/day | 32 | lymphosarcoma (stem cell) | 5 | 0 |
| BALB/c | 32 | TB | 0.05 ml CFA/2 weeks[f] | Azathioprine | 15 mg/kg day | 20 | lymphosarcoma (stem cell) | 3 | 0 |
| BALB/c | 64 | BSA[g] | 0.2 ml 10% sol./day | Azathioprine | 15 mg/kg/day | 20 | lymphosarcoma (stem cell) | 4 | 0 |
| BALB/c | 32 | LDV[h] | $1 \times 10^{8.5}$ $ID_{50}$ | ALS[i] | 0.25 ml/weeks | 0[b] | — | — | 0 |
| BALB/c | 32 | TB | 0.05 ml CFA/2 weeks[f] | ALS[i] | 0.25 ml/weeks | 0[b] | — | — | 0 |
| DBA | 34 | BSA[g] | 0.2 ml 10% sol./day | Azathioprine | 15 mg/kg/day | 66 | lymphosarcoma (stem cell) | 5 | 12[c] |
| DBA | 34 | BSA[g] | 0.2 ml 10% sol./day | Azathioprine | 5 mg/kg/day | 16[d] | lymphosarcoma (stem cell) | 6[d] | 3[c] |
| DBA | 34 | BSA[g] | 0.2 ml 10% sol./day | Methotrexate | 3 mg/kg/day | 12 | lymphosarcoma (stem cell) | 6 | 0 |
| DBA | 34 | BSA[g] | 0.2 ml 10% sol./day | TEM[e] | 0.3 mg/kg/day | 0 | — | — | 0 |

[a] Either antigenic stimulation or immunosuppression alone. [b] 40% of the mice showed a generalized immature plasmacytosis; all were dead before the end of the latent period. [c] Azathioprine treatment alone. [d] Experiment unfinished. [e] Triethylene melamine. [f] CFA: complete Freund's adjuvant. [g] BSA: bovine serum albumin. [h] Lactic dehydrogenase elevating virus. [i] ALS: Antilymphocyte serum.

a single infection with Pl. berghei. His experiments, however, are documented in a way that does not allow a clear comparison between control and test animals.

The effect on tumor induction of producing both antigenic stimulation and immunologic suppression in mice was investigated using a variety of agents [42, 44]. Such manipulation and alteration of the immune system in mice has indeed resulted in a significantly increased incidence of lymphomas. The results of these studies are summarized in Table 1.

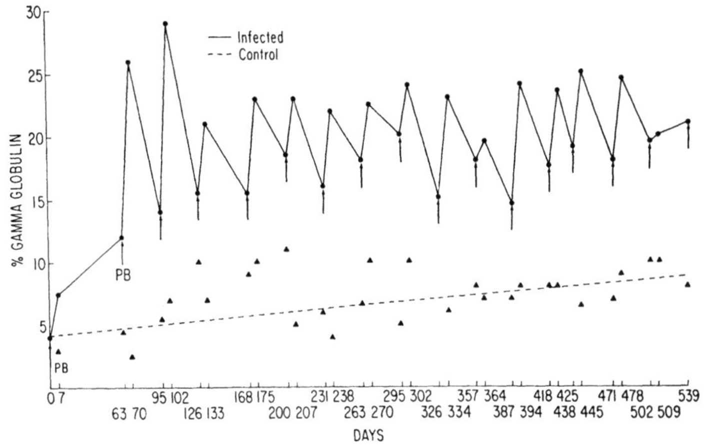


Fig. 7. Chart showing the persistent hypergammaglobulinemia in mice with repeated (i.e. chronic) malaria infection (Courtesy of Sizaret *et al.*, 1971)

Tumor incidence in animals stimulated with Lacticdehydrogenase virus (LDV), tuberculin (TB) or bovine serum albumin (BSA) and suppressed with azathioprine ranged from 12 to 66%. No tumors were seen in control animals given antigenic stimulation alone. In two groups which received azathioprine alone without antigenic stimulation there was a 3 and 12% tumor incidence but this contrasts with an incidence of 16 and 66% respectively in the comparable test groups. When antilymphocyte serum (ALS) or triethylene melamine (TEM) was the immunosuppressant no lymphomas were observed but in the case of ALS the experiments were inconclusive.

All induced lymphomas developed in an atrophic thymus and subsequently spread to involve the remaining lymphoreticular and hemoreticular tissues, as well as nearly all other organs. Tumor cells are growing in tissue culture and can be isotransplanted. They all carry the theta-antigen that identify them as thymus-derived [43, 44, 45].

The induced lymphomas resembled histologically Burkitt's lymphoma (Figs. 8, 9, 10). However, this histological type of tumor is not uncommon in mice and is usually observed in AKR and C 58 strains. Similar tumors induced by a variety of agents have been described by Butler *et al.* [46], Rappaport [47], Kaplan [48] and others [49].

In our experiments non-oncogenic antigens were intentionally used for persistent stimulation, yet malignant lymphomas developed in high frequency. C-type particles

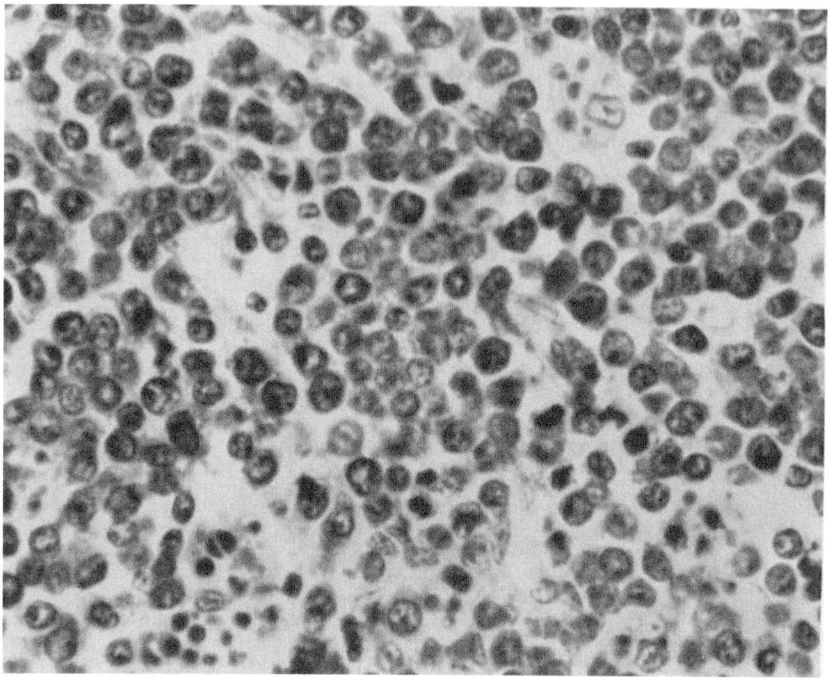

Fig. 8. Section of the mouse lymphosarcoma induced in a BALB/c mouse with azathioprine and BSA. H & E, ×375

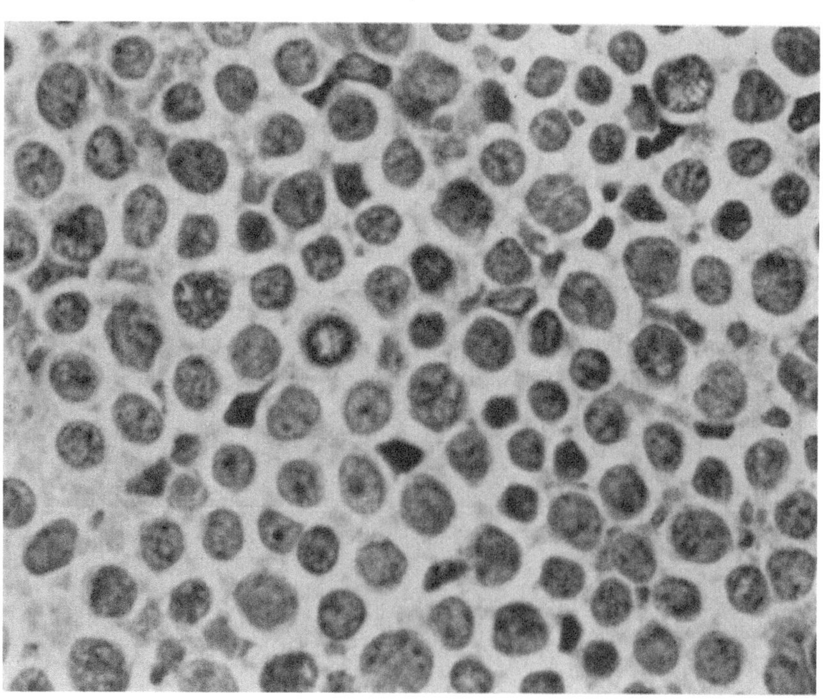

Fig. 9. Imprint of the same tumor shown in Fig. 8. Wright-Giemsa, ×675

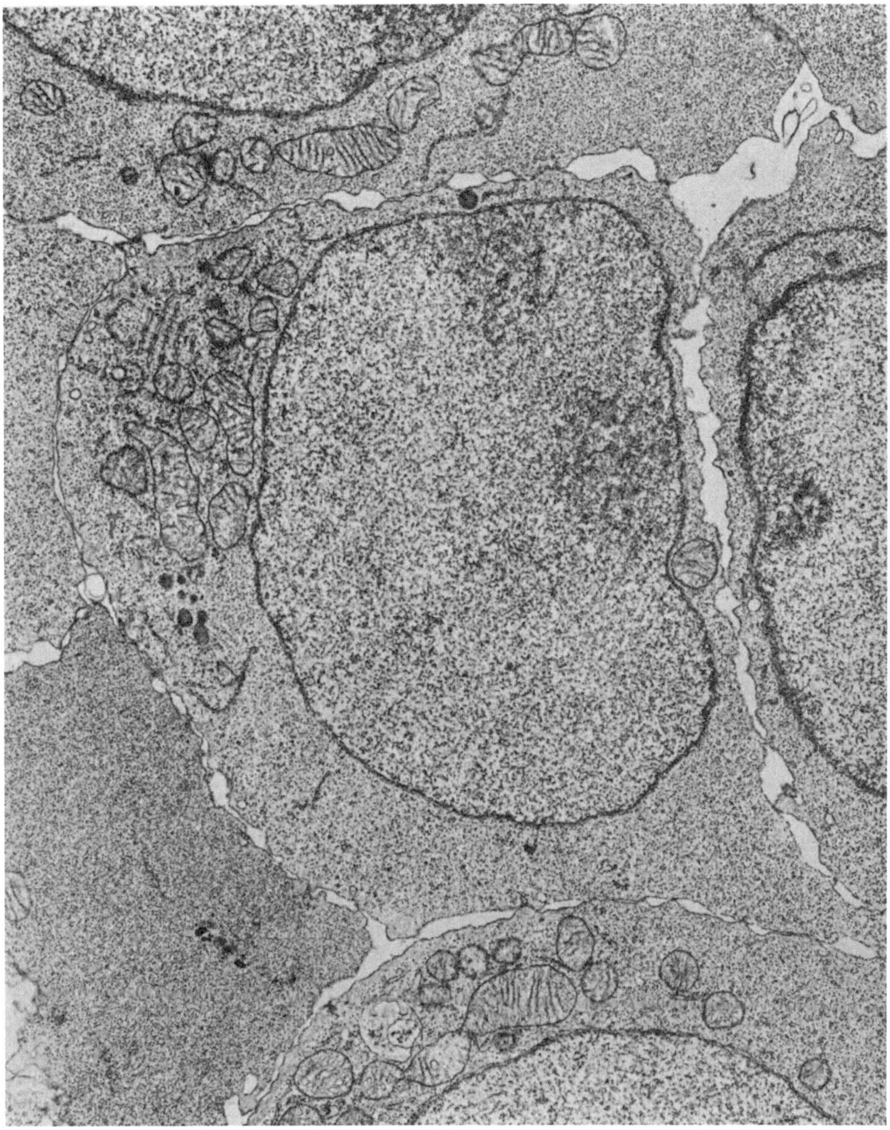

Fig. 10. Electron microgram of the tumor shown in Fig. 8. Uranyl acetate, ×16000

were observed only in occasional lymphomas, and cell-free transplantation of these tumors remained always unsuccessful. No tumor-specific immunologic cross-reactivity could be demonstrated in our lymphomas [45]. We, therefore, assume that the role of virus in the induction of these tumors, whether the virus was introduced or was a passenger, is one of immunologic stimulation rather than direct oncogenicity.

The immunologic capacity of the experimental mice during the latent period of lymphoma development showed some variation. While the cellular immune response, as measured by foot pad tests with the inducing antigen (TB or BSA) and by histological evaluation, was constantly negative, the humoral immune response varied between marked suppression and moderate enhancement [50, 43, 45] (Fig. 11). Humoral antibody production against BSA was measured by the passive hemagglutination method using tanned erythrocytes, and by the coprecipitation method using $^{125}$I-labeled BSA. The variation in the humoral antibody response probably is caused by [1] differences in mouse strains, by [2] differences in the type and dose of the immunosuppressant, and by [3] a variation in the relative concentration of BSA complexes in the injected antigen solution.

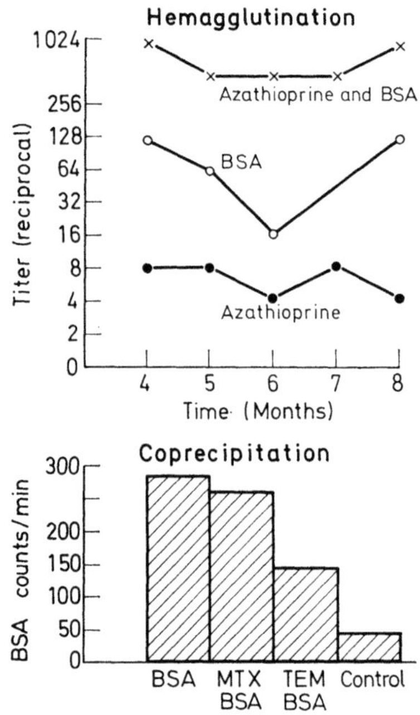


Fig. 11. Chart showing the average anti-BSA antibody titer from experimental and control mice during the latent period and during the period of early tumor formation (a). Chart b showing representative anti-BSA antibody titers in experimental mice receiving as immunosuppressant methotrexate (MTX) or triethylene melamine (TEM) together with the antigen. Control mice were unimmunized and received one immunosuppressant, respectively

The Epstein-Barr virus is a DNA herpes-type virus and like other viruses of this group may possess oncogenic properties [51, 52, 53]. At least some of the C-type RNA viruses in animals are clearly oncogenic [54, 55, 56]. Although both the EBV and C-type viruses are ubiquitous in nature [51, 57, 58] tumor development is relatively uncommon. This had led to the "oncogene theory" of Huebner and Todaro [59] which states that a vertically transmitted viral genome or portion thereof results in tumor induction when "switched on" in some way. The "switch-on mechanism" however, still needs elucidation. From the results of our experiments one may suggest that in the case of lymphoreticular neoplasms a coincidence of persistent antigenic stimulation and immunosuppression represents part of this switch-on mechanism: a large pool of undifferentiated proliferating cells which are especially susceptible to viral infection and transformation are provided at a time when normal immunological surveillance is disturbed [39, 60]. Atypical cells or mutant clones thus may easily grow and invade the host's tissues. Immunosupression related to human tumor induction may be a result of chronic infection, inherited immune deficiency, or immunosuppressive chemotherapy. Persistent antigenic stimulation results from many viral infections, especially those caused by slow viruses. Other, even non-pathogenic organisms or non viable antigens can have the same effect as demonstrated in our experiments.

Oncogenic viruses or viruses with a cell-transforming capacity may have an additional aptitude for the induction of lymphoreticular malignancies because of their immunosuppressive capacities [61, 62, 63, 64]. It would seem from our results as well as from those of others [65, 66] that the suppression of cellular immunity is more important for lymphoma development than is the inhibition of antibody formation. In Burkitt's tumor patients high titers of anti-Epstein-Barr virus antibodies are usually present but a depression of this antibody titer sometimes follows progessive tumor growth [67, 68]. The antibody status in patients prior to development of Burkitt's tumor—during the latent period—is not yet known, nor is there adequate information concerning their cellular immune response. FASS and coworkers [69] studied the delayed cutaneous hypersensitivity reaction to autologous Burkitt's tumor extract and reported positive and negative reactions that correlated with late and early recurrences, respectively. This information, however, allows no conclusion as to the function of cellular immune reactions with respect to tumor pathogenesis. Assuming that malaria parasites and Epstein-Barr viruses both are important antigens and/or immunosuppressive agents active during the induction period of Burkitt's tumor, the cellular immune reactions against these organisms should be screened in a susceptible population.

In conclusion, it appears that the unique coincidence of abnormal environmental and immunological conditions is responsible, at least in Africa, for the development of the malignant lymphoma known as Burkitt's tumor. The epidemiological studies directed to this tumor have suggested laboratory models and investigations which tend to confirm certain pathogenetic concepts relating to lymphoma induction in man. Extension of investigations of this type both in man and in animals hold promise for additional etiological information and generate considerable optimism that prevention and control are indeed possible.

## References

1. MOVAT, H. Z., FERNANDO, N. V.: The fine structure of lymphoid tissue during antibody formation. Exp. Molec. Path. **4**, 155—188 (1965).
2. World Health Organization. Histopathological definition of Burkitt's Tumour. Bull. Wld. Health Org. **40**, 601—607 (1969).
3. LENNERT, K., CAESAR, R., MULLER, H. K.: Electron microscopic studies of germinal centers in man. pp. 49—59 in Germinal Centers in Immune Responses. Eds.: H. COTTIER, N. ODARTCHENKO, R. SCHINDLER, and C. C. CONGDON. Berlin-Heidelberg-New York: Springer 1967.
4. MORI, I., LENNERT, K.: Electron Microscopic Atlas of Lymph Node Cytology and Pathology. Berlin-Heidelberg-New York: Springer 1969.
5. DAMASHEK, W.: Immunoblasts and Immunocytes — An attempt at a functional nomenclature. Blood **21**, 243—245 (1963).

6. Burkitt, D. P., O'Conor, G. T.: Malignant lymphoma in African children. I. A clinical syndrome. Cancer (Philad.) **14**, 258—269 (1961).
7. O'Conor, G. T.: Malignant lymphoma in African children. II. A pathological entity. Cancer (Philad.) **14**, 270—283 (1961).
8. Burkitt, D. P.: A lymphoma syndrome dependent on environment. Part II. Epidemiological features. Symp. Lymph. Tumours in Africa, Paris 1963. Basel: Karger 1964, pp. 119—136.
9. Booth, K., Burkitt, D., Bassett, D. J., Cooke, R. A., Budddulph, J.: Burkitt lymphoma in Papua, New Guinea. Brit. J. Cancer **21**, 657 (1967).
10. Burkitt, D. P.: Recent developments in geographical distribution. pp. 36—41 in Treatment of Burkitt's Tumour. Eds.: J. H. Burchenal and D. P. Burkitt. Berlin-Heidelberg-New York: Springer 1967.
11. Burkitt, D. P., Davies, J. N. P.: Lymphoma syndrome in Uganda and tropical Africa. Afr. Med. Press **245**, 367 (1961).
12. Bell, T. M.: Viruses associated with Burkitt's tumor. Progr. med. Virol. **9**, 1—34 (1967).
13. Epstein, M. A., Achong, B. G., Barr, Y. M.: Virus particles in cultured lymphoblasts from Burkitt's lymphoma. Lancet **1964 I**, 702.
14. Henle, G., Henle, W.: Immunofluorescence in cells derived from Burkitt's lymphoma. J. Bact. **91**, 1248 (1966).
15. Old, L. J., Boyse, E. A., Oettgen, H. F., De Harven, E., Geering, G., Williamson, B., Clifford, P.: Precipitating antibody in human serum to an antigen present in cultured Burkitt's lymphoma cells. Proc. nat. Acad. Sci. (Wash.) **56**, 1699—1704 (1966).
16. Klein, G., Clifford, P., Klein, E., Stjernswärd, J.: Search for tumor-specific immune reactions in Burkitt lymphoma patients by the membrane immunofluorescence reaction. Proc. nat. Acad. Sci. (Wash.) **55**, 1628—1635 (1966).
17. Goetz, O., Lampert, F., Peller, P., Prechtel, K.: Histologisch und virologisch gesicherter Burkitt-Tumor bei einem 10jährigen Knaben. Münch. med. Wschr. **112**, 1373—1376 (1970).
18. Gallmeier, W. M., Göbel, F. W., Hartung, W., Schmidt, C. G.: Studien an einem Burkitt-Lymphom. Klin. Wschr. **48**, 537—542 (1970).
19. Levine, P. H., O'Conor, G. T., Berard, C. W.: Antibodies to Ebstein-Barr virus (EBV) in American patients with Burkitt's lymphoma. Abstract, Spring Meeting, American Association for Cancer Research, St. Louis (1971).
20. Henle, W., Henle, G.: The relation between the Epstein-Barr virus and infectious mononucleosis, Burkitt's lymphoma and cancer of the postnasal space. Afr. med. J. **46**, 402—413 (1969).
21. Levine, P. H., Ablashi, D. V., Berard, C. W., Carbone, P. P., Waggoner, D. E., Malan, L.: Elevated antibody-iters to Epstein-Barr virus in Hodgkin's disease. Cancer (Philad.) **27**, 416—421 (1971).
22. Stevens, D. A., Fink, M. A., Pry, T. W., Maestri, N. E.: Prevalence of precipitating antibody to antigens derived from Burkitt's lymphoma cultures infected with herpes type virus. Blood (in press).
23. Rauscher, F. J.: Virologic studies in human leukemia and lymphoma: The herpes-type virus. Cancer Res. **28**, 1311 (1968).
24. O'Connor, G. T., Davies, J. N. P.: Malignant tumours in African children with special reference to malignant lymphoma. J. Pediat. **56**, 526—535 (1960).
25. Daldorf, G., Linsell, C. A., Barnhart, F. E., Martyn, R.: An epidemiologic approach to the lymphomas of African children and Burkitt's sarcoma of the jaws. Perspect. Biol. Med. **7**, 435—449 (1964).
26. Linsell, A.: Epidemiology of Burkitt's tumour. Lancet **1967 I**, 54.
27. Burkitt, D. P.: Etiology of Burkitt's lymphoma — an alternative hypothesis to a vectoral virus. J. nat. Cancer Inst. **42**, 19—28 (1969).
28. O'Conor, G. T.: Persistent immunologic stimulation as factor in oncogenesis, with special reference to Burkitt's tumor. Amer. J. Med. **48**, 279—285 (1970).
29. Kafuko, G. W., Burkitt, D. P.: Burkitt's lymphoma and malaria. Int. J. Cancer **6**, 1—9 (1970).
30. Bell, T. M.: Review of the evidence for a viral aetiology for Burkitt's lymphoma. In: Treatment of Burkitt's Tumour. Eds.: J. H. Burchenal and D. P. Burkitt. Berlin-Heidelberg-New York: Springer 1967, pp. 52—58.

31. STANLEY, N. F.: Reovirus type 3 and the etiology of Burkitt's lymphoma. In: Treatment of Burkitt's Tumour. Eds.: J. H. BURCHENAL and D. P. BURKITT. Berlin-Heidelberg-New York: Springer 1967, pp. 59—63.
32. WEDDERBURN, N.: Effect of concurrent malarial infection on development of virus-induced lymphoma in BALB/c mice. Lancet **1970 II**, 1114—1116.
33. KRÜGER, G.: Versuch einer immunologischen Deutung der Lymphomentstehung. Dtsch. Med. J. **21**, 28—34 (1970).
34. MCGREGOR, T. A., BARR, M.: Antibody response to tetanus toxoid inoculation in malarious and non-malarious Gambian children. Trans. roy. Soc. trop. Med. Hyg. **56**, 364—367 (1962).
35. SALAMAN, M. H.: Immunodepression by mammalian viruses and plasmodia. Proc. roy. Soc. Med. **63**, 11—15 (1970).
36. GREENWOOD, B. M., PLAYFAIR, J. H. L., TORRIGIANI, G.: Burkitt lymphoma and malaria. Lancet **1970 II**, 418.
37. BARKER, L. R.: Immune responses in malaria. Lancet **1970 II**, 819—820.
38. MICHAUX, J. L.: Les immunoglobulins des Bantous a l'etat normal et pathologique. Ann. Soc. belge Méd. trop. **46**, 483—674 (1966).
39. KRÜGER, G.: Pathogenesis of lymphoreticular neoplasms in transplant recipients. Verh. dtsch. path. Ges. **54**, 175—181 (1970).
40. SIZARET, P., O'CONOR, G. T., KRETSCHMAR, W., BEAUMONT, R., LAVAL, M.: Serum protein patterns in mice following primary and challenge infection with plasmodium berghei. Accepted for publication, Z. Tropenmed. Parasitol. (1971).
41. JERUSALEM, C.: Relationship between malaria infection (plasmodium berghei) and malignant lymphoma in mice. Z. Tropenmed. Parasitol. **19**, 94—108 (1968).
42. KRÜGER, G., MALMGREN, R. A., BERARD, C. W.: Malignant lymphomas and plasmacytosis in mice under prolonged immunosuppression and persistent antigenic stimulation. Transplant. **11**, 138—144 (1971).
43. KRÜGER, G.: Impaired immunologic reactivity as pacemaker for lymphoma development. Verh. dtsch. path. Ges. **55**, 200—204 (1971).
44. KRÜGER, G., HEINE, U.: Morphogenesis of two immunologically induced mouse lymphomas. Submitted for publication (1971).
45. KRÜGER, G.: Host response during the latent period and the growth of an immunologically induced mouse lymphoma. Beitr. Path. Anat. (In print.)
46. BUTLER, J. J., SZAKACS, A., SINKOVICS, J. G.: Virus-induced murine lymphoma resembling Burkitt's tumor. Amer. J. Path. **51**, 629—637 (1967).
47. RAPPAPORT, H., BARONI, C.: A study of the pathogenesis of malignant lymphoma induced in the Swiss mouce by 7, 12-dimethylbenz (a) anthracene injected at birth. Cancer Res. **22**, 1067 to 1074 (1962).
48. KAPLAN, H. S.: Radiation-induced lymphoid tumors of mice. Acta Unio. Internat. Contra Cancr. **7**, 849—859 (1952).
49. RESKE-NIELSEN, E.: Neurologiske og neuropatologiske forandringer hos mus med transplantabelt reticulosarcom. Aarhus: Universitetsforlaget 1961.
50. KRÜGER, G.: Continuous immunologic stimulation, immunosuppression, and lymphomagenesis. Abstract, 3rd Internat. Congress of the Transplant. Soc., The Hague, Sept. 1970.
51. GOODHEART, C. R.: Herpesviruses and cancer. J. Amer. med. Ass. **211**, 91—96 (1970).
52. GERBER, P., WHANG-PENG, J., MONROE, J. H.: Transformation and chromosome changes induced by Epstein-Barr virus in normal human leukocyte cultures. Proc. nat. Acad. Sci. **63**, 740—747 (1969).
53. MELENDEZ, L. V.: Herpesvirus: II. Experimentally induced malignant lymphoma in primates. Lab. Animal Care **19**, 378—386 (1969).
54. HUEBNER, R. J., TODARO, G. J., SARMA, P., HARTLEY, J. W., FREEMAN, A. E., PETERS, R. L., WHITMIRE, C. E., MEIER, H., GILDEN, R. V.: "Switched-off" vertically transmitted C-type RNA tumor viruses as determinants of spontaneous and induced cancer: A new hypothesis of viral carcinogenesis. In: Defectiveness, Rescue and Stimulation of Oncogenic Viruses, pp. 33—57. (2nd Internat. Sympos. on Tumor Viruses, Royaumont, June 1969.) Editions du Centre National de la Recherche Scientifique, Paris 1970.
55. RAUSCHER, F. J.: A virus-induced disease of mice characterized by Erythocytopoiesis and lymphoid leukemia. J. nat. Cancer Inst. **29**, 515—543 (1962).

56. Theilen, G. H., Dungworth, D. L., Kawakami, T. G.: Experimental induction of lymphosarcoma in the cat with "C"-type virus. Cancer Res. **30**, 401—408 (1970).
57. (Editorial) E.B. virus, infectious mononucleosis, and Burkitt lymphoma. Lancet **1969 II**, 887 to 888.
58. Myers, D. D., Meier, H., Huebner, R. J.: Prevalence of murine C-type virus group specific antigen in inbred strains of mice. Life Sci. **9**, 1071—1080 (1970).
59. Huebner, R. J., Todaro, G. J.: Oncogenes of RNA tumor viruses as determinants of cancer. Proc. nat. Acad. Sci. **64**, 1087—1094 (1969).
60. Krüger, G.: Morphology of chemical immunosuppression. Adv. Pharmacol. Chemother. **10**, 1—90 (1972).
61. Ceglowski, W. S., Friedman, H.: Immunosuppressive effects of Friend and Rauscher leukemia disease viruses on cellular and humoral antibody formation. J. nat. Cancer Inst. **40**, 983—995 (1968).
62. Salaman, M. H.: The effect of some leukemogenic viruses on immune reactions. In: Symp. Comp. Leukemia Res., Paris 1967, pp. 92—96. Bibl. haemat. 31. Basel: Karger 1968.
63. Wedderburn, N., Salaman, M. H.: The immunodepressive effect of Friend virus. II. Reduction of splenic hemolysin-producing cells in primary and secondary responses. Immunology **15**, 439—454 (1968).
64. Seidel, H. J., Lauenstein, K.: Zur immunosuppression durch Leukämieviren. Untersuchungen mit dem Rauscher-Virus an einem Leukämie-Resistenten Mäusestamm. Z. Krebsforsch. **72**, 219—225 (1969).
65. Dent, P. B., Peterson, R. D. A., Good, R. A.: A defect in cellular immunity during the incubation period of passage: A leukemia in $C^3H$ mice. Proc. Soc. exp. Biol. (N.Y.) **119**, 869—871 (1965).
66. Doell, R. G., de Vaux, St., Cyr, C., Grabar, P.: Immune reactivity prior to development of thymic lymphoma in C57B1 mice. Int. J. Cancer **2**, 103—108 (1967).
67. Klein, G., Clifford, P., Henle, G., Henle, W., Geering, G., Old, L. J.: EBV-Associated serological patterns in a Burkitt lymphoma patient during regression and recurrence. Int. J. Cancer **4**, 416—421 (1969).
68. Ziegler, J. L., Cohen, M. H., Morrow, R. H., Kyalwazi, S. K., Carbone, P. P.: Immunologic studies in Burkitt's lymphoma. Cancer (Philad.) **25**, 734—739 (1970).
69. Fass, L., Herberman, R. B., Ziegler, J.: Delayed cutaneous hypersensitivity reactions to autologous extracts of Burkitt-lymphoma cells. New Engl. J. Med. **282**, 776—780 (1970).

# Etiology of Burkitt's Lymphoma[1]

Guy de-Thé

Biological Carcinogenesis Unit, International Agency for Research on Cancer, Lyon, France

The epidemiology of Burkitt's lymphoma (BL) strongly favours the hypothesis of a vector transmitted factor playing a role in the development of the tumour (Burkitt, 1963). The serological association between a new herpes virus, discovered by Epstein *et al.* (1964), and this disease makes this virus an obvious canditate for etiology, although the ubiquitous presence of such an agent in all populations all around the world prevents from considering this virus as the only possible cause of the tumour. Two questions can be put forward:

1. Is the Epstein-Barr virus (EBV) oncogenic? As discussed elsewhere (de-Thé *et al.*, 1972b) the EBV appears to have oncogenic potential *in vitro* when uninfected lymphocytes are used as target cells.

2. Is the EBV a *necessary factor* for the development of BL? To answer that critical question, we are implementing a large prospective sero-epidemiological study in Uganda, East Africa. Our aim is to distinguish between three hypotheses regarding the relationship between EBV and BL.

*Hypothesis* 1. There is no causal relationship between EBV and BL. According to this hypothesis, EBV antibody status of those who subsequently develop BL will in no way be different from the EBV status of those who do not develop BL.

*Hypothesis* 2. EBV infection is necessary for the development of BL, which appears clinically after a fairly short and constant latent period (18 ± 6 months). This hypothesis implies that the EBV antibody titre is negative two years or more before the manifestation of the tumour.

*Hypothesis* 3. BL develops in children who have a long and heavy exposure to EBV. This implies continued high antibody titres in the pre-illness sera of BL patients.

A fourth hypothesis implies a causal relationship but of such complicated nature that long and variable latent periods are expected and that it cannot be tested within the proposed framework. However, the role of malaria as possible co-factor can and will be investigated.

Details of the rationale and the implementation of such study were described earlier (Geser and de-Thé, 1972; de-Thé and Geser, 1972a). The field work involved is considerable (follow-up of 35,000 children) but as no other approach

---

1 Supported by Contract No 702076 within the Special Virus Cancer Program of the National Institutes of Health, Dept. of Health, Education and Welfare, United States of America.

seems available to test the hypothesis of viral oncogenicity in humans, the effort appears justified.

## References

BURKITT, D.: A children's cancer dependent on environment. In viruses nucleic acids and cancer. pp. 615—629. Baltimore: The Williams and Wilkins Company 1963.

EPSTEIN, M. A., ACHONG, B. G., BARR, Y. M.: Virus particles in cultured lymphoblasts from Burkitt's lymphoma. Lancet **1964 I**, 702—703.

GESER, A., DE-THÉ, G.: Does the Epstein-Barr virus play an etiological role in Burkitt's lymphoma? (The planning of a longitudinal sero-epidemiological survey in the West Nile district, Uganda). In: Oncogenesis and Herpesviruses. BIGGS, P. M., DE-THÉ, G., and PAYNE, L. N., eds. IARC, Lyon, 1972, pp. 372—375.

DE-THÉ, G., GESER, A.: A prospective sero-epidemiological study to investigate the role of EBV in Burkitt's lymphoma. Proceedings of the Vth Symposium on Comparative Leukemia Research, Padova, September 1971. Bibl. Haemat. (in press), 1972a.

DE-THÉ, G., GESER, A., DAY, N. E.: Problems raised by the association of a herpes virus with two different human tumours: Burkitt's lymphoma and nasopharyngeal carcinoma. Proceedings of the International Cancer Conference, Sydney, March 1972. In: The nature of leukaemia, pp. 65 to 67. P. G. VINCENT (ed.). 1972b.

# Epidemics of Hodgkin's Disease [1]

J. N. P. DAVIES

Department of Pathology Albany Medical College of Union University, Albany, New York, USA

The purpose of this meeting I am informed is to discuss recent work and developments. In March of this year I did not believe epidemics of Hodgkin's Disease existed. I am speaking of work done since March by my colleagues and myself. I am a classic old fashioned morbid anatomist interested in the epidemiology of cancer. Dr. GREENWALD is Director of the New York State Health Departments Cancer Bureau which registers cancer in the state excluding the metropolitan area of New York City. The catalyst was my young colleague Dr. NICHOLAS VIANNA who is a physician with special interests in infectious disease and he persuaded us to join him in a community study of Hodgkin's Disease. He pointed out that many had noted that Hodgkin's Disease had some of the features of an infectious disease. He had the startlingly simple idea of studying the disease in the *community as if it were an infectious disease* [1, 2, 3]. That chance sometimes favours the unprepared mind is shown by the fact that on April 10th this year we published a paper [2] in which we said "There has been no satisfactory evidence of clustering and the low familial and close case concentration are well established". How wrong we were for the day after the proofs of this paper were sent for publication a colleague referred us to an epidemic of Hodgkin's Disease right in our own city and when our findings were publicized [4] we soon found ourselves with more epidemic situations on hand than time has allowed us to investigate fully. However, we have investigated three such situations and all show exactly the same features.

Let us first consider a small outbreak (up-state) involving persons in three different cities. Three of those involved are students. The first case (B 1) while in school had shared a room with another girl we term Contact BA. In June 1970 Case B 1 was diagnosed by biopsy. In January 1971 Case B 2 developed the disease. He was a classmate and close friend of Case B 1, and also associated closely in work with her exroommate, Contact BA. But he was also very friendly with a girl we call Contact BB, and had a limited acquaintance with her father. He, Case B 3, developed Hodgkin's Disease in June 1971 while his daughter Contact BB remains well. Meanwhile in another city lives a lady who is a friend of Case B 3, has a son who was a roommate in college with the son of Case B 3. This lady in 1967 developed

1 Personal Research support has come from the Damon Runyon Memorial Fund for Cancer Research (D.R.G. 1053) and from the Brown Hazen Fund, and from N.I.H. Contract Award No. N.I.H. 71-2426 from the National Cancer Institute. I am grateful to my colleagues Dr. P. GREENWALD and Dr. N. J. VIANNA with whom these investigations are made and to my research assistant Mrs. J. BRADY.

a mixed histiocytic lymphocytic nodular lymphoma. Meanwhile Contact BA had gone to another state and at the university there had shared a room for several months with a girl who developed Hodgkin's Disease in January 1971.

Now you can regard this as an interesting but non significant anecdote but in it I invite you to see the basic features that are repeated in other epidemics. A small closely associated group of students, some develop Hodgkin's Disease, some are contacts and in their household relatives or those they room with Hodgkin's Disease or perhaps some other solid lymphoma develops. Note that Case B 4 and probably Case B 3 would deny that they had Hodgkin's Disease in their family or that they knew anyone with Hodgkin's Disease. We have recently heard that the father of Case B 2 developed a solid lymphoma, not Hodgkin's Disease in 1959. Thus in this outbreak we have 4 interlinked cases of Hodgkin's Disease.

But now consider a situation in a school in down state New York. This school takes in 250 students per year divided into classes of 25 each. The total enrollment is 1,000. In September 1962 a new teacher of English joined the staff which includes 5 other English teachers so that not all students are ever taught by all the English teachers, they teach certain classes only. In January 1963 this teacher, Case C1, was diagnosed as having Hodgkin's Disease. Between March 1965 and June 1971 five students developed Hodgkin's Disease, in one case the disease has been variously diagnosed as a Hodgkin Sarcoma or a histiocytic sarcoma but the remainder are typical Hodgkin's Disease cases. These are the only cases of Hodgkin's Disease that have developed in students of this school over a 10 year period. All save one (Case C6) were in classes taught by this teacher. But Case C6 it then transpired was the editor of the school newspaper. The teacher, Case C1, was the faculty advisor and Case C6 and C1 were in daily contact over several years. But on further inquiry an even more intriguing situation was seen. Case C6 lived at home with her elder sister. Her sister was a close friend of Case C2, and she was being dated by Case C3. But Case C6 was also being dated herself by Case C5 and was working in the same house as Case C4. Thus by the time Case C6 developed the disease she had been in contact with 5 cases of Hodgkin's Disease. In the 1965 class, and therefore classmates and friends with Cases C4 and C5 was a girl who remains well and lived with her mother at home. Her mother developed Hodgkin's Disease in 1968. We have at least one other home contact who develops Hodgkin's Disease. Here I suggest, but on a larger scale we have repeated every feature of the upstate outbreak that I have suggested; the student clique, the close intermingling over a long period, cases and contacts carrying the disease to their relatives in the houses they are living in, and the occurrence of solid lymphomas other than Hodgkin's Disease.

I have chosen to deal first with these small epidemic outbreaks of Hodgkin's Disease, and other solid lymphomas because they manifest every major aspect of the Albany epidemic to which our attention was first drawn. The Albany picture is so complex that to deal with it fully in the time available is impossible. A detailed report is being published [4, 5]. We, at first, tended to think it primarily involved the 1954 graduating class of the Albany High School. It is impossible to speak too highly of the cooperation extend to us by members of this class. The graduating class totalled 317. We have interviewed to time of writing 228 class members, 160 to their knowledge had never encountered a case of Hodgkin's Disease, 61 knew of only a case or cases in the involved school clique (53 of these knew of Case 2 who was

Table 1. Cases and contacts and relationships — Albany epidemic

| A-Albany Cases | | | | | | |
|---|---|---|---|---|---|---|
| Number | Sex | Age at Diagnosis | Year of Diagnosis | Type | Cases Associated with | Contacts Associated with |
| 1 | M | 16 | 1948 | MC | | |
| 2 | M | 15 | 1952 | Gr | 3, 4, 17, 27, 30 | B, C, E, F, I, M, P, W, Z, [AA |
| 3 | M | 22 | 1957 | MC | 2, 4, 30 | F, S, W |
| 4 | M | 22 | 1960 | NS | 2, 3, 30 | J, N, R, W |
| 5 | M | 17 | 1970 | LD | 7 | C |
| 6 | M | 67 | 1967 | MC | | B |
| 7 | F | 16 | 1968 | MC | 5 | D |
| 8 | F | 16 | 1953 | NS | | E, F, G, W |
| 9 | F | 17 | 1958 | NS | 12 | G, U |
| 10 | F | 15 | 1970 | LP | 11 | D, W |
| 11 | M | 74 | 1957 | MC | 10 | D, W |
| 12 | M | 14 | 1955 | NS | 9, 34 | C, H, U |
| 13 | F | 18 | 1951 | MC | | K |
| 14 | F | 61 | 1960 | MC | | R |
| 15 | M | 25 | 1958 | MC | 4 | I, R |
| 16 | M | 49 | 1964 | MC | | N, O |
| 17 | M | 16 | 1953 | MC | 2 | P |
| 18 | F | 18 | 1961 | MC | | O |
| 19 | M | 23 | 1951 | MC | | M |
| 20 | M | 39 | 1962 | MC | | Q |
| 21 | M | 32 | 1957 | MC | | L |
| 22 | F | 37 | 1966 | NS | | T |
| 23 | M | | 1957 | MC | | S |
| 24 | F | 20 | 1953 | NS | | V |
| 25 | M | 40 | 1970 | MC | | H, Y |
| 26 | M | 65 | 1970 | | | A |
| 27 | M | 30 | 1968 | NS | 2 | C |
| 28 | F | 26 | 1957 | | | X |
| 29 | M | 37 | 1970 | NS | | H |
| 30 | M | 26 | 1962 | * | 2, 3, 4 | |
| 31 | F | | 1963 | | | Z |
| 32 | M | | 1957 | * | | AA |
| 33 | M | | 1971 | | | H |
| 34 | M | 24 | 1970 | * | 12 | |

* Lymphoma other than Hodgkin's.

class vice-president) and only 7, including 2 physicians and one priest had personally encountered Hodgkin's Disease outsite this school.

We were originally told of 7 possible persons involved in the school and these included Cases 2, 3, and 4. When the school made available the individual files of these students we found that the names of their close friends were noted on themles. Cases 2, 3, and 4 had been friends long before they entered the school and fro fi the files it was clear that the same names of friends recurred over and over again. We thus defined a clique of close knit friends who associated all together over a period of years and a larger group who associated with one or two members of the clique but not with the others. The clique was not confined to the one school but included

Table 1 (continued)

B-Albany Contacts

| Contact | Sex | Year of Graduation | Cases in Contact with and Relationship |
|---|---|---|---|
| A | F | 1952 | 26-father* |
| B | F | 1954 | 6-father* |
| C | M | 1954 | 5-cousin*, 12-friend, 27-friend |
| D | M | 1968 | 7-friend, 10-sister*, 11-uncle |
| E | M | 1954 | 2-friend, 8-dated |
| F | M | 1953 | 2-same club, 3-classmate, 8-sister* |
| G | F | 1954 | 8-friend, 9-sister* |
| H | F | 1952 | 12-brother*, 25-co-worker, 29-friend, 33-co-worker |
| I | F | 1954 | 2-dated, 15-brother* |
| J | F | 1955 | 4-classmate, 15-brother* |
| K | F | 1954 | 13-first cousin |
| L | M | 1955 | 21-uncle* |
| M | M | 1954 | 2-close friend, 19-first cousin |
| N | F | 1956 | 16-father* |
| O | F | 1957 | 16-uncle, 18-friend |
| P | M | 1954 | 2-close friend, 17-close friend |
| Q | F | 1957 | 20-father* |
| R | F | 1955 | 4-classmate, 14-mother* |
| S | M | 1954 | 2-classmate, 3-close friend, 23-grandfather* |
| T | F | 1952 | 22-sister-in-law |
| U | M | 1963 | 9-sister*, 12-friend |
| V | M | 1954 | 3-same club, 24-dated |
| W | M | 1955 | 2-friend, 3-friend, 10-cousin, 11-grandfather, 8-friend |
| X | F | 1952 | 28-sister-in-law |
| Y | F | 1954 | 8-classmate, 25-brother* |
| Z | M | 1954 | 2-classmate, 31-co-worker |
| AA | F | 1954 | 2-classmate, 32-uncle* |

* Lived in same house prior to diagnosis.

boys and girls attending other schools but living in the area. Put briefly from this clique and group, which numbers about 30 persons, we have so far interlinked via direct association, or via one contact who remains well, no less than 38 other cases comprising 32 cases of Hodgkin's Disease and 6 of other solid lymphomas. Of these, 13 cases occurred in persons living in the same house as a member of the group or clique.

In brief summary we know that when the majority of those who formed the clique or group with which we are concerned there was in the Albany High School one boy with established Hodgkin's Disease (Case 1) and two girls developed the disease in 1951 (Cases 13) and 1953 (Cases 24). These latter two girls though not themselves in the clique had relatives and friends in the clique. In 1951 the disease was diagnosed in a boy in another school (Case 19) who also had relatives and friends in the clique. By December 1952 Hodgkin's Disease had developed in 4 students, one a clique member and the group included 3 close contacts and relatives of established cases. From 1953—1960 thirteen cases of Hodgkin's Disease developed.

Thus by 1960 of 18 cases, 7 had developed in Albany High School students, 5 in student friends in other schools, and 6 in non-school individuals, 4 of these living in the same house as a group contact. By 1960 all clique and group members had left their schools (Fig. 1) but from then to the present cases of Hodgkin's Disease have continued to develop in members and associates of this clique and in their household contacts and those they roomed with in other educational institutions. Thus we know of two subsidiary microepidemics of Hodgkin's Disease set off by the migration of clique or group members to other colleges and are on the trail of others. Moreover, other lymphomas, (and one case of acute lymphatic leukemia) have occurred in the exstudents and their household associates and we have at least two instances, in which a contact who remains well, seems to have carried the disease to several other persons over a period of years.

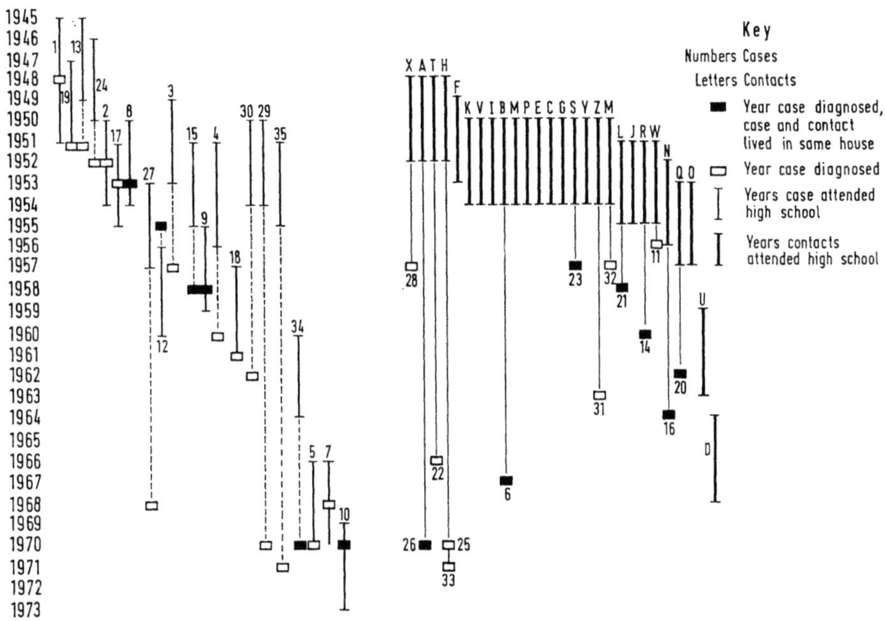


Fig. 1. School Attendance Periods of Interlinked Cases of Hodgkin's Disease and Other Lymphomas in Albany

This investigation is still in active progress and fresh information is being added weekly so that this is no more than an interim report. If the results and conclusions to date are summarised they are as follows:

As regards the Albany epidemic

1. For the years 1953—1959 the incidence rates for Hodgkin's Disease in Albany County based on reported cases were above the average rates of reported cases in the other 56 upstate counties of New York State and after 1960 the rates were generally below the average of the other counties. Thus the use of the term epidemic is justified.

2. When the incidence rates per 100,000 are calculated for Albany County for Hodgkin's Disease by year of diagnosis the increased incidence of the disease is

again seen, extending to even higher rates for the period 1953—1961 but then there was a period of 4 years of low incidence.

3. To this increased incidence a small group of young school students contributed a quite disproportionate number of cases of Hodgkin's Disease, both directly and via their close associates and by members who acted as contacts involving further cases in their houses or work fellows.

4. All ages from 14—74 years were involved, save for more rapid progression in the elderly the disease seemed to behave similarly at all ages.

5. All histological subtypes [6] of Hodgkin's Disease were seen in these patients.

6. In all the epidemic situations we have studied we have noted the formation of a clique of young students who associated closely over a period of years, the disease develops in several of the clique members, in their associates and in their families, other solid lymphomas also develop. When the clique splits up subsidiary micro-epidemics occur.

7. In the more than 50 cases of Hodgkin's Disease studied in these epidemics only 2 intra-familial cases have been noted [7].

8. With one dubious exception the disease seemed to spread to the older persons from the younger but not from old persons to the young.

9. In the community Hodgkin's Disease behaves, at least on occasion, like an infective disease with a long incubation period. The similarities to the epidemiologic features of leprosy are very close.

10. These disease can be spread by case to case transmissio n or by case to contact to case transmission, the contacts remain in good health but some of these seem to be capable of transmitting the disease for many years.

11. Transmission is probably by the oral route.

12. While within the clique contacts are repetitive and prolonged we have some evidence that contact need not be prolonged for transmission to occur.

13. At present no satisfactory method of statistical approach to the interlinkings we have described is known to us or those we have consulted. We have found no evidence of clustering in the usual sense of the word. To the questions—have you any Hodgkin's Disease in your family or in your friends—most of our cases, especially the household cases, could rightly have answered no. The disease was present in the friends of their young housemates often unknown to them.

14. Our evidence suggests that Hodgkin's Disease is a unitary disease [7], is due to an infectious agent or agents, is spread by case—case or case-contact-case transmission and that the histologic sub types indicate different reactions to a single disease process.

One final comment is worth consideration. When at an earlier stage our evidence was scrutinised by two experienced radiotherapists—both separately made in virtually identical terms a remark we now consider highly significant—it was, "You know I have never seen an unattractive girl with Hodgkin's Disease".

## References

1. Vianna, N. J., Greenwald, P., Davies, J. N. P.: Tonsillectomy and Hodgkin's Disease: The Lymphoid Tissue Barrier. Lancet **1971 I**, 431.

2. Vianna, N. J., Greenwald, P., Davies, J. N. P.: Nature of the Hodgkin's Disease Agent. Lancet **1971 I**, 733.

3. VIANNA, N. J., GREENWALD, P., POLAN, A., DAVIES, J. N. P.: Epidemiologic Survey of Hodgkin's Disease in Children and Young Adults. In Preparation. 1972.
4. VIANNA, N. J., GREENWALD, P., DAVIES, J. N. P.: Extended Epidemic of Hodgkin's Disease in High School Students. Lancet **1971 I**, 1209.
5. VIANNA, N. J., GREENWALD, P., BRADY, J., DWORK, A., POLAN, A., MAURO, T., DAVIES, J. N. P.: Hodgkin's Disease: Cases with Features of a Community Outbreak. Ann. Int. Med. **77**, 169—180 (1972).
6. LUKES, R. J., BUTLER, J. J., HICKS, E. B.: Natural History of Hodgkin's Disease as related to its Pathologic Picture. Cancer (N.Y.) **19**, 317 (1966).
7. SMITHERS, D. W.: Hodgkin's Disease: One Entity or Two? Lancet **1970 II**, 1285.

# Hodgkin's Disease in Childhood — An Epidemiological Study in Northern Germany[1]

H. DÖRKEN and H. SINGER-BAKKER

I. Medizinische Universitätsklinik Hamburg, Germany

Beginning with clinical observations, we followed in Hamburg three main paths of investigation of Hodgkin's disease.

First, there was the unique age distribution with two ["bimodality"] or even three modes. LENNERT has already mentioned this pattern 1953 [15] and MACMAHON has analysed it in his well-known papers [19, 21]. Hodgkin's disease is separated by this specific age distribution from other lymphomas and neoplasms and the question of several entities in it seems justified [19, 22, 26]. We could add a detail: The origin of the second (or third resp.) peak is located one or two 5-years-age groups earlier in the male sex [5] (Fig. 1, 2).

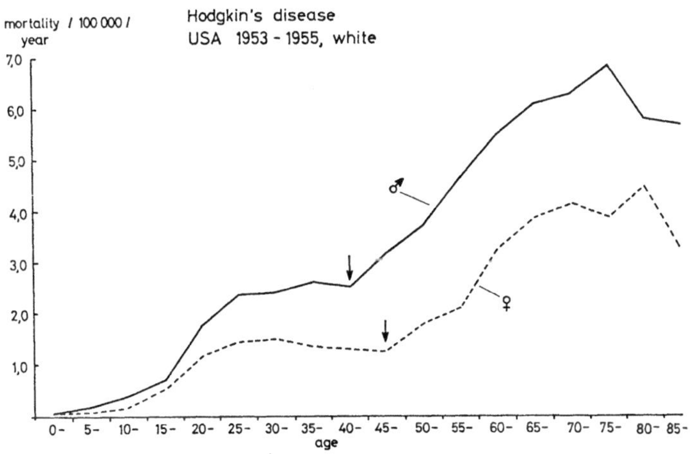


Fig. 1. Hodgkin's disease — age- and sex-specific death rates

Secondly, we found, like others, manifestation of Hodgkin's disease more frequent in the cold season (Fig. 3). This behaviour is similar to that in some infectious diseases [6, 13, 28]. Deaths—in contrast—are evenly distributed (Fig. 4).

---

1 Supported by a grant of the Siemers-Stiftung.

Thirdly and surprisingly we saw in our town a greater number of patients coming from rural districts. Perhaps this is due to chance alone, for Hamburg is surrounded by rural districts.

Therefore we investigated this point by a survey of the 272,000 original death certificates of Northern Germany (Schleswig-Holstein, Niedersachsen, the States of Hamburg and Bremen) for the years 1964—1965 [7]. This area comprises one quarter of the Federal Republic of Germany with one third of its population. We found 344 cases of Hodgkin's disease (all ages) with histological proof (112 postmortems). The age-adjusted death rates were comparable with the known values of other European countries and of a similar study based on the material of the "lymph

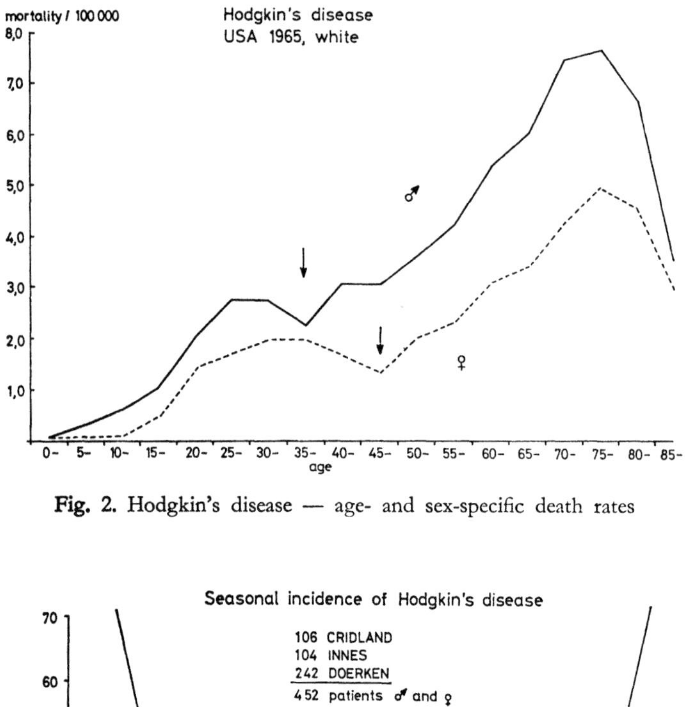


Fig. 2. Hodgkin's disease — age- and sex-specific death rates

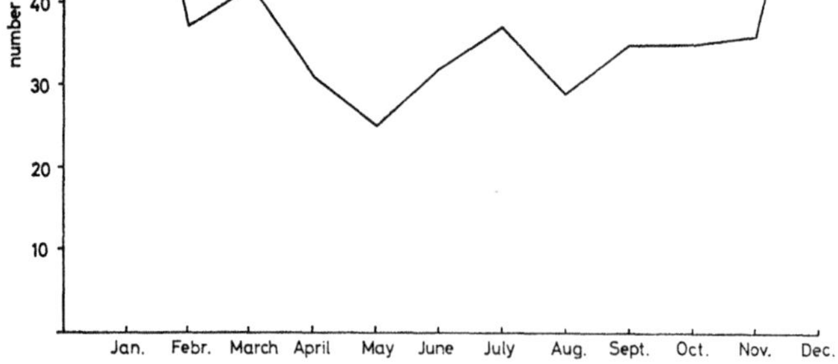


Fig. 3. Hodgkin's disease — incidence by season (three curves of the literature plotted together)

node registry" [16]. There was only chance variation in the 101 counties—similar e.g. to those in Norway [3]—and no evidence of "clustering" in these two years. Furthermore, the rates were nearly equal in urban and in rural areas. With this so called "urban/rural-ratio" [17] of about 1.0 Hodgkin's disease can once again be separated from most other neoplasms, as is evident in the age-adjusted ratios calculated from the wellknown Danish Cancer Registry [4].

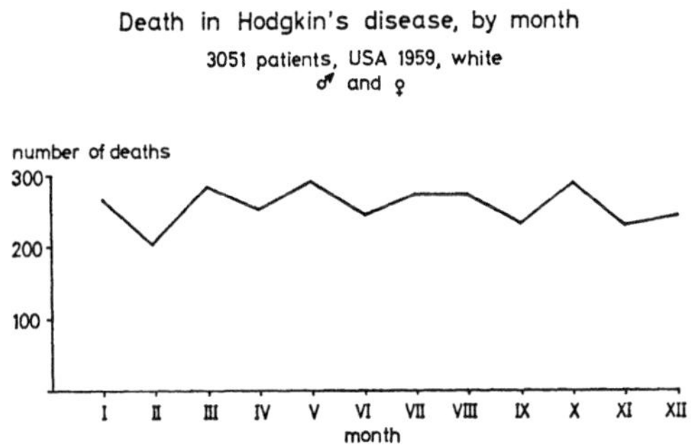


Fig. 4. Hodgkin's disease — death by season

A further analysis of the age-specific rates revealed a small but distinct prevalence of the younger rural victims (until 30 years of age), but only for males. The same was found in the two neighbouring countries Norway and Denmark [4, 7, 23]. Now the question for the values in childhood arises. I should like to remind you that these "rural factors" were already discussed in some older papers over forty years ago [18, 27, 31].

We have also studied Hodgkin's disease (and leukemia) in the most rural part of the State of Hamburg, in Finkenwerder. We found rather high values for both diseases, some neighbourhood-cases and some patients in small farm-houses. A higher mortality of farm residents in California has been described [10].

We also payed attention everywhere to cattle leukosis, which is a problem in Northern Germany. We found no evidence for a correlation.

Venice has no air pollution—but yet lung cancer enough—and has no agriculture. We found in Venice rather high values for Hodgkin's disease (and leukemia) and no visible clustering. We found tremendous numbers of cats and pigeons, only one or two pigs, but no cattle or sheep indeed.

Epidemiological investigations with childhood populations seem to be valuable for three reasons: The life span is still short, important factors (like occupational influences or tobacco) can be neglected and the parents cooperate well.

We collected 125 children with histological proven Hodgkin's disease, manifested before the age of 15 in whole Northern Germany since World War II. There were 86 deaths, and survival of the remainder up to 16 years until now. To avoid selection as well as possible we contacted all 44 childrens hospitals in this area. The Clinic of Bremen has the largest numbers (25 children). Hamburg is somewhat overrepresented especially because of our own cancer registry, which we contacted too.

The clinical picture of Hodgkin's disease, the distribution of the affected lymph nodes, the differential diagnosis seems to be the same like in older age-groups

[8, 9, 15, 25]. We find the very special symptoms of Hodgkin's disease—periodic fever, itching, diazo reaction—in childhood also. Hodgkin-sarcoma was described in 8%. There was no therapy with X-rays and no therapy with hydantoins, known predisposing factors, in the histories. So far we contacted and interviewed the families of 95 cases. No second case in relatives could be found. The family background was rather uniform. Remarkable perhaps a "Zinsser-Cole-Engman-Syndrome" (dyskeratosis congenita) in a brother of a young girl with Hodgkin's disease. Concordant twins with Hodgkin's disease are very rare [14], we found no instance.

The estimation of the morbidity rate for boys and girls together was 0.16/100,000/year.

The resulting urban/rural distribution of these 125 children (with the limit for "urban" of 20,000 inhabitants) showed a clear preponderance of the rural cases in 5 of the 6 age groups, significant at the 99% confidence level (method in [1]). This preponderance is more marked in boys than in girls (Fig. 5).

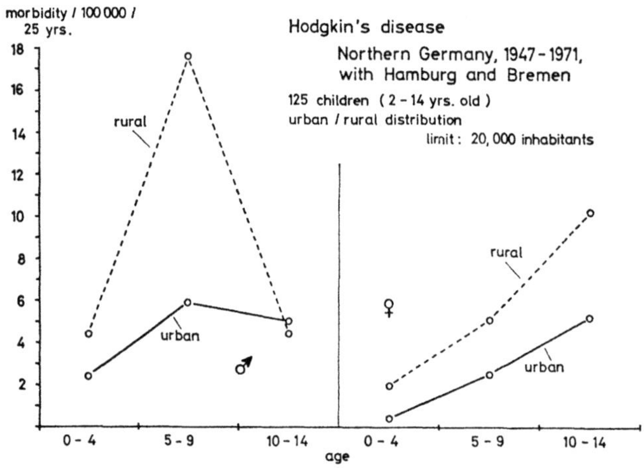


Fig. 5. Hodgkin's disease — urban/rural-distribution in Northern Germany (limit: 20,000 inhabitants)

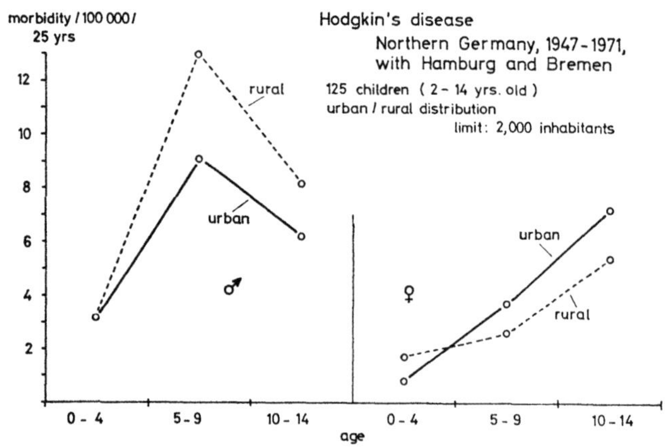


Fig. 6. Hodgkin's disease — urban/rural-distribution in Northern Germany (limit: 2,000 inhabitants)

If we reduce the limit down to only 2,000 inhabitants, there remains still a preponderance for the boys, but not for the girls (Fig. 6).

Looking at the geographical distribution of the individual cases, we see the bulk besides the towns. We found no clustering, but some neighbourhood-cases, especially at the coast, which warrant further investigation. Also in adults we saw very seldom local aggregations of Hodgkin's disease in Hamburg, and we are still studying clusters. Non is as impressive as those of doctor Davies and doctor Vianna in New York [29, 30].

I come to the end. Despite all success in diagnosis and therapy the prognosis of Hodgkin's disease is uncertain in every patient, even up to 20 and more years. Moreover, there appears to be an increase in the 20th Century [2], but it is very difficult to proof. With new and concerted efforts we should study the clustering (the "Krebshäuser" and "Krebsdörfer" of the literature some 80 years ago) with its statistical problems [12]. We should analyse the factors in the rural environment. Perhaps we will look here at the domestic animals and their products soon and first of all. The retrospective case-control study referring to this is in progress.

We wish to thank the many colleagues in Northern Germany who added their efforts to our studies.

We wish to thank for much advice and help Dr. Clemmesen (Kopenhagen), Prof. Dr. Ferrari (Venedig), Prof. Dr. MacMahon (Boston), Dr. Miller, Dr. Fraumeni (Bethesda), Dr. Keding (Hamburg), Prof. Dr. Lennert (Kiel) and Dr. Franks (London).

## References

1. Bailar, C., Ederer, F.: Significance factors for the ratio of a Poisson variable to its expectation. Biometrics **20**, 639—643 (1964).
2. Begemann, H.: Klinische Hämatologie. Stuttgart: Thieme 1970.
3. Bjelke, E.: Hodgkin's disease in Norway — Mortality trends, incidence, and survival. Acta med. scand. **185**, 73—81 (1969).
4. Clemmesen, J.: Statistical studies in the aetiology of malignant neoplasms. Kopenhagen: Munksgaard 1965.
5. Dörken, H.: Über die Altersverteilung der Lymphogranulomatose. Klin. Wschr. **38**, 944—947 (1961).
6. Dörken, H., Buss, H., Müller, G., Fliessbach, R., Rauchenberger, B.: Die Epidemiologie der Lymphogranulomatose (M. Hodgkin). Arch. Geschwulstforsch. **34**, 322—335 (1969).
7. Dörken, H., Fliessbach, R., Buss, H.: Die geographische Verteilung der Lymphogranulomatose (M. Hodgkin) und ihre Stadt/Land-Relation in Norddeutschland. Z. Krebsforsch. **74**, 190—199 (1970).
8. Eckler, E.: Pathogenese, Diagnose und Therapie der Lymphogranulomatose im Kindesalter. Verh.-Ber. dtsch. Arbeitsgemeinsch. Leukämieforsch. Behandl. Kindesalter, 6. Tagg., Frankfurt 1968.
9. Falk, W., Waltersdorfer-Hinrichs, R.: Betrachtungen zur Diagnose und Differentialdiganose der Lymphknotentoxoplasmose im Kindesalter. Ann. paediat. (Basel) **201**, 349—364 (1963).
10. Fasal, E., Jackson, E. W., Klauber, M. R.: Leukemia and lymphoma mortality and farm residence. Amer. J. Epidem. **87**, 267—274 (1968).
11. Fraumeni, J. F., Li, F. P.: Hodgkin's disease in childhood: An epidemiological study. J. nat. Cancer Inst. **42**, 681—691 (1969).
12. Glass, A. G., Hill, J. A., Miller, R. W.: Significance of leukemia clusters. J. Pediat. **73**, 101—107 (1968).
13. Hartwich, G., Schlabeck, H.: Lymphogranulomatose — Jahreszeitliche Verteilung der Erstmanifestation. Dtsch. med. Wschr. **95**, 1387—1389 (1970).

14. JÖRGENSEN, G.: Lymphogranulomatose bei Zwillingen. Dtsch. med. Wschr. **95**, 716 (1970).
15. LENNERT, K.: Über die Berechtigung der Unterscheidung von drei Lymphogranulomatoseformen von Jackson und Parker. Verh. dtsch. path. Ges. **37**, 174—180 (1953).
16. LENNERT, K.: Die derzeitige Häufigkeit der einzelnen Lymphknotenerkrankungen in Schleswig-Holstein. Dtsch. med. Wschr. **94**, 2194—2202 (1969).
17. LINDEN, L. L.: The reconciliation of census and national center for health statistics definitions of urban and rural populations. Techn. Inform. Notes No. 17, Nat. Center for Health Statistics, Washington 1965.
18. LITTECK, I.: Die regionäre Verteilung des malignen Granuloms in Ostpreußen. Dtsch. med. Wschr. **54**, 960—962 (1928).
19. MACMAHON, B.: Epidemiology of Hodgkin's disease. Cancer Res. **26**, 1189—1200 (1966).
20. MUSSHOFF, K., BOUTIS, L.: Therapy results in Hodgkin's disease. Freiburg i. Br., 1948—1966. Cancer (Philad.) **21**, 1100—1113 (1968).
21. NEWELL, G. R., COLE, S. R., MIETTINEN, O. S., MACMAHON, B.: Age differences in the histology of Hodgkin's disease. J. nat. Cancer Inst. **45**, 311—317 (1970).
22. NOVAK, D., HILWEG, D.: Häufigkeit und Formen intrathorakaler Manifestation maligner Lymphome. Dtsch. med. Wschr. **96**, 230—234 (1971).
23. PEDERSEN, E.: Cancer registration in Norway; the incidence of cancer in Norway 1959—1961. Norwegian Cancer Soc., Oslo 1964.
24. OBRECHT, P.: Die Lebenserwartung Hämoblastosekranker. Dtsch. Röntgenkongress 1966, Teil B, Sonderbd. Strahlentherapie **64**, 252—264 (1967).
25. SCHUSTER, W., DOMULA, M., BREIDENBACH, H.: Zur Lymphogranulomatose im Kindesalter. Kinderärztl. Prax. **38**, 481—486 (1970).
26. SMITHERS, D. W.: Hodgkin's disease: One entity or two? Lancet **1970 II**, 1285—1288.
27. UDDSTRÖMER, M.: On the occurence of lymphogranulomatosis (Sternberg) in Sweden 1915—31 and some considerations as to its relation to tuberculosis. Acta tuberc. scand., Suppl. **I** (1934).
28. UHL, N., HUNSTEIN, W.: Jahreszeitliche Schwankungen in Auftreten der Lymphogranulomatose. Dtsch. Arch. klin. Med. **216**, 355—370 (1969).
29. VIANNA, N. J., GREENWALD, P., DAVIES, J. N. P.: Nature of Hodgkin's disease agent. Lancet **1971 I**, 733—735.
30. VIANNA, N. J., GREENWALD, P., DAVIES, J. N. P.: Extended epidemic of Hodgkin's disease in high-school students. Lancet **1971 I**, 1209—1211.
31. ZECHNALL, W.: Über die Lymphogranulomatose in Südbaden. Dtsch. Arch. klin. Med. **179**, 38—50 (1936/37).
32. Vital statistics of the United States (annual). Washington: U.S. Government Printing Office.
33. Volks- und Berufszählung vom 6. Juni 1961: Statistisches Bundesamt, Wiesbaden 1966; Fachserie A, Bevölkerung und Kultur, Heft 4, Bevölkerung nach Alter und Familienstand.
34. Amtliches Gemeindeverzeichnis für die Bundesrepublik Deutschland. Statistisches Bundesamt; Ausgabe 1961. Stuttgart u. Mainz: Kohlhammer 1963.

# Subject Index

*Monographs already Published*

1 SCHINDLER, R., Lausanne: Die tierische Zelle in Zellkultur
2 Neuroblastomas — Biochemical Studies. Edited by C. BOHUON, Villejuif (Symposium)
3 HUEPER, W. C., Bethesda: Occupational and Environmental Cancers of the Respiratory System
4 GOLDMAN, L., Cincinnati: Laser Cancer Research
5 METCALF, D., Melbourne: The Thymus. Its Role in Immune Responses, Leukaemia Development and Carcinogenesis
6 Malignant Transformation by Viruses. Edited by W. H. KIRSTEN, Chicago (Symposium)
7 MOERTEL, CH. G., Rochester: Multiple Primary Malignant Neoplasms. Their Incidence and Significance
8 New Trends in the Treatment of Cancer. Edited by L. MANUILA, S. MOLES, and P. RENTCHNICK, Geneva
9 LINDENMANN, J., Zürich, and P. A. KLEIN, Gainesville/Florida: Immunological Aspects of Viral Oncolysis
10 NELSON, R. S., Houston: Radioactive Phosphorus in the Diagnosis of Gastrointestinal Cancer
11 FREEMAN, R. G., and J. M. KNOX, Houston: Treatment of Skin Cancer
12 LYNCH, H. T., Houston: Hereditary Factors in Carcinoma
13 Tumours in Children. Edited by H. B. MARSDEN and J. K. STEWARD, Manchester
14 ODARTCHENKO, N., Lausanne: Production cellulaire érythropoïétique
15 SOKOLOFF, B., Lakeland/Florida: Carcinoid and Serotonin
16 JACOBS, M. L., Duarte/California: Malignant Lymphomas and their Management
17 Normal and Malignant Cell Growth. Edited by R. J. M. FRY, Argonne, M. L. GRIEM, Argonne, and W. H. KIRSTEN, Chicago (Symposium)
18 ANGLESIO, E., Torino: The Treatment of Hodgkin's Disease
19 BANNASCH, P., Würzburg: The Cytoplasm of Hepatocytes during Carcinogenesis
20 Rubidomycin. A new Agent against Leukemia. Edited by J. BERNARD, R. PAUL, M. BOIRON, C. JACQUILLAT, and R. MARAL, Paris
21 Scientific Basis of Cancer Chemotherapy. Edited by G. MATHÉ, Villejuif (Symposium)
22 KOLDOVSKÝ, P., Philadelphia: Tumor Specific Transplantation Antigen
23 FUCHS, W. A., Bern, J. W. DAVIDSON, Toronto, and H. W. FISCHER, Ann Arbor: Lymphography in Cancer
24 HAYWARD, J. L., London: Hormonal Research in Human Breast Cancer
25 ROY-BURMAN, P., Los Angeles: Analogues of Nucleic Acid Components. Mechanisms of Action
26 Tumors of the Liver. Edited by G. T. PACK and A. H. ISLAMI, New York
27 SZYMENDERA, J., Warsaw: Bone Mineral Metabolism in Cancer
28 MEEK, E. S., Bristol: Antitumour and Antiviral Substances of Natural Origin
29 Aseptic Environments and Cancer Treatment. Edited by G. MATHÉ, Villejuif (Symposium)

30 Advances in the Treatment of Acute (Blastic) Leukemias. Edited by G. MATHÉ, Villejuif (Symposium)
31 DENOIX, P., Villejuif: Treatment of Malignant Breast Tumors: Indications and Results
32 NELSON, R. S., Houston: Endoscopy in Gastric Cancer
33 Experimental and Clinical Effects of L-Asparaginase. Edited by E. GRUNDMANN, Wuppertal-Elberfeld, and H. F. OETTGEN, New York (Symposium)
34 ENDO, H., Fukuoka, T. ONO, Tokyo, and T. SUGIMURA, Tokyo: Chemistry and Biological Actions of 4-Nitroquinoline 1-oxide
35 PENN, I., Denver: Malignant Tumors in Organ Transplant Recipients
36 Current Concepts in the Management of Leukemia and Lymphoma. Edited by J. E. ULTMANN, M. L. GRIEM, W. H. KIRSTEN, and R. W. WISSLER, Chicago (Symposium)
37 CHIAPPA, S., R. MUSUMECI, and C. USLENGHI, Milano: Endolymphatic Radiotherapy in Malignant Lymphomas
38 KOLLER, P. C., London: The Role of Chromosomes in Cancer Biology
39 Current Problems in the Epidemiology of Cancer and Lymphomas. Edited by E. GRUNDMANN, Münster, and H. TULINIUS, Lyon (Symposium)

Special Supplement: Biology of Amphibian Tumors. Edited by M. MIZELL, New Orleans

## *In Production*

40 LANGLEY, F. A., and A. C. CROMPTON, Manchester: Epithelial Abnormalities of the Cervix Uteri
41 Tumours in a Tropical Country. A Survey of Uganda (1964—1968). Edited by A. C. TEMPLETON, Minneapolis

## *In Preparation*

BOIRON, M., Paris: The Viruses of the Leukemia-Sarcoma Complex

CAVALIERE, R., A. ROSSI-FANELLI, B. MONDOVI, and G. MORICCA, Roma: Selective Heat Sensitivity of Cancer Cells

GARATTINI, S., FRANCHI, G., Milano: Chemotherapy of Cancer Dissemination: Methods and Results

GRUNDMANN, E., Münster: Morphology and Cytochemistry of Carcinogenesis

GRUNDMANN, E., Münster: Recent Results in Carcinogenesis (Symposium)

KOLDOVSKY, P., Philadelphia: Canceroembryoantigens

LEVIN, A., Nairobi: Human Tumour Immunology for Clinicians and Experimentalists

MATHÉ, G., Villejuif: Immunotherapy of Cancers

MATHÉ, G., Villejuif: Standardisation of Nomenclature and Methodology for Clinical Trials in Acute Leukemia (Symposium)

MERKOW, L., and M. SLIFKIN, Pittsburgh: Oncogenic Simian Adenoviruses

OETTGEN, H. F., New York: Tumor Immunology

PARKER, J. W., and R. J. LUKES, Los Angeles: Lymphocyte Transformation in Neoplastic Disease

WEIL, R., Lausanne: Biological and Structural Properties of Polyoma Virus and its DNA

WISSLER, R. W., Chicago: Breast Cancer: A Challenging Problem (Symposium)